THE YEAR IN
SMALL ANIMAL MEDICINE

VOLUME 1

THE YEAR IN
SMALL ANIMAL
MEDICINE

VOLUME 1

EDITED BY

JILL E MADDISON and **MARK G PAPICH**

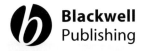

© 2005 Atlas Medical Publishing Ltd

Blackwell Publishing

Editorial Offices:

Blackwell Publishing Ltd, 9600 Garsington Road, Oxford OX4 2DQ, UK

Tel: +44 (0)1865 776868

Blackwell Publishing Professional, 2121 State Avenue, Ames, Iowa 50014-8300, USA

Tel: +1 515 292 0140

Blackwell Publishing Asia, 550 Swanston Street, Carlton, Victoria 3053, Australia

Tel: +61 (0)3 8359 1011

First published 2005

Library of Congress Cataloguing-in-Publication Data is available

ISBN-13: 978-14051-3194-0
ISBN-10: 1-4051-3194-2

A catalogue record for this title is available from the British Library

The publisher makes no representation, express or implied, that the dosages in this book are correct. Readers must therefore always check the product information and clinical procedures with the most up-to-date published product information and data sheets provided by the manufacturers and the most recent codes of conduct and safety regulations. The authors and the publisher do not accept any liability for any errors in the text or for the misuse or misapplication of material in this work.

Project conceived and developed by Clinical Publishing, the medical imprint of Atlas Medical Publishing Ltd, Oxford Centre for Innovation, Mill Street, Oxford OX2 0JX, UK

Commissioning Editor: Jonathan Gregory
Project Manager: Rosemary Osmond
Typeset by Footnote Graphics Limited, Warminster, Wiltshire, UK
Printed by Biddles Limited, King's Lynn, Norfolk, UK

The publisher's policy is to use permanent paper from mills that operate a sustainable forestry policy, and which has been manufactured from pulp processed using acid-free and elementary chlorine-free practices. Furthermore, the publisher ensures that the text paper and cover board used have met acceptable environmental accreditation standards.

For further information on Blackwell Publishing, visit our website:
www.blackwellpublishing.com

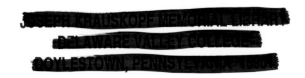

Contents

Editors and contributors

Editors

Jill E Maddison, BVSC, PHD, FACVSC, MRCVS
Beaumont Animals' Hospital, The Royal Veterinary College, London, UK

Mark G Papich, DVM, MS, DIPLOMATE ACVCP
Professor of Clinical Pharmacology, College of Veterinary Medicine, North Carolina State University, Raleigh, North Carolina, USA

Contributors

Linda Barton, DVM, DAVECC
Head, Emergency/Critical Care Service, The Animal Medical Center New York, New York, USA

Adrian Boswood, MA, VETMB, DVC, DIPECVIM-CA(CARDIOLOGY), ILTM, MRCVS
Senior Lecturer in Internal Medicine/Cardiology, Department of Veterinary Clinical Sciences, The Royal Veterinary College, London, UK

Jonathan Bray, MVSC, MACVSC(SURGERY), CERTSAS, MRCVS, DIPLECVS
Soft Tissue Surgeon, Davies Veterinary Specialists, Manor Farm Business Park, Higham Gobion, Hertfordshire, UK

Dennis J Chew, DVM DIPLOMATE, ACVIM(INTERNAL MEDICINE)
Full Professor, Department of Veterinary Clinical Sciences, College of Veterinary Medicine, The Ohio State University, Columbus, Ohio, USA

Cécile Clercx, DVM, PHD, DIPECVIM-CA
Professor of Small Animal Internal Medicine, Department of Clinical Sciences, Faculty of Veterinary Medicine, University of Liège, Sart Tilman, Belgium

Michael J Day, BSC, BVMS(HONS), PHD, FASM, DIPLECVP, FRCPATH, FRCVS
Professor of Veterinary Pathology, Director, Langford Veterinary Diagnostics, Division of Veterinary Pathology, Infection and Immunity, School of Clinical Veterinary Science, University of Bristol, Langford, UK

Linda M Fleeman, BVSC, MACVSC(CANINE MED)
Nestlé Purina PetCare Lecturer in Small Animal Nutrition, Centre for Companion Animal Health, School of Veterinary Science, The University of Queensland, St Lucia, Australia

Ann E Hohenhaus, DVM, DIPLOMATE, ACVIM(ONCOLOGY AND INTERNAL MEDICINE)
Chairman, Department of Medicine, The Animal Medical Center, New York, New York, USA

Kenneth A Johnson, MVSC, PHD, FACVSC, DIPLOMATE ACVS, DIPLOMATE ECVS
Professor of Orthopaedics, The Ohio State University, College of Veterinary Medicine, Columbus, Ohio, USA

Annette Litster, BVSC, PHD, FACVSC(FELINE MED)
Research Manager, Centre for Companion Animal Health, School of Veterinary Science, The University of Queensland, St Lucia, Australia

Ralf S Müller, DR.MED.VET, DR.MED.VET.HABIL, MACVSC, DIPACVD, FACVSC, DIPECVD
Chief of Dermatology and Allergy, Medizinische Kleintierklinik, Ludwig-Maximilians-University Munich, Munich, Germany

Reto Neiger, PROF.DR.MED.VET, PHD, DIPLACVIM, DIPLECVIM-CA
Professor of Small Animal Internal Medicine, Head, Small Animal Clinic (Internal Medicine and Surgery), Justus-Liebig University Giessen, Giessen, Germany

Karine Onclin, DVM, PHD, DECAR
Lecturer, University of Florida Veterinary College LACS, SARC, Gainesville, Florida, USA

Mark G Papich, DVM, MS, DIPLOMATE ACVCP
Professor of Clinical Pharmacology, College of Veterinary Medicine, North Carolina State University, Raleigh, North Carolina, USA

Simon Platt, BVM&S, MRCVS, DIPLACVIM(NEUROLOGY), DIPLECVN, RCVS SPECIALIST IN VETERINARY NEUROLOGY
Head of Neurology and Neurosurgery Unit, Centre for Small Animal Studies, Animal Health Trust, Lanwades Park, Newmarket, Suffolk, UK

Jacquie S Rand, BVSC, DVSC, DIPACVIM(INT MED)
Professor Companion Animal Health, School of Veterinary Science, University of Queensland, St Lucia, Australia

Patricia A Schenck, DVM, PHD
Assistant Professor, Diagnostic Center for Population and Animal Health, Endocrinology Section, Michigan State University, Lansing, Michigan, USA

John Verstegen, DVM, MSC, PHD, DECAR
Professor, University of Florida Veterinary College LACS, SARC, Gainesville, Florida, USA

David L Williams, MA, VETMB, PHD, CERTVOPHTHAL, MRCVS
Associate Lecturer in Veterinary Ophthalmology, Department of Clinical Veterinary Medicine, University of Cambridge; and Director of Studies, Pathology and Veterinary Medicine, College Lecturer in Pathology, St John's College, Cambridge, UK

1

Dermatology

RALF MÜLLER

Introduction

Dermatology is an integral part of small animal practice. Many patients presented to the practitioner have skin problems. Skin diseases in veterinary medicine frequently are syndromes that may be managed but cannot be cured. Thus, a good diagnostic approach to the patient with skin disease and a thorough knowledge of the therapeutic options and prognoses of the most common cutaneous disorders are essential for the small animal practitioner. In the last 12–15 months more than 250 articles on veterinary dermatology have been published, covering topics from allergic dermatitis to zygomycosis. Skin diseases may be caused by allergies, ectoparasites, microorganisms, endocrine abnormalities, abnormal immune responses and many others. Because of editorial constraints, we will only examine a small selection of the many valuable papers published in this field. Articles were chosen based on their scientific quality, relevance to small animal practice today and perceived relevance to changes in veterinary dermatology in the future. Of course, choices were difficult, but the author hopes to highlight some of the exciting changes in this field. As animals with allergies pose one of the biggest challenges in small animal dermatology due to the chronicity of allergic disorders and the frequency with which they occur worldwide, a number of studies have been selected that concentrate on atopic dermatitis (AD) and food adverse reactions. These papers are followed by studies focusing on less common skin diseases that nevertheless have contributed significantly to our understanding of the pathogenesis, diagnosis and/or treatment of these skin diseases.

Evidence-based veterinary dermatology: a systematic review on the pharmacotherapy of canine atopic dermatitis

Olivry T, Mueller RS, and the International Task Force on Canine Atopic Dermatitis. *Vet Dermatol* 2003; **14**(3): 121–46

BACKGROUND. The efficacy of pharmacological interventions used for treatment of canine AD, excluding fatty acid supplementation and allergen-specific

Table 1.1 Trials reporting treatment with oral glucocorticoids

Citation (reference)	Paradis, 1991 [1]	Reddy, 1992 [2]	Guaguère, 1996 [3]	Ferrer, 1999 [4]	Olivry, 2002 [5]	Steffan, 2003 [6]
Quality of evidence	B2	C1	C1	A3	A3	A1
Randomization (allocation generation)	unclear	none	none	adequate	adequate	adequate
Randomization (allocation concealment)	unclear	none	none	adequate	adequate	adequate
Masking of outcome assessor	adequate	inadequate	inadequate	adequate	adequate	adequate
Intention-to-treat analyses	no statistical analyses	no statistical analyses	no statistical analyses	inadequate	adequate	adequate
Quality of inclusion of study subjects	fairly characterized	poorly characterized	fairly characterized	well characterized	well characterized	well characterized
No. of dogs entered in trial (total)	30	120	80	40	30	176
No. of dogs entered in trial (AD only)	21	9	17	40	30	176
No. of dogs with AD treated with GC	21	9	17	10; 10	15	59
Length of trial (length GC treatment) (wks)	9 (1) + 2 to verify sustained efficacy	not specified	3 (3)	4 (4)	6 (6)	16 (16)
Pharmacological intervention	prednisone 0.2–0.4 mg kg⁻¹ BID	prednisolone 0.5 mg kg⁻¹ BID, then QD then BID EOD	methylprednisolone 0.4–0.8 mg kg⁻¹ QD then EOD	prednisone 0.25mg kg⁻¹ BID then QD, EOD; 0.5 mg kg⁻¹ BID	prednisolone 0.5 mg kg⁻¹ QD	methylprednisolone 0.5–1.0 mg kg⁻¹ QD, then EOD, then dosage tapered by 50 and 75%
Mean/median % reduction in lesional scores	NA	NA	NA	67%*; 83%*	69%	45%
Mean/median % reduction in pruritus scores	NA	NA	NA	58%*; 67%*	81%	33%
% dogs with ≥50% reduction in lesional score	NA	NA	NA	70%*; 60%*	86%	58%
% dogs with ≥50% reduction in pruritus scores	57%	NA	NA	60%*; 60%*	71%	42%
Other outcome measures		'good-to-excellent' response in 100% of dogs with atopy	86% 'very good results' (>75% improvement) assessed by clinician	*data calculated using 'last-value-carry-forward' rule	NA	60–63% 'good-to-excellent' global assessment of efficacy by owner and clinician

BID, twice daily; EOD, every other day; QD, once daily; NA, not available.
Source: Olivry et al. (2003).

Table 1.2 Trials reporting treatment with the calcineurin-inhibitor CsA

Citation (reference)	Fontaine, 2001 [7]	Olivry, 2002 [5]	Olivry, 2002 [8]		Steffan, 2003 [6]
Quality of evidence	C3	A3	A2		A1
Randomization (allocation generation)	none	adequate	adequate		adequate
Randomization (allocation concealment)	none	adequate	adequate		adequate
Masking of outcome assessor	inadequate	adequate	adequate		adequate
Intention-to-treat analyses	adequate	adequate	adequate		adequate
Quality of inclusion of study subjects	well characterized	well characterized	well characterized		well characterized
No. dogs entered in trial (total)	14	30	91		176
No. dogs entered in trial (AD only)	14	30	91		176
No. dogs with AD treated with active drug	14	15	30	31	117
Length of trial (length drug treatment) (wks)	2(2)	6 (6)	6 (6)		16 (16)
Pharmacological intervention	CsA proemulsion concentrate	CsA proemulsion concentrate	CsA proemulsion concentrate		CsA proemulsion concentrate
	5.0 mg kg^{-1} QD	5.0 mg kg^{-1} QD	2.5 mg kg^{-1} QD	5.0 mg kg^{-1} QD	5.0 mg kg^{-1} QD, EOD or TW
Mean/median % reduction in lesional scores	60%	58%	41%	67%	52%
Mean/median % reduction in pruritus scores	100%	78%	31%	45%	36%
% dogs with ≥50% reduction in lesional scores	79%	69%	47%	71%	66%
% dogs with ≥50% reduction in pruritus scores	86%	77%	33%	48%	40%
Other outcome measures	86% 'good-to-excellent' global assessment by owner	NA	33–40% 'good-to-excellent' global assessment of efficacy by owner and clinician	61% 'good-to-excellent' global assessment of efficacy by owner and clinician	75–76% 'good-to-excellent' global assessment of efficacy by owner and clinician

EOD, every other day; QD, once daily; TW, twice weekly; NA, not available.
Source: Olivry et al. (2003).

immunotherapy, was evaluated based on the systematic review of prospective clinical trials published between 1980 and 2002. Studies were compared in regards to design characteristics (randomization generation and concealment, masking, intention-to-treat analyses and quality of enrolment of study subjects), benefit (improvement in skin lesions or pruritus scores) and harm (nature, severity and frequency of adverse drug events) of the various interventions.

INTERPRETATION. Meta-analysis of pooled results was not possible because of heterogeneity of the drugs evaluated. Forty trials enrolling 1607 dogs were identified. There is good evidence for recommending the use of oral glucocorticoids (Table 1.1) and cyclosporin A (CsA) (Table 1.2) for the treatment of canine AD, and fair evidence for using topical triamcinolone spray, topical tacrolimus lotion, oral pentoxifylline or oral misoprostol. Insufficient evidence is available for or against recommending the prescription of oral first- and second-generation type-1 histamine receptor antagonists, tricyclic antidepressants, cyproheptadine, aspirin, Chinese herbal therapy, a homeopathic complex remedy, ascorbic acid, AHR-13268, papaverine, immune-modulating antibiotics or tranilast and topical pramoxine or capsaicin. Finally, there is fair evidence against recommending the use of oral arofylline, leukotriene synthesis inhibitors and cysteinyl leukotriene receptor antagonists.

Comment

This paper introduces the concept of evidence-based medicine in the evaluation of pharmacotherapy for canine skin diseases and is as such a milestone in veterinary dermatology. This approach tries to increase objectivity in the assessment of useful therapies. As AD is a common disease in small animal practice, every practitioner is interested in treatment options and their efficacy. Based on the above study, oral glucocorticoids and CsA are effectively treating canine AD. Interestingly, 'good evidence' of patient benefit is lacking for many treatment modalities used in canine AD. However, in the context of evidence-based medicine, this does not necessarily mean that these medications are worthless, but rather that randomized, double-blinded, controlled trials are lacking. These randomized, controlled and blinded trials are difficult to perform over longer periods of time. Most of the studies only assess relatively short treatment periods, and thus long-term adverse effects are often not adequately assessed and placebo effects are overestimated. Nevertheless, the paper sets a new standard in the evaluation of pharmacotherapy in veterinary dermatology and highlights the need for good scientific studies assessing drugs such as type 1 histamine receptor antagonists, tricyclic antidepressants and other drugs commonly used in practice.

Comparison of cyclosporine A with methylprednisolone for treatment of canine atopic dermatitis: a parallel, blinded, randomized controlled trial dermatitis

Steffan J, Alexander D, Brovedani F, Fisch RD. *Vet Dermatol* 2003; **14**: 11–22

BACKGROUND. The objective of this multicentre, parallel, blinded, randomized controlled study was to evaluate the efficacy and safety of CsA (117 dogs) in comparison with methylprednisolone (MP group, 59 dogs) in the treatment of AD for 4 months. Mean induction dose of both drugs (5 mg/kg CsA, 0.75 mg/kg MP) was tapered over time according to the clinical response.

INTERPRETATION. There was a significant improvement in clinical scores over time (Fig. 1.1). At the end of the study, the mean estimated percentage reduction from baseline (confidence interval [CI] of lesion scores was 52% (44–59) and 45% (35–56), and the reduction in pruritus score was 36% (27–43) and 33% (23–43) in dogs in the CsA and MP groups, respectively (Table 1.3). These percentages were not significantly different between groups. A significantly better overall assessment of efficacy was obtained in the CsA-treated dogs (76 vs 63% responses excellent or good in the CsA compared with the MP group). CsA-treated dogs presented a higher frequency of gastrointestinal (GI) disorders, mainly vomiting, but MP dogs tended to be more susceptible to infections. There was no remarkable change over baseline of the haematological and biochemical parameters in the two groups.

Comment

Double-blinded and randomized studies with larger numbers of dogs should be the gold standard for drug evaluation. This study was a multicentre study with a well-thought out protocol evaluating MP and CsA for the treatment of canine AD and including more than 170 dogs. It was randomized and blinded, thus trying to minimize subjective bias and the duration of the study (4 months) was sufficient to detect

Table 1.3 Percentage improvement over baseline for Canine AD Extent and Severity Index (CADESI) lesional scores and owner pruritus scores

	Week 4	8	12	16
CADESI				
CsA	44 (40–49)	53 (47–59)	50 (43–57)	52 (44–59)
MP	44 (38–51)	45 (36–53)	41 (31–51)	45 (35–56)
Pruritus				
CsA	34 (27–41)	39 (32–46)	32 (25–39)	36 (27–43)
MP	46 (36–56)	38 (28–48)	33 (23–43)	33 (23–43)

Data presented as mean estimates (95% confidence intervals).
Source: Steffan *et al.* (2003)

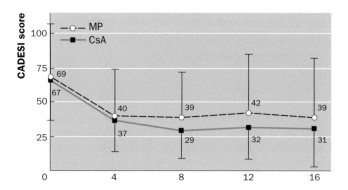

Fig. 1.1 Evolution of mean CADESI lesional scores during the course of the study. The dogs received CsA (5 mg/kg daily) or MP (0.5–1 mg/kg daily for 1 week then every other day for 3 weeks) for a month. The dose was then tapered according to the clinical response (see text). Means for all dogs included in the study (*n* = 117 in the CsA group and 59 in the MP group, intent-to-treat analysis). Source: Steffan *et al.* (2003).

mid-term adverse effects. The study showed that CsA was at least equivalent in efficacy to MP, one of the accepted and most efficacious drugs used to treat AD in dogs. Together with a couple of preceding studies |**5,7**|, these results make CsA one of the most thoroughly evaluated drugs in veterinary dermatology. Although vomiting and diarrhoea are seen in 20–40% of the patients, they necessitate cessation of CsA in only a small number of patients. The use of this drug will be limited by the expense, particularly in larger dogs. Long-term adverse effects in the dog after years of therapy are not known as of yet. However, CsA is a valuable alternative to glucocorticoid therapy and is approved for the use of canine AD in many countries.

 ## A randomised, controlled study to evaluate the steroid sparing effect of essential fatty acid supplementation in the treatment of canine atopic dermatitis
Sævik BK, Bergvall K, Holm BR, *et al. Vet Dermatol* 2004; **15**: 137–45

BACKGROUND. A randomized, double blind, placebo-controlled multicentre clinical trial of 12 weeks' duration was undertaken in 60 dogs with AD to evaluate the steroid sparing effect of essential fatty acid supplementation. The dogs were randomly assigned to either receive a combination of borage seed oil and fish oil or a placebo in addition to prednisolone tablets. All dogs received a standardized basal diet. Owners of the dogs recorded pruritus daily using a 10-cm visual analogue scale and the dosage of prednisolone was established based on pruritus score, according to written instructions. The dosage of prednisolone and the use of any concurrent treatment (shampoo and/or ear cleanser) were recorded by the owners on a daily basis. The investigators graded the skin lesions at days 0, 42 and 84.

INTERPRETATION. The use of prednisolone during the test period was lower in the active group, but the difference was not statistically significant ($P = 0.32$). The test period was sequentially divided into 43–84, 50–84, 57–84, 64–84, 71–84 and 78–84 days. On day 64, the difference between the active group and the placebo group reached statistical significance ($P = 0.04$) with an increasing difference towards the end of the study (Table 1.4). A statistically significant reduction in the pruritus scores and the total clinical scores from day 0 to day 84 was apparent in both groups ($P < 0.0001$) (Table 1.5). At the end of the study, both the pruritus score and the total clinical score were lower in the active group. These findings indicate a steroid sparing effect of essential fatty acid supplementation in canine AD and furthermore, that there is a time lag before it is achieved.

Comment

This study confirmed anecdotal information and a couple of non-controlled studies regarding the benefit of essential fatty acid supplementation to reduce the require-

Table 1.4 The use of prednisolone (mg/kg^{-1}) expressed as the area under the curve (AUC) for different time periods in the active ($n = 28$) and placebo group ($n = 29$)

	Active group		Placebo group		P values
	Mean	95% CI	Mean	95% CI	
AUC_{1-84}	17.9	(13.2–20.1)	21.5	(15.2–27.8)	0.324
AUC_{43-84}	6.7	(4.9–8.5)	10.2	(6.3–14.1)	0.094
AUC_{50-84}	5.4	(3.9–6.8)	8.4	(5.1–11.7)	0.081
AUC_{57-84}	4.0	(2.8–5.1)	6.6	(4.1–9.7)	0.059
AUC_{64-84}	2.7	(1.9–3.5)	4.9	(3.1–6.8)	0.037
AUC_{71-84}	1.7	(1.1–2.2)	3.2	(2.0–4.4)	0.024
AUC_{78-84}	0.7	(0.5–1.1)	1.5	(0.9–2.1)	0.018

Data are given as mean with 95% CI.
Source: Sævik et al. (2004).

Table 1.5 The pruritus scores in the active group ($n = 28$) and the placebo group ($n = 29$) on days 0, 41 and 83

		Mean	95% CI
Day 0	Active group	52.0	(46.3–57.8)
	Placebo group	51.2	(44.5–57.9)
Day 41	Active group	26.0	(19.2–32.7)
	Placebo group	25.2	(19.8–30.6)
Day 83	Active group	19.6	(14.0–25.2)
	Placebo group	27.8	(22.3–33.2)

Data are given as mean with 95% CI.
Source: Sævik et al. (2004).

ment for glucocorticoids in the treatment of canine AD. As glucocorticoids are the most commonly used and one of the most effective drugs for the treatment of AD, but are frequently associated with adverse effects, the scientific confirmation of this benefit hopefully will change our treatment habits and induce many veterinarians to add fatty acids to their treatment protocol on a regular basis. However, it is still unclear if n-3 fatty acids from fish oil or flax oil or n-6 fatty acids derived from evening primrose, borage or sunflower oil are preferable in the treatment of canine allergic skin disease. In addition, it is not clear what the ideal dose for these fatty acids is and if increasing the intake above the recommended doses is of clinical benefit. Further large studies such as this one are eagerly awaited to guide the small animal practitioner in the choice of fatty acid supplement and its dose.

The clinical effect of environmental control of house dust mites in 60 house dust mite-sensitive dogs
Swinnen C, Vroom M. *Vet Dermatol* 2004; **15**: 31–6

BACKGROUND. The purpose of this study was to evaluate the effects of benzyl benzoate, an acaricide for the control of house dust mites, in 60 house dust mite-sensitive dogs. All dogs showed positive reactions on intradermal testing for house dust mites (*Dermatophagoides farinae, Dermatophagoides pteronyssinus*) alone or house dust mites with storage mites (*Acarus siro, Tyrophagus putrescentiae, Glycophagus domesticus*). House dust samples from the owners' houses were collected and sent to the clinic where the authors performed a test (Acarex® test) to semiquantify the amount of guanine, a house dust mite product. Treatment with benzoyl benzoate was repeated until the house dust samples were negative for house dust mite guanine.

INTERPRETATION. After treatment, 29 of 60 house dust mite-sensitive dogs (48%) showed no skin lesions or pruritus (Table 1.6). Moderate results were achieved in 22 dogs (36%) with reduced pruritus and minimal skin lesions, but still requiring medication. In 13 dogs, this required regular treatment (three to four times a year) with antibiotics and antiyeast medication, and in eight dogs, immunotherapy was used. One dog was controlled with essential fatty acids as monotherapy and one dog was controlled with immunotherapy and essential fatty acids. In the remaining nine dogs (15%), the pruritus remained the same, and these dogs were controlled with oral corticosteroids. These results indicate that house dust mite elimination is a useful tool in the management of house dust mite-sensitive dogs.

Comment

House dust mite is by far the most common allergen involved in human and canine atopy |9|. In human medicine, avoidance of these mites by environmental control is a controversial topic with a number of studies showing benefit of such environmental control and an equally high number demonstrating no statistically significant benefit. In veterinary dermatology, a number of studies evaluate the success of dust mite-specific immunotherapy |**10–12**|, but the success of allergen avoidance has not been

Table 1.6 Summary of signalment, intradermal test results and clinical response in 60 house dust mite-sensitive dogs from homes with a positive house dust mite test

No.	Breed	Age	Sex	DF	DP	AS	T	G	PB	PA
1	WHW terrier	8 years	F	+					P	P (pred.)
2	WHW terrier	6 years	F	+					P	M (Ab + yeast)
3	WHW terrier	8 years	M	+	+				P	M (Ab + yeast)
4	Jack Russell terrierr	4 years	M	+					P	P (pred.)
5	Griffon Bruxelles	3 years 1 month	F	+					P	E
6	Giant schnauzer	3 years	M	+					P	E
7	German shepherd dog	3 years 5 months	F	+	++				P	P (pred.)
8	English cocker spaniel	4 years 1 month	F	+					P	E
9	Airedale terrier	2 years	F	+	+++				P	P (pred.)
10	Basset hound	2 years	F	+					P	E
11	Berner serner	3 years 5 months	M	+					P	M (Ab + yeast)
12	Cairn terrier	6 years 6 months	F	+					P	M (Ab + yeast)
13	American Staffordshire terrier	5 years 5 months	M	+		+			P	E
14	Berner serner	5 years 5 months	F	+		+	+++		P	M (desen. + Ab)
15	Boxer	3 years 8 months	F	+		+			P	P (pred.)
16	Boxer	2 years	M	+		+		+	P	E
17	Boxer	1 year	M	+		+			P	E
18	Border collie	4 years 6 months	F	+	+	+	+		P	E
19	Cross breed	1 year 6 months	M	+		+	+		P	E
20	Cross breed	3 years 9 months	M	+	+	+	+	+++	P	E
21	Cross breed	6 years 2 months	F	+		+	+		P	E (antihist.)
22	Cross breed	4 years 4 months	M	+		+	+	+	P	M (desen. + EFA)
23	Cross breed	4 years 9 months	F	+		+	+		P	E
24	Cross breed	5 years 11 months	M	+		+			P	E
25	Cross breed	5 years 1 month	F	+		+	+	+	P	M (Ab + yeast)
26	Cavalier King Charles	5 years 6 months	F	+		+			P	E (antihist.)
27	Dachshund	3 years 8 months	M	+		+			P	M (Ab + yeast)
28	Dachshund	4 years	F	+		+		+	P	M (Ab + yeast)
29	German short hair pionter	5 years 10 months	M	+		+	+++		P	E
30	German short-hair pointer	2 years 7 months	F	+		+		+	P	P (pred.)
31	English cocker spaniel	4 years 7 months	F	+		+			P	E
32	English springer spaniel	6 years 4 months	F	+		+			P	E

Table 1.6 (Continued)

No.	Breed	Age	Sex	DF	DP	AS	T	G	PB	PA
33	Fox terrier	5 years 6 months	F	+		+			P	E
34	German shepherd dog	4 years 7 months	F	+		+	+		P	M (Ab + yeast)
35	Golden retriever	6 years 9 months	F	+		+	+++		P	E
36	Golden retriever	4 years 10 months	F	+	+	+	+++	+	P	E
37	Golden retriever	4 years 4 months	F	+		+	+++		P	E
38	Golden retriever	1 year 2 months	M	+		+	+++		P	E
39	Golden retriever	6 years 10 months	M	+	+	+	+++	+	P	E
40	Jack Russell terrier	7 years 5 months	M	+		+	+++		P	P (pred.)
41	Jack Russell terrier	4 years 4 months	M	+		+	+++	+	P	P (pred.)
42	Jack Russell terrier	5 years 10 months	M	+	+	+	+++		P	E
43	Jack Russell terrier	3 years 10 months	F	+		+			P	P (pred.)
44	Labrador retriever	6 years	M	+		+	+++	++	P	M (Ab + yeast)
45	Labrador retriever	3 years 10 months	F	+	+	+	+++		P	E
46	Labrador retriever	4 years 8 months	F	+		+	+++		P	M (desen.)
47	Labrador retriever	2 years 5 months	F	+		+	++		P	M (desen.)
48	Labrador retriever	5 years 10 months	M	+		+	+++	+	P	M (Ab + yeast)
49	Labrador retriever	1 year 10 months	M	+		+	+++		P	M (desen. + Ab)
50	Labrador retriever	3 years 6 months	M	+		+			P	E
51	Labrador retriever	5 years 2 months	F	+		+			P	M (desen. + Ab)
52	Labrador retriever	6 years 11 months	M	+		+	+++	+	P	M (desen. + Ab)
53	Labrador retriever	3 years 6 months	M	+		+	+++	++	P	M (EFA + Ab+ yeast)
54	Labrador retriever	4 years 4 months	M	+		+	+++		P	E
55	Labrador retriever	6 years 2 months	F	+		+	+++		P	M (Ab + yeast)
56	Labrador retriever	3 years 8 months	M	+		+	+++		P	M (Ab + yeast)
57	Petit Basset Griffon	8 years	M	+		+			P	M (desen.)
58	Polsky Owezarek	3 years 8 months	F	+		+			P	E
59	Rottweiler	4 years 6 months	M	+		+	+++		P	E
60	Shetland sheepdog	4 years 11 months	M	+		+		+	P	M (Ab + yeast)

DF, *Dermatophagoides farinae*; DP, *Dermatophagoides pteronyssinus*; AS, *Acarus siro*; T, *Tyrophagus putrescentiae*; G, *Glycophagus domesticus*.
+, positive result; PB, pruritus grade before benzyl benzoate; PA, pruritus grade after benzyl benzoate and (prescribed treatment); pred, prednisolone treatment;
Ab, antibiotic treatment; desen, allergen-specific immunotherapy; antihist, antihistamine treatment; EFA, essential fatty acid treatment.
P = poor response, M = moderate response and E = excellent response.
Source: Swinnen and Vroom (2004).

demonstrated so far. This study showed a remission rate similar to or higher than the success rates reported with immunotherapy. Although no follow-up period was stated and the study was not controlled and not blinded (and thus the results have to be interpreted with caution), it is a landmark study that hopefully will trigger further double-blinded, placebo-controlled studies with longer follow-up to confirm these findings.

Evaluation of serum obtained from atopic dogs with dermatitis attributable to *Malassezia pachydermatis* for passive transfer of immediate hypersensitivity to that organism

Morris DO, DeBoer DJ. *Am J Vet Res* 2003; **64**: 262–6

BACKGROUND. This study determined the functionality of canine anti-*Malassezia* IgE via the passive transfer of immediate hypersensitivity localized to the skin from atopic dogs with dermatitis attributable to overgrown *Malassezia pachydermatis* (*Malassezia* dermatitis [MD]) to healthy recipient dogs by use of the Prausnitz-Küstner (P-K) technique. Seven clinically normal dogs were used to determine concentrations of crude *Malassezia* extract for intradermal testing. Serum from atopic dogs with MD was used for P-K tests on three normal dogs. Serial dilutions of untreated, heat-inactivated, IgE-absorbed and bovine serum albumin-absorbed aliquots of serum were injected intradermally in triplicate for dermal sensitization. Twenty-four, 48 and 72 h later, a crude extract of *M. pachydermatis* was injected intradermally into the sites used for sensitization injections, and immediate hypersensitivity reactions were graded on a four-point scale. Using a monoclonal anticanine IgE antibody, enzyme-linked immunosorbent assay testing was performed on the serum of seven normal dogs and 32 atopic dogs with or without MD/otitis.

INTERPRETATION. Untreated serum of an atopic dog with MD and cutaneous reactivity to intradermal testing with *Malassezia* crude extract and of an atopic dog with high concentrations of anti-*Malassezia* IgE determined by enzyme-linked immunosorbent assay testing caused P-K reactivity beginning 24 h after passive sensitization and persisting through 72 h (titres 1:32 to 1:64). Heat inactivation and IgE absorption of serum eliminated P-K reactivity, whereas treatment of serum with bovine serum albumin did not. There was no difference in the concentration of serum anti-*Malassezia* IgE between normal dogs, atopic dogs with *Malassezia* infection and atopic dogs without evidence of yeast infection.

Comment

MD has been recognized as a clinical problem for some years. In normal dogs *Malassezia* organisms are found in low numbers. However, under special circumstances, the opportunistic pathogen can proliferate secondary to changes in the barrier function of the stratum corneum or increased lipid content of the skin surface. In the dog, MD is particularly common secondary to atopic disease. Type 1 hypersensitivity reactions to crude extracts of *M. pachydermatis* and increased concentrations of

Malassezia-specific IgE have been identified in allergic dogs |**13,14**|. However, the link between the presence of IgE and intradermal reactions has hitherto not been determined. This study elegantly shows that *Malassezia*-specific IgE is indeed present in dogs and can be transferred to intradermal mast cells, where it leads to degranulation and weal formation after intradermal injection of *Malassezia* extract. Thus, a hypersensitivity to *Malassezia* antigens can occur and contribute to the clinical signs of canine AD. Future studies will hopefully establish if, and to what degree, *Malassezia* antigen-specific immunotherapy is of therapeutic benefit in these dogs and if dogs with *Malassezia* hypersensitivity respond differently to topical or systemic anti-*Malassezia* therapy than dogs with MD not based on immunological hypersensitivity.

Serum IgE and IgG responses to food antigens in normal and atopic dogs and dogs with gastrointestinal disease

Foster AP, Knowles TG, Moore AH, Cousings PDG, Day MJ, Hall EJ. *Vet Immunol Immunopathol* 2003; **92**: 113–24

BACKGROUND. In human food allergy, with or without concurrent atopy, there may be significant increases in serum allergen-specific IgE. Serological methods have been tried but are not currently recommended for diagnosis of suspected food allergy in dogs. The aim of this study was to investigate humoral immune responses to food antigens in dogs. Serum IgG and IgE antibodies specific for food antigens were measured by enzyme-linked immunosorbent assay using polyclonal antidog IgG and IgE reagents. Antigens tested were beef, chicken, pork, lamb, chicken, turkey, white fish, whole egg, wheat, soybean, barley, rice, maize corn, potato, yeast and cow's milk. Three groups were examined: normal dogs, dogs with AD and dogs with one of four types of GI disease (small intestinal bacterial overgrowth, inflammatory bowel disease, food-responsive disease and infectious diarrhoea).

INTERPRETATION. Statistically significant differences in food-specific antibodies were not detected between the GI subgroups. There were statistically significant differences in the IgG (Table 1.7) and IgE concentrations (Table 1.8) between the normal dogs, and dogs with atopic or GI disease, for all of the antigens tested (except IgG against egg and yeast). The relationship of antigen responses for pooled data was analysed using principal components analysis and cluster plots. Some clustering of variables was apparent for both IgE and IgG. For example, all dogs (normal and diseased) made a similar IgG antibody response to chicken and turkey. Compared with other groups, atopic dogs had more food allergen-specific IgE and this would be consistent with a T-helper 2 humoral response to food antigens. Dogs with GI disease had more food allergen-specific IgG compared with the other groups. This may reflect increased antigen exposure due to increased mucosal permeability, which is a recognized feature of canine intestinal disease.

Comment

A number of papers have evaluated the use of intradermal testing and serum testing for allergen-specific IgE in dogs with food adverse reactions resulting in skin or GI

Table 1.7 Summary of the IgG responses to food antigens showing the mean ln(IgG) serum concentration within each group of dogs, the standard error of the mean and the F value and the P value from the analysis of variance

	Atopic dermatitis (n = 91)		Gastrointestinal (n = 72)		Normal (n = 91)		F value	P value
	Mean	Standard error of mean	Mean	Standard error of mean	Mean	Standard error of mean		
Barley	3.5788[a]	0.0552	3.4167[a,b]	0.1578	3.1103[b]	0.0684	6.721	0.001
Beef	2.6470[a]	0.0446	3.5223[b]	0.0693	3.3001[c]	0.0608	61.360	0.000
Chicken	3.0022[a]	0.0474	3.1590[a]	0.0796	4.1235[b]	0.0441	123.253	0.000
Corn	3.4965[a]	0.0594	4.0946[b]	0.0977	3.2081[a]	0.1129	22.195	0.000
Egg	3.7960[a]	0.0549	3.7120[a]	0.0769	3.9138[a]	0.0883	1.780	0.171
Fish	3.2761[a]	0.0759	3.9370[b]	0.0777	3.2403[a]	0.0537	29.559	0.000
Lamb	2.9455[a]	0.0532	3.3262[b]	0.0752	2.6324[c]	0.0852	21.787	0.000
Milk	3.0090[a]	0.0573	3.6535[b]	0.1597	3.5404[b]	0.0570	13.685	0.000
Pork	3.1741[a]	0.0377	3.5397[b]	0.0583	2.9778[c]	0.0486	33.372	0.000
Potato	3.5768[a]	0.0698	3.6636[a]	0.1242	1.9342[b]	0.1088	96.071	0.000
Rice	2.3958[a]	0.0846	3.1267[b]	0.0683	2.0098[c]	0.0926	41.942	0.000
Soy	3.0457[a]	0.0685	3.6091[b]	0.0897	3.2637[a,c]	0.0773	12.491	0.000
Turkey	3.0655[a]	0.0587	3.7522[b]	0.0756	3.8590[b]	0.0642	45.157	0.000
Wheat	4.0160[a]	0.0515	3.4387[b]	0.1055	3.6592[b]	0.0657	15.320	0.000
Yeast	2.5191[a]	0.1097	2.6165[a]	0.1544	2.3885[a]	0.0893	0.925	0.398

Means with different superscripts across rows were significantly different ($P < 0.05$).
Source: Foster et al. (2003).

Table 1.8 Summary of the IgE responses to food antigens

	Percentage positive ELISA result			Pearson Chi-square value	Exact two-sided significance
	Atopic dermatitis (n = 91)	Gastrointestinal (n = 72)	Normal (n = 40)		
Barley	80.2[a]	98.4[b]	100[b]	19.613	0.000
Beef	76.9[a]	46.9[b]	67.5[a]	15.062	0.000
Chicken	60.4[a]	50.0[a]	87.5[b]	15.108	0.000
Corn	78[a]	71.9[a]	55[b]	7.211	0.025
Egg	79.1[a]	39.1[b]	57.5[b]	25.821	0.000
Fish	92.3[a]	31.3[b]	42.5[b]	67.656	0.000
Lamb	71.4[a]	37.5[b]	92.5[c]	36.031	0.000
Milk	69.2[a]	31.3[b]	75[a]	28.247	0.000
Pork	81.3[a]	21.9[b]	55[c]	54.036	0.000
Potato	83.5[a]	62.5[b]	65[a,b]	9.940	0.007
Rice	91.2[a]	39.1[b]	52.2[b]	49.822	0.000
Soy	80.2[a]	46.9[b]	55[b]	19.967	0.000
Turkey	91.2[a]	40.6[b]	62.5[c]	45.630	0.000
Wheat	78[a]	68.8[a,b]	52.5[b]	8.622	0.014
Yeast	82.4[a]	34.4[b]	47.5[b]	38.986	0.000

The percentage of dogs positive for IgE within each group are shown together with the Chi-square statistic and an exact P value for the test of association between response/non-response and the groups of dog. Different superscripts across rows indicate which groups differed when tested in pairs.
Source: Foster et al. (2003).

disease and currently neither is recommended or helpful for the diagnosis of food adverse reaction |**15–17**|. This study showed the propensity of atopic dogs to produce more IgE in an environment characterized by T-helper 2 cytokines, such as interleukins 4 and 5, promoting isotype switching to IgE and in contrast an increase in food allergen-specific IgG in dogs with GI disease. There were no differences in antibody production in the dogs with food-responsive GI disease versus dogs with infectious diarrhoea; both groups had increases in IgG rather than IgE. This may be due to the fact that IgE-mediated food allergy predominantly causes cutaneous signs and a non-allergic pathogenesis is present in the dogs with food-responsive GI disease. However, it could also be an indication for a non-specific and clinically not relevant increase in IgE production in atopic dogs. In the latter scenario, serum testing for food allergen-specific IgE may not be clinically relevant for many years to come while with the former scenario IgE testing may become a useful diagnostic tool for dogs with skin disease in the future. However, based on this study, it seems that IgE testing for dogs with GI signs is not rewarding in clinical practice.

Evaluation of the clinical and allergen-specific serum immunoglobulin E responses to oral challenge with cornstarch, corn, soy and a soy hydrolysate diet in dogs with spontaneous food allergy

Jackson HA, Jackson W, Coblentz L, Hammerberg B. *Vet Dermatol* 2003; **14**: 181–7

BACKGROUND. Fourteen dogs with known clinical hypersensitivity to soy and corn were maintained on a limited antigen duck and rice diet until cutaneous manifestations of pruritus were minimal after 11 weeks. Sequential oral challenges with cornstarch, corn and soy were then performed. Subsequently the dogs were fed a diet containing hydrolysed soy protein and corn starch. Throughout the study period the dogs were examined for cutaneous manifestations of pruritus and additionally serum was collected for measurement of allergen-specific and total IgE concentrations. Intradermal testing with food antigens was performed prior to entry into the study and after 12 weeks.

INTERPRETATION. A statistically significant improvement was measured between days 0 and 83 (Fig. 1.2). Significant pruritus was induced after oral challenge with cornstarch, corn and soy ($P = 0.04$, 0.002, 0.01, respectively) but not with the hydrolysed diet ($P = 0.5$). The positive predictive value of the skin test for soy and corn allergy was reduced after feeding a soy- and corn-free diet. Although increases in soy- and corn-specific serum IgE concentrations were measured in individual dogs postchallenge, they were not statistically significant and could not be used to predict clinical hypersensitivity.

Comment

Food adverse reaction is a controversial topic in veterinary dermatology. Owner compliance with the currently only accepted diagnostic standard, a home-cooked

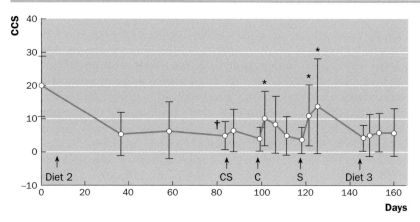

Fig. 1.2 Mean cutaneous clinical scores (CCS) throughout the study period. Error bars represent the standard deviation from the mean. At time 0 the dogs were receiving diet 1. CS, cornstarch; C, corn; S, soy. † A significant reduction at day 83 compared with day 0 ($P = 0.001$).* Significant increases post-challenge ($P = 0.009$, 0.0028 and 0.0001), compared with day 83. Source: Jackson *et al.* (2004).

elimination diet, is suboptimal. Thus, commercial elimination diets such as hydrolysed diets or diets using unusual proteins, have been marketed as an easier way to diagnose the disease. Unfortunately, neither hydrolysed diets nor diets with unusual proteins are reliable in the diagnosis of food adverse reaction [18,19]. Similarly, intradermal testing and serum testing for food antigen-specific IgE is commercially available to facilitate the diagnosis. Unfortunately, neither of these tests has been proven to be associated with an acceptable positive or negative predictability [15–17]. The above study tried to evaluate scientifically a hydrolysed diet and serum testing for food antigen-specific IgE in a colony of atopic research dogs with documented adverse reactions to foods. Results of intradermal testing and serum IgE testing were disappointing in this study, and confirmed previous findings that, so far, neither of these tests is suitable for the diagnosis of food adverse reaction in the dog. However, based on these results, hydrolysed diets may be an interesting alternative to home-cooked elimination diets. As complete resolution of pruritus with these diets has not been reported, a home-cooked elimination diet may be initiated after improvement (albeit not complete resolution) on the hydrolysed food.

Feline pemphigus foliaceus: a retrospective analysis of 57 cases

Preziosi DE, Goldschmidt MH, Greek JS, *et al.* *Vet Dermatol* 2003; **14**: 313–21

BACKGROUND. Fifty-seven cases of feline pemphigus foliaceus were identified from biopsy specimens submitted to a pathology laboratory by veterinary

dermatologists from 1991 to 2002. Results of physical examination, skin biopsy and treatment and prognosis were recorded.

INTERPRETATION. Age of onset ranged from less than 1 to 17 years (median 5 years). At the time of biopsy, distribution of lesions varied, but included some combination of face, head, paws, dorsum or ventrum and consisted of crusts, erosions, scale and alopecia (Fig. 1.3). The histological features of 208 biopsy specimens included acantholytic cells in both intact and degenerating pustules. The proportion of diagnostic samples was significantly higher in cats not pretreated with glucocorticoids ($P = 0.0027$). The diagnosis could be made by examination of crusts in the absence of pustules in a number of cats. Forty-four cases were followed for 1–54 months (median 9 months). Triamcinolone was more successful at inducing remission without significant adverse effects than prednisone alone or in combination with chlorambucil. Only four of 44 cats died from their disease or therapy during the study period.

Comment

Pemphigus foliaceus is the most common immune-mediated skin disease in small animals. It is surprising, that prior to the above study, only 11 feline cases were reported in the literature. In essence, the study emphasizes points that were anecdotally well known among veterinary dermatologists. Avoidance of glucocorticoid administration prior to biopsy increased the chance for diagnostic results. Several sites should be sampled, and if primary lesions such as pustules are not present, fresh crusts offer a good chance to be diagnostic histopathologically. Triamcinolone showed less adverse effects and higher efficacy than prednisone. It is unfortunate

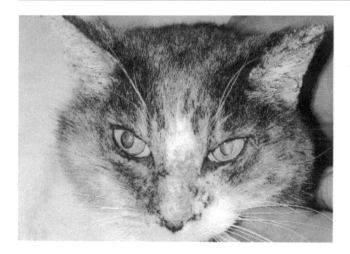

Fig. 1.3 Face of cat with pemphigus foliaceus. Crusts and erosions can be seen on the face, margins of the pinnae, dorsal nose and periocular area. Source: Preziosi *et al.* (2003).

that no cat was treated with prednisolone, which may have led to a different outcome than prednisone in at least some patients. The prognosis for this disease is good with appropriate therapy and this fact, not necessarily widely known in small animal practice, was nicely demonstrated in this study. However, all of the cats in the study were biopsied and subsequently treated by board-certified veterinary dermatologists and referral may be considered if the general practitioner has no experience with this particular disease.

MDR 1-deficient genotype in collie dogs hypersensitive to the P-glycoprotein substrate ivermectin
Roulet A, Puel O, Gesta S, *et al. Eur J Pharmacol* 2003; **460**: 85–91

BACKGROUND. Multidrug resistance (MDR) phenotypes in cancer cells are associated with overexpression of the drug carrier P-glycoprotein. The antiparasitic drug ivermectin, one of its substrates, abnormally accumulates in the brain of transgenic mice lacking the P-glycoprotein, resulting in neurotoxicity. Similarly, an enhanced sensitivity to ivermectin has been reported in certain dogs of the collie breed. To explore the basis of this phenotype, the authors analysed the canine P-glycoprotein-encoding MDR 1 gene.

INTERPRETATION. cDNA for wild-type (beagle) P-glycoprotein was characterized for the first time. The corresponding transcripts from ivermectin-sensitive collies revealed a homozygous 4-bp exonic deletion (Fig. 1.4). The authors demonstrated, by genetic testing, that the MDR 1 frameshift is predictable. Accordingly, no P-glycoprotein was detected in the homozygote-deficient dogs. This unique case of naturally occurring gene invalidation provides a putative novel model that remains to be exploited in the field of human therapeutics and that might significantly affect tissue distribution and drug bioavailability studies.

Comment

It has long been known that administration of ivermectin to sensitive collie dogs results in severe neurotoxicity and death |20|. This can also occasionally occur in individual dogs of other breeds |21| and presumably was due to a defect of the blood–brain barrier in these animals. Subsequently, evidence was presented, that P-glycoprotein, a drug carrier protein, was responsible for the protection of the nervous system against ivermectin and that a deficiency in the MDR 1 gene encoding this protein was associated with neurotoxicity in mice receiving ivermectin |22|. In this study, the gene was sequenced and a homozygous mutation in sensitive collie dogs demonstrated. Owing to the homology between the human and canine P-glycoprotein, the collies were proposed as a suitable animal model for drug bioavailability studies. However, the antibody used to show the lack of polypeptide in tissue specimens may possibly be used to identify ivermectin-sensitive canine patients prior to therapy, allowing veterinarians to minimize adverse effects with this drug.

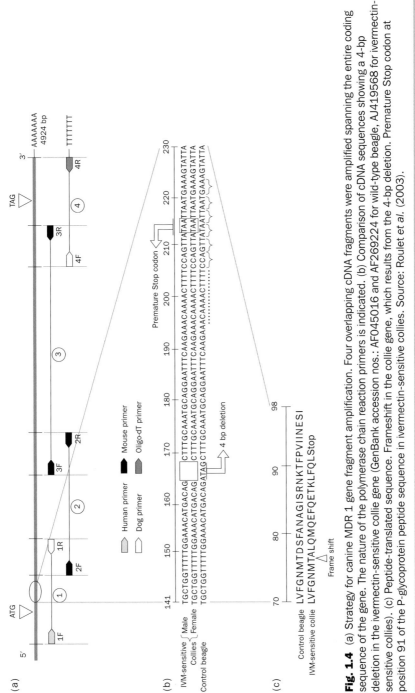

Fig. 1.4 (a) Strategy for canine MDR 1 gene fragment amplification. Four overlapping cDNA fragments were amplified spanning the entire coding sequence of the gene. The nature of the polymerase chain reaction primers is indicated. (b) Comparison of cDNA sequences showing a 4-bp deletion in the ivermectin-sensitive collie gene (GenBank accession nos.: AF045016 and AF269224 for wild-type beagle, AJ419568 for ivermectin-sensitive collies). (c) Peptide-translated sequence. Frameshift in the collie gene, which results from the 4-bp deletion. Premature Stop codon at position 91 of the P-glycoprotein peptide sequence in ivermectin-sensitive collies. Source: Roulet et al. (2003).

Retrospective evaluation of sex hormones and steroid hormone intermediates in dogs with alopecia

Frank LA, Hnilica KA, Rohrbach BW, Oliver JW. *Vet Dermatol* 2003; **14**: 91–7

BACKGROUND. The purpose of this study was to determine if there are specific steroid hormone aberrations associated with suspect endocrine alopecia in dogs in whom hypothyroidism and hyperadrenocorticism have been excluded. Steroid hormone panels submitted to the University of Tennessee College of Veterinary Medicine endocrinology laboratory over a 7.5-year period (783 samples) from dogs with alopecia were reviewed. During this period, 276 dogs met the criteria for inclusion and were comprised of 54 different breeds.

INTERPRETATION. Approximately 73% of dogs had at least one baseline or post-adrenocorticotrophic hormone (ACTH) stimulation steroid hormone intermediate greater than the normal range (Table 1.9). The most frequent hormone elevation noted was for progesterone (57.6% of the samples). When compared with normal dogs, oestradiol was significantly greater in keeshond dogs and progesterone was significantly greater in pomeranian and Siberian husky dogs. Not all individual dogs had hormonal abnormalities. Chow chow, samoyeds and malamutes had the greatest percentage of normal steroid intermediates of the dogs in this study. Baseline cortisol concentrations were significantly correlated with progesterone, 17-hydroxyprogesterone and androstenedione. Results of this study suggest that the pathomechanism of the alopecia, at least for some breeds, may not relate to steroid hormone intermediates and emphasizes the need for breed-specific normals.

Comment

In the past, a number of alopecias have been identified that responded to a variety of hormonal treatments. Oestrogen-responsive, testosterone-responsive, growth hormone-responsive, and castration-responsive dermatoses are examples [23]. All of these diseases had similar clinical presentation of hyperpigmentation and alopecia without any systemic signs or demonstrable hormonal abnormalities on the classical assays. The exception was growth hormone-responsive dermatosis, where xylazine- or clonidine-response tests showed abnormalities in some (but not all) dogs. Unfortunately, some normal dogs also showed these abnormalities, making an interpretation of the tests difficult. A partial deficiency in 21-hydroxylase enzyme (as described in people with congenital adrenal hyperplasia) was postulated in a group of pomeranians with elevation of 17-hydroxyprogesterone [24]. However, normal pomeranians showed the same results of steroid hormone intermediates on baseline and post-ACTH stimulation as affected dogs. Subsequently, due to their common clinical presentations, these dermatoses all were grouped together and named alopecia X for the lack of a demonstrated aetiology. This study used a large number of dogs evaluating the concentration of steroid hormone intermediates at baseline and post-ACTH stimulation. Although some statistically significant differences between dogs of different breeds became evident, no uniform abnormality was identified

Table 1.9 Percentage of dogs with steroid hormone intermediates greater than the normal range

Hormone	Base (%)†	Post (%)‡	Base or post (%)§
Oestradiol	34/276 (12.3)	34/276 (12.3)	43/276 (15.6)
Progesterone	122/276 (44.2)	100/276 (36.2)	159/276 (57.6)
17-OHP¶	49/276 (17.8)	19/276 (6.9)	57/276 (20.7)
DHEAS**	15/276 (5.4)	16/276 (5.8)	17/276 (6.2)
Androstenedione	49/276 (17.8)	6/276 (2.2)	50/276 (18.1)

† Percentage of dogs with increases in baseline hormone concentrations.
‡ Percentage of dogs with increases in post-ACTH stimulation hormone concentrations.
§ Percentage of dogs with increases in baseline or post-ACTH stimulation hormone concentrations.
¶ 17-Hydroxyprogesterone.
** Dihydroepiandrosterone sulfate.
Source: Frank et al. (2003).

for any breed. The need for breed-specific normals was emphasized. Based on these results, it seems unlikely that the pathogenesis is due to an abnormality of steroid hormone intermediates and testing for such hormonal abnormalities at this point of time seems ineffective. Further research may focus on hair follicles, receptors on the surface of follicular cells and interaction between these cells and various hormones at a follicular level.

Multicenter case–control study of risk factors associated with development of vaccine associated sarcomas in cats

Kass PH, Spangler WL, Hendrick MJ, et al. J Am Vet Med Assoc 2003; **223**: 1283–92

BACKGROUND. This study tried to determine whether particular vaccine brands, other injectable medications, customary vaccination practices, or various host factors were associated with the formation of vaccine-associated sarcomas in cats. It was a prospective multicentred case–control study using cats in the United States and Canada with soft tissue sarcomas or basal cell tumours. Veterinarians submitting biopsy specimens from cats with a confirmed diagnosis of soft tissue sarcoma or basal cell tumour were contacted for patient medical history. Time window statistical analyses were used in conjunction with various assumptions about case definitions.

INTERPRETATION. No single vaccine brand or manufacturer within antigen class was found to be associated with sarcoma formation. Factors related to vaccine administration were also not associated with sarcoma development, with the possible exception of vaccine temperature prior to injection. Two injectable medications (long-acting penicillin and methylprednisolone acetate) were administered to case cats more frequently than to control cats. These findings do not support the hypotheses that specific brands or types of vaccine within antigen class, vaccine practices such as reuse of syringes, concomitant viral infection, history of trauma, or residence either increase or decrease the risk of vaccine-associated sarcoma formation in cats. There was evidence to suggest that certain long-acting injectable medications may also be associated with sarcoma formation.

Comment

Some diseases are relatively rare or influenced by many environmental factors. In human medicine, large, multicentred epidemiological studies with many thousand patients try to establish relevant pathogenetic epidemiological and environmental factors through the large number of patients and various statistical evaluations. This study tries to achieve the same goal evaluating feline sarcomas suspected to be induced by vaccinations due to their location. When 'vaccine-induced' sarcomas were first reported some years ago |25|, a number of hypotheses regarding the pathogenesis of these sarcomas were presented. However, based on this study the induction of sarcomas seems to be possible with any injection, independent of manufacturer and exact content.

Conclusion

Small animal dermatology is a rapidly developing field and cutaneous diseases have a widely variable pathogenesis. The most prominent skin disorders seen in practice are allergies. The prevalence of atopic diseases in human medicine has dramatically increased over the last half a century and, although specific epidemiological studies showing such an increase have not been published in veterinary medicine, allergic diseases and associated secondary infections are very frequently encountered in practice. Studies in these areas were equally prominent during the last year and this emphasis is mirrored in the selection of articles for this chapter. Olivry *et al.* showed in their evidence-based review on the treatment of canine AD, how much of clinical dermatology is based on anecdotal reports and that scientific proof for the efficacy of many frequently used drugs is still lacking. However, there is good evidence for the use of some drugs such as glucocorticoids and CsA and against the use of others such as leukotriene inhibitors or receptor antagonists. Steffan *et al.* documented the efficacy of CsA for canine AD in comparison with MP over 4 months of therapy. Sævik *et al.* reported the steroid-sparing effect of fatty acid supplementation for atopic dogs in a multicentre study. The most common allergen involved in canine AD is a house dust mite antigen and Swinnen and Vroom for the first time in veterinary medicine showed that environmental reduction of allergen load can ameliorate clinical signs of disease in dogs allergic to house dust mites. Secondary infection with *Malassezia* organisms is frequently seen in allergic animals. Evidence for a hypersensitivity reaction against these organisms in some dogs was provided recently. Now Morris and DeBoer documented that *Malassezia*-specific IgE can be transferred to normal dogs by the use of the Prausnitz-Küstner technique and can elicit a cutaneous reaction, providing the link between intradermal reactions to yeast antigen and IgE production. Food adverse reaction is a controversial topic in veterinary dermatology and little is known about details of the pathogenesis. It is not as frequent as AD, but due to the similar clinical picture a common differential diagnosis. Foster *et al.* evaluated food-specific antibody production in normal dogs and dogs with AD and GI disease. They showed that atopic dogs had increased concentrations of food-specific IgE compared with normal dogs. In contrast, food-specific IgG was increased in dogs with GI disease independent of the pathogenesis. This provides evidence against clinical GI problems due to increased IgE production, but still could not answer the question of how relevant food-specific IgE is clinically in atopic dogs. Jackson *et al.* could not measure significant antigen-specific IgE increases in food-allergic dogs after rechallenge with the offending antigen, further questioning the value of serum food-allergen-specific IgE in the diagnosis of canine food reactions.

Pemphigus foliaceus is one of the most common immune-mediated skin diseases in small animals. Particularly in cats, published studies are absent and case reports scarce. Preziosi *et al.* published a large retrospective study evaluating this disease in cats and confirmed the good prognosis for pemphigus foliaceus with appropriate treatment. In addition, triamcinolone was identified as the treatment of choice.

Ectoparasites are another part of veterinary dermatology and ivermectin has been used in the past for many of these, even though it is not registered in small animals for this use at the appropriate doses. Ivermectin toxicity is well known in collies, but has also been seen in a number of other dog breeds and cats. Roulet *et al.* have identified a homozygous 4-bp exonic deletion of the gene for P-glycoprotein, a drug carrier protein, as the reason for the occurrence of clinical toxicity and showed the lack of this polypeptide in tissue specimens of affected dogs with an antibody-based assay.

Hormonal diseases also may cause cutaneous signs and one of the more puzzling entities in cutaneous endocrinology is alopecia X, an alopecia associated with hyperpigmentation, but lacking inflammation and systemic signs. Abnormalities in growth hormone concentrations have been hypothesized some years ago. Adrenal hormone production was the centre of attention recently. Frank *et al.* evaluated blood samples from pre- and post-ACTH stimulation in a large number of dogs with alopecia X for hormonal abnormalities and measured a number of steroid hormone intermediates. They failed to show any consistent abnormality for any of the breeds examined. Based on these results, an actual abnormality in steroid intermediate hormone blood concentrations seems to be unlikely as a cause for alopecia X and further research should probably focus more on the hair follicle itself.

Feline fibrosarcomas are common tumours in the cat and an association between fibrosarcomas in the shoulder areas and vaccination has been hypothesized. Initially, aluminium (used as adjuvant in many vaccines) had been identified in the centre of fibrosarcomas in three cats. Kass *et al.* performed a large epidemiological study evaluating many different factors and could not identify any correlation between fibrosarcoma development and vaccine type or manufacturer. However, there was a possible influence of long-acting injectable drugs contributing to the sarcoma development.

References

1. Paradis M, Scott DW, Giroux D. Further investigations on the use of non-steroidal and steroidal anti-inflammatory agents in the management of canine pruritus. *J Am Anim Hosp Assoc* 1991; **27**: 44–8.

2. Reddy NRJ, Umesh KG, Rao M, Rai T. Therapeutic evaluation of pheneramine maleate and prednisolone as antipruritic agents in dogs. *Ind Vet J* 1992; **69**: 259–61.

3. Guaguère E, Lasvergeres F, Arfi L. Efficacy of oral methylprednisolone in the symptomatic treatment of allergic dermatitis (in French). *Prat Méd Chir Anim Comp* 1996; **31**: 171–5.

4. Ferrer L, Alberola J, Queralt M, Brazis P, Rabanal R, Llenas J, Puigdemont A. Clinical anti-inflammatory efficacy of arofylline. A new selective phosphodiesterase-4 inhibitor, in dogs with atopic dermatitis. *Vet Rec* 1999; **145**: 191–4.

5. Olivry T, Steffan J, Fisch RD, Prelaud P, Guaguere E, Fontaine J, Carlotti DN; European Veterinary Dermatology Cyclosporine Group. Randomized controlled trial of the efficacy of cyclosporine in the treatment of atopic dermatitis in dogs. *J Am Vet Med Assoc* 2002; **221**: 370–7.

6. Steffan J, Alexander D, Brovedani F, Fisch RD. Comparison of cyclosporine A with methylprednisolone for treatment of canine atopic dermatitis: a parallel blinded random-ized controlled trial. *Vet Dermatol* 2003; **14**: 11–22.

7. Fontaine J, Olivry T. Treatment of canine atopic dermatitis with cyclosporine: a pilot clinical study. *Vet Rec* 2001; **148**: 662–3.

8. Olivry T, Rivierre C, Jackson HA, Murphy KM, Davidson G, Sousa CA. Cyclosporine decreases skin lesions and pruritus in dogs with atopic dermatitis: a blinded randomized prednisolone-controlled trial. *Vet Dermatol* 2002; **13**: 77–87.

9. Mueller RS, Bettenay SV, Tideman L. Aero-allergens in canine atopic dermatitis in south-eastern Australia based on 1000 intradermal skin tests. *Aust Vet J* 2000; **78**: 392–9.

10. Scott KV, White SD, Rosychuk RAW. A retrospective study of hyposensitization in atopic dogs in a flea-scarce environment. In: Ihrke PJ, Mason IS, White SD (eds). *Advances in veterinary dermatology*. New York: Pergamon Press, 1993; pp. 79–87.

11. Willemse A, Van den Brom WE, Rijnberk A. Effect of hyposensitisation on atopic dermatitis in dogs. *J Am Vet Med Assoc* 1984; **184**: 1277–80.

12. Mueller RS, Bettenay SV. Long-term immunotherapy of 146 dogs with atopic der-matitis—a retrospective study. *Aust Vet Practit* 1996; **26**: 128–32.

13. Morris DO, Olivier NB, Rosser EJ. Type-1 hypersensitivity reactions to Malassezia pachy-dermatis extracts in atopic dogs. *Am J Vet Res* 1998; **59**: 836–41.

14. Nuttall TJ, Halliwell RE. Serum antibodies to Malassezia yeasts in canine atopic der-matitis. *Vet Dermatol* 2001; **12**: 327–32.

15. Jeffers JG, Shanley KJ, Meyer Ek. Diagnostic testing of dogs for food allergy. *J Am Vet Med Assoc* 1991; **198**: 245–50.

16. Kunkle G, Horner S. Validity of skin testing for the diagnosis of food allergy in dogs. *J Am Vet Med Assoc* 1992; **200**: 677–80.

17. Mueller RS, Tsohalis J. Evaluation of serum allergen-specific IgE for the diagnosis of food adverse reactions in the dog. *Vet Dermatol* 1998; **9**: 167–71.

18. Leistra MHG, Markwell PJ, Willemse T. Evaluation of selected-protein-source diets for management of dogs with adverse reactions to foods. *J Am Vet Med Assoc* 2001; **219**: 1411–14.

19. Beale KM, LaFlamme DP. Comparison of a hydrolyzed soy protein diet containing corn starch with a positive and a negative control diet in corn or soy sensitive dogs. Annual Meeting of the American Academy of Veterinary Dermatology/American College of Veterinary Dermatology 2001.

20. Paul AJ, Tranquilli WJ, Seward RL, Todd KS Jr, DiPietro JA. Clinical observations in Collies given ivermectin orally. *Am J Vet Res* 1987; **48**: 684–5.

21. Mueller RS, Bettenay SV. A proposed new therapeutic protocol for the treatment of canine mange with ivermectin. *J Am Anim Hosp Assoc* 1999; **35**: 77–80.

22. Schinkel AH, Smit JJ, van Tellingen O, Beijnen JH, Wagenaar E, van Deemter L, Mol CA, van der Valk MA, Robanus-Maandag EC, te Riele HP. Disruption of the mouse mdr1a P-glycoprotein gene leads to a deficiency in the blood–brain barrier and to increased sensitivity to drugs. *Cell* 1994; **77**(4): 491–502.

23. Scott DW, Miller W, Griffin CE. Endocrine and metabolic diseases. *Muller's and Kirk's Small Animal Dermatology*. 6th ed. Philadelphia: W.B. Saunders, 2001; 780–885.

24. Schmeitzel LP, Lothrop CD. Hormonal abnormalities in Pomeranians with normal coat and in Pomeranians with growth hormone-responsive dermatosis. *J Am Vet Med Assoc* 1990; **197**: 1333–41.

25. Hendrick MJ, Goldschmidt MH, Shofer FS, Wang YY, Somlyo AP. Postvaccinal sarcomas in the cat: epidemiology and electron probe microanalytical identification of aluminum. *Cancer Res* 1992; **52**: 5391–4.

2

Immunology

MICHAEL DAY

Introduction

The science of immunology underlies many aspects of companion animal clinical practice. The single best example of this is the impact of serological testing and vaccination on the prevalence of infectious disease. Most veterinarians in clinical practice would use these practical applications of immunology on a daily basis, and clear understanding of the immunological principles underlying these techniques is crucial. This is particularly so in a climate where the adverse effects of vaccination receive more attention than the profound benefit for animal welfare that these products have brought.

Another example is the probable increasing frequency with which we deal with the spectrum of immune-mediated diseases in dogs and cats—particularly the allergic or autoimmune disorders. New diagnostic approaches to the investigation of these diseases have been introduced in recent times, and the practising veterinarian must often decide on the most appropriate of an array of test modalities.

Finally, immunomodulatory agents, used either alone or in combination, are widely administered to companion animals and novel products of this type continue to come to market. There has never been a time when pet owners have greater knowledge or expectation of what is possible for the management of small animal disease, and veterinarians need to be able to critically evaluate both new licensed products and the growing range of alternative immunomodulatory therapies.

Against this background, I have chosen 12 papers accepted into the peer-reviewed scientific literature during the year 2003–2004 to illustrate the pivotal role that immunology currently plays in companion animal practice. These papers have been grouped under four themes.

Advances in basic companion animal immunology

The first set of papers covers a selection of basic scientific advances in our knowledge of the immune system of dogs and cats as it pertains to disease. There is no more exciting time to be involved in such research, as we have unprecedented access to new laboratory tools to enable dissection of the companion animal immune system. Most of these new techniques have come from the application of molecular biology to companion animal immunology research. The ability to characterize canine and feline gene sequences on the basis of using 'consensus sequence' from other species (including humans and laboratory rodents) has been revolutionary. Coupled with the recent availability of the entire canine genome, it means that rapid advances are likely in the near future.

Cytokine profiles of peripheral blood mononuclear cells from dogs experimentally sensitized to Japanese cedar pollen

Fujiwara S, Yasunaga S, Iwabuchi S, Masuda K, Ohno K, Tsujimoto H.
Vet Immunol Immunopathol 2003; **93**: 9–20

BACKGROUND. In Japan, a major aeroallergen in humans and dogs is pollen from the Japanese cedar (*Cryptomeria japonica*). These authors have previously reported an experimental model of sensitization of beagle dogs to this allergen, and shown that sensitized dogs develop allergen-specific IgE antibodies and positive intradermal tests. This study aimed to determine whether sensitized dogs also had evidence of underlying T-helper (Th) 2 immunity.

INTERPRETATION. Beagle dogs were sensitized by two subcutaneous injections of Japanese cedar pollen in alum. Control dogs were not sensitized. Two weeks after the second injection, blood was taken and the peripheral blood mononuclear cells (PBMC) collected. A fraction of these cells was immediately snap-frozen, and the remainder was cultured for 24 h with pollen allergen before snap-freezing. Control cultures were also established using an irrelevant allergen (*Dermatophagoides pteronyssinus* house dust mite extract). RNA was isolated from the frozen cells and subjected to quantitative reverse transcriptase–polymerase chain reaction (RT–PCR). mRNA encoding the cytokines interleukin (IL)-1β, IL-2, IL-4, IL-6, IL-8, IL-10, IL-18, interferon-γ, transforming growth factor-β and tumour necrosis factor-α was quantified relative to that encoding β-actin as a 'housekeeper'. The most significant finding was that the Japanese cedar cultured PBMC from sensitized dogs expressed markedly increased IL-4 mRNA compared with cells from controls (Fig. 2.1), indicating that the sensitization of the dogs with allergen had induced Th2 lymphocytes. This was further supported by the observation that the non-stimulated PBMC of sensitized dogs had significantly less mRNA encoding the Th1 cytokine interferon-γ than control unstimulated PBMC. Other parameters were also measured in the dogs. Sensitized dogs all had a positive intradermal test to Japanese cedar pollen extract and developed serum allergen-specific IgE. A standard 72-h lymphocyte proliferation test using Japanese cedar pollen extract showed significant proliferative responses in the majority of the sensitized dogs.

Comment

A fundamental concept in modern immunology is that there are subpopulations of T lymphocytes that have either enhancing or suppressive effects on the immune response. Although often phenotypically similar, the subpopulations are defined

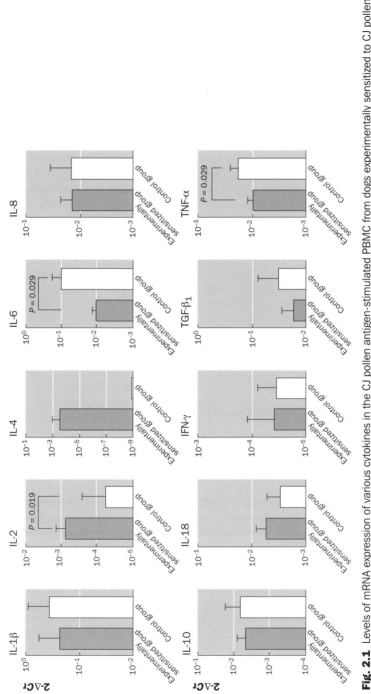

Fig. 2.1 Levels of mRNA expression of various cytokines in the CJ pollen antigen-stimulated PBMC from dogs experimentally sensitized to CJ pollen extract and control dogs. The amounts of mRNA are expressed relative to the amount of beta-actin mRNA in each sample and are shown as the mean ± SD values. Grey columns, experimentally sensitized group; white columns, control group. Significant differences between the groups are expressed as P values. Source: Fujiwara et al. (2003).

functionally by the type of soluble mediators (cytokines) that they secrete. These
T cells are often cross-regulatory, and the relative balance of the effects of 'helper' or
'regulatory' cells determines the nature of any immune response. Two important
T-cell subsets are the Th1 and Th2 'helper' cells, which basically enhance either
cell-mediated (cytotoxic) or humoral (antibody-mediated) immunity respectively.

This paper addresses this concept with respect to the dog, and confirms that as in
humans and experimental rodents, the allergic response is produced by activity of the
Th2 subset. The gene encoding the 'signature' Th2 cytokine IL-4 was activated in the
PBMC of dogs experimentally sensitized to develop allergy to Japanese cedar pollen.
Although other investigators have shown that allergic dogs have a Th2 dominated
immune response |1|, this is one of the first companion animal studies to demon-
strate cytokine mRNA production by 'real-time' quantitative RT–PCR. We cannot
yet reliably measure the majority of canine and feline cytokine proteins, but it is now
possible to quantify indirectly activation of the genes that encode them via this new
methodology. This has wide application to studies of disease in companion animals.
Indeed, in our laboratory, we have recently completed similar work investigating
cytokine mRNA expression by quantitative RT–PCR in the gut mucosa of dogs
and cats with inflammatory bowel disease |2|, and the skin of cats with allergic
dermatopathy |3|.

The clinical relevance of such studies is significant. The ability to relate disease
phenotype to cytokine profile may have diagnostic potential, and more significantly
there are numerous approaches whereby cytokine profile can be manipulated *in vivo*
to 'restore balance' in an immune response. There are now numerous anticytokine
monoclonal antibodies licensed for use in human medicine that have precisely this
effect via neutralizing the cytokine for which they are specific |4|.

Isotype determination of circulating autoantibodies in canine autoimmune subepidermal blistering dermatoses

Favrot C, Dunston SM, Paradis M, Olivry T. *Vet Dermatol* 2003; **14**: 23–30

BACKGROUND. Humans and dogs are both affected by a range of autoimmune
subepidermal blistering dermatoses that includes the individual entities bullous
pemphigoid, mucous membrane pemphigoid and epidermolysis bullosa acquisita.
These diseases are characterized by the presence of autoantibodies directed against
specific molecules within the basement membrane zone that separates the
epidermis from dermis. In recent years, it has been shown that these autoantibodies
may be demonstrated in the serum of affected dogs using techniques such as
enzyme-linked immunosorbent assay or indirect immunofluorescence. In affected
humans, the IgG autoantibodies are predominantly of the IgG1 and IgG4 subclasses.
The aim of the present study was to determine the immunoglobulin class and IgG
subclass profile of the equivalent canine autoantibodies.

INTERPRETATION. Serum samples were collected from dogs with bullous pemphigoid
(*n* = 5), mucous membrane pemphigoid (*n* = 15) or epidermolysis bullosa acquisita

($n = 11$) for testing by indirect immunofluorescence using salt-split normal canine gingiva as substrate tissue. Normal dog serum was used as a negative control. The exposure of gingival tissue to a specific salt formulation results in separation of the epidermis and dermis via clefting through the centre of the lamina lucida of the basement membrane zone. This process enhances exposure of relevant autoantigens such that when sections of the salt-split tissue are overlaid with patient serum, there will be binding of the circulating autoantibodies to the target antigens. In bullous pemphigoid and mucous membrane pemphigoid the autoantibodies localize to the epidermal side of the split, whereas in epidermolysis bullosa acquisita there is binding to the dermal side. Autoantibody binding is detected via the use of secondary reagents—in this study antisera specific for canine IgG, IgM, IgA, IgE and the IgG subclasses (IgG1–IgG4). All sera were screened at an initial dilution of 1:10, and positive samples were fully titrated.

IgG autoantibodies were detected in all canine sera tested, whereas autoantibodies of other immunoglobulin classes were less frequently found. Overall, IgE autoantibodies were more commonly detected than those of the IgA or IgM class. IgG1 and IgG4 autoantibodies were more common overall than those of the IgG2 or IgG3 subclasses (Fig. 2.2). This pattern of a predominant IgG1, IgG4 and IgE autoantibody response mimics that seen in human patients with the homologous diseases.

Comment

There are several important immunological points that are illustrated by this publication. This study is the latest in a series by these authors that have fundamentally defined a range of canine and feline autoimmune dermatoses in terms of the specific cutaneous molecules that are the target autoantigens in these diseases. Knowledge of target autoantigens is key to being able to develop specific immunotherapy designed to selectively inhibit an autoimmune response while leaving the remainder of the immune system unimpaired and able to provide body defences. In addition to these autoimmune dermatoses, we have some understanding of target autoantigens in immune-mediated haemolytic anaemia (IMHA) |5| and thrombocytopenia |6|, but have much to learn for the majority of companion animal autoimmune diseases. In experimental rodents and humans it has been clearly shown that administration of peptides derived from such target autoantigens via the oral or nasal mucosa can selectively impair the autoimmune response |7|. Such targeted immunotherapy is at a clinical trial stage in human medicine, and there is potential for equivalent studies in companion animals.

The identification of IgG1, IgG4 and IgE as dominant autoantibodies in these diseases may also have more immediate clinical benefit. In humans, the relative proportions of these antigen-specific immunoglobulins alter with the phase of clinical disease or treatment-induced clinical remission. This may also apply to canine patients, and the stated aim of the authors is to investigate this area in follow-up studies.

The final point raised by this paper relates to the fundamental immunological question of why particular immune responses tend to be dominated by specific subclasses of IgG. This phenomenon is best defined in mice, where an immune response

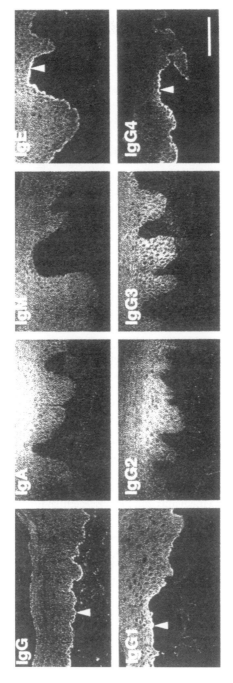

Fig. 2.2 Indirect IF staining profile in canine MMP. Serum from a dog with MMP (case MMP5) was tested by indirect IF, at 1:10 dilution, for detection of basement membrane-specific autoantibodies. IgG, IgG1, IgG4 and IgE autoantibodies bound to the epithelial side of the splits (*arrowheads*) (bar = 90 μm). Source: Favrot et al. (2003).

regulated by Th2 lymphocytes (see above) is associated with IgE and IgG1 produc-
tion, while a Th1-driven, cell-mediated response is linked to IgG2a synthesis |8|. Such
bias in IgG subclass usage in immune responses has been a concept difficult to apply
to other species, where the IgG subclass nomenclature also varies considerably. In
humans, there are clinical data suggesting that IgG1 and IgG4 antibodies are more
often produced during allergy or autoimmune diseases such as those discussed here.

The canine IgG subclasses were defined by our laboratory on the basis of their
equivalence to the human counterparts in terms of relative serum concentration and
electrophoretic mobility |9|, but there has been much confusion in canine immun-
ology regarding whether there is subclass bias in specific immune responses. This
confusion has largely come from a series of studies of the immune response in infec-
tious diseases such as leishmaniasis or ehrlichiosis |10,11| where the failure to find
consensus likely relates to the use of flawed reagents that do not conform to current
nomenclature. Indeed, work from our laboratory has clearly shown that there is no
IgG subclass skewing in canine leishmaniasis |12|, but further studies are needed to
correlate IgG subclass usage with T-cell cytokine production in canine disease.

Concurrent bartonellosis and babesiosis in a dog with persistent thrombocytopenia

Tuttle AD, Birkenheuer AJ, Juopperi T, Levy MG, Breitschwerdt EB. *J Am Vet Med Assoc* 2003; **223**: 1306–10

BACKGROUND. This study describes the clinical presentation and diagnostic
procedures applied to a dog coinfected with *Bartonella* and *Babesia.*

INTERPRETATION. A 12-year-old, west highland white terrier was referred with a 1-year
history of syncopal episodes and a range of secondary disease. The major haematological
features were a poorly regenerative anaemia and marked thrombocytopenia. The dog was
Coombs' test negative and bone marrow aspiration revealed active erythropoiesis and
thrombopoiesis. A coagulation profile was normal suggesting platelet destruction as the
mechanism underlying thrombocytopenia. There was ultrasonographic evidence of a range of
tissue changes. Serological testing revealed the presence of antibody specific for *Bartonella
vinsonii (ss berkhoffii)* but *Bartonella* DNA was not identified by PCR. The syncopal episodes,
anaemia and thrombocytopenia were attributed to bartonellosis and the dog was treated with
doxycycline and prednisone.

On day 40 the dog presented with a history of extreme lethargy and hind limb weakness.
At this time the anaemia and thrombocytopenia had largely resolved and the dog was
seronegative to *Bartonella*. The clinical signs were attributed to glucocorticoid-induced
myopathy. The dog developed further signs related to long-term glucocorticoid therapy;
however, on day 123 thrombocytopenia was again present and azathioprine was added to
the treatment regimen in order to work towards substituting this drug for prednisone. On day
151 the dog was again anaemic and thrombocytopenic. *Bartonella* antibody titre was not
clinically significant, but on this occasion large-form *Babesia* were noted on the blood film
and confirmed by PCR testing to be *B. canis vogeli*. Retrospective PCR testing revealed
B. canis DNA in blood samples from days 1 and 40. Imidocarb dipropionate was added to the

treatment regimen and the dog showed clinical improvement, subsequently becoming seronegative to *Bartonella* and PCR negative for *Babesia*.

Comment

I have chosen only one individual case report in this selection of literature, as the case in question is an excellent example of a recently emerging and important area of companion animal clinical immunology. This relates to the fascinating and complex relationship between arthropod-transmitted pathogens, their vectors and the immune system of the animal that plays host to the ectoparasite and microbial pathogens. It would appear that some arthropod salivary factors, released into the host dermal microenvironment while these parasites take in a blood meal, have potent immuno-regulatory function. These factors may modulate the host immune response to permit infection and establishment of the microbe that is transmitted during feeding. Moreover, these factors and the microbe itself interact with the host immune system in a way that allows persistence of the infection and the onset of a spectrum of secondary immune-mediated phenomena |**13**|.

Arthropod-transmitted organisms such as *Bartonella*, *Babesia*, *Ehrlichia*, *Leishmania*, *Anaplasma*, *Rickettsia* and *Borrelia* are considered emerging pathogens in both humans and companion animals. As part of their pathogenesis, these agents are known to trigger immune complex formation and autoantibody production in addition to their specific tissue pathologies. Clinically, these infections can mimic primary, idiopathic (autoimmune) disease, and have therefore become important differential diagnoses for autoimmunity in companion animals. This group of infectious agents is also characterized by being exceedingly difficult to diagnose by standard means, and by producing chronic and sometimes latent, subclinical infections. The organisms and their arthropod vectors appear to be extending their traditional geographical range—permitted by changes such as freedom of companion animal travel, climate change and altered environmental usage. This is exemplified by the recent emergence of leishmaniasis and small form babesiosis in the United States, and the occurrence of these infections in northern Europe as pet animals move more freely within the European Union |**14**|.

The present case report provides a timely example of these concepts. A dog presenting with primary haemolytic anaemia and destructive thrombocytopenia in an area non-endemic for arthropod-borne infection might once have been considered to have autoimmune disease. In this case, the clinical presentation was related to coinfection with two microbes that are likely to cause disease in part by engendering erythrocyte and platelet-bound antibodies. Veterinarians in geographical areas considered non-endemic for arthropod-borne infections will increasingly need to consider these agents in the clinical work-up of companion animals with apparent immune-mediated disease. Successful treatment of this patient required the use of appropriate antimicrobials in addition to immunosuppressive agents. The difficulty in diagnosing these infections, and the possibility of latent infection is demonstrated by the fact that PCR was required to identify *Babesia* in early samples—a diagnosis that was only made retrospectively. The new clinical association between babesiosis and thrombocytopenia highlights how much we have to learn about the interplay between these organisms and the host immune system, particularly when coinfections occur when the microbes share an arthropod vector.

Advances in immunodiagnosis

This second group of papers gives clear examples of how advances in laboratory methodology, led by the molecular revolution, can be directly translated into new diagnostic approaches for canine disease. The sensitivity of molecular diagnosis has altered our approach to the diagnosis of infection, and will shortly broaden the range of diagnostic tests available. Moreover, as genetic associations with disease become documented, molecular screening tests will become increasingly important in animal breeding and the elimination of diseases involving genetic mutation.

Diagnosis of canine lymphoid neoplasia using clonal rearrangements of antigen receptor genes
Burnett RC, Vernau W, Modiano JF, Olver CS, Moore PF, Avery AC. *Vet Pathol* 2003; **40**: 32–41

BACKGROUND. The diagnosis of lymphoma or lymphoid leukaemia currently relies on the microscopic examination of cytological or biopsy samples, and increasingly on the application of monoclonal antibodies to detect a range of cell membrane antigens via immunocytochemistry or immunohistochemistry. In the majority of cases these methodologies are adequate for diagnostic purposes, but in a proportion of animals the diagnosis is not straightforward. Without obvious hallmarks of malignancy, it can sometimes be difficult to distinguish between a reactive lymphoid hyperplasia and neoplasia, and in some situations (e.g. feline alimentary lymphoma) there is thought to be a progression between reactive and neoplastic change. Moreover, traditional diagnostic methods have limited ability to detect residual neoplastic populations following successful chemotherapy. This study applies molecular analysis of the clonality of lymphocytes in a sample as a novel diagnostic procedure. As neoplastic lymphocytes are clonal, gene rearrangements within a neoplastic population should be uniform, whereas in an inflammatory lesion with lymphocytes of a range of antigen specificity such clonal rearrangements will not be present.

INTERPRETATION. Samples were collected from 77 dogs with lymphoid neoplasia (20 lymphoma, 54 lymphoid leukaemia, two myeloma, one plasmacytoma) and 24 dogs that were either clinically normal ($n = 4$) or had a range of other diseases. The samples included tissue, bone marrow, blood or cellular aspirates. The majority of lymphoid tumours were immunophenotyped to determine whether they were of T- or B-cell origin.

   The targets for assessment of clonal rearrangement were the most variable regions of the B-cell immunoglobulin receptor and the γ chain of the T-cell receptor (TCR) molecules, areas that contact the antigenic molecules that the receptors are designed to bind. These regions are known as the third 'complementarity determining regions' (CDR3) and are formed by recombination of genes encoding variable, diversity and joining regions of the immunoglobulin, or variable and joining genes of the γ chain of the TCR. Consequently, for the PCR reactions used in this study, primers were designed against a selection of V and J regions of either immunoglobulin or TCR-γ chain. Following PCR, the amplified products were separated on gels. In this assay, clonality was defined by the presence of one (monoclonal), two (biclonal) or more (oligoclonal) discrete bands irregularly spaced on the gel, whereas amplification from a polyclonal sample gave discrete bands that were evenly spaced on the gel (Fig. 2.3).

The PCR test demonstrated clonality in 70 of the 77 lymphoid neoplasms examined (91%). Of these, 40 tumours had clonal rearrangement of immunoglobulin genes, 29 of TCR-γ genes and one of both sets of genes. Only one of the 24 control tissues (4%) had clonal rearrangements of TCR-γ genes, and this dog had ehrlichiosis. Where immunophenotyping was performed, there was agreement with the rearrangements detected in all cases but one T-cell leukaemia, which had both TCR and immunoglobulin rearrangements.

In order to test the sensitivity of the assay for detecting small numbers of neoplastic cells in a background of normal cells, DNA from a B-cell leukaemia was serially diluted into a constant amount of DNA extracted from a normal liver. The clonal rearrangement was still detected at 0.1 ng of DNA, where the tumour DNA comprised only 0.1% of the total DNA in the sample. This sensitivity did vary dependent upon the tissue from which the DNA used for dilution was obtained.

The results of this study indicate that this methodology has important clinical application in the detection and characterization of canine lymphoma. The sensitivity of the test for tumour detection in a clinical setting is likely to be less than the 91% reported here with selected well-characterized tumour samples. The test is likely to be able to detect small numbers of clonal cells within otherwise non-neoplastic tissue. The presence of two immunoglobulin or TCR gene rearrangements within a single tumour was thought to reflect either the presence of two neoplastic clones, or the presence of rearrangements on both chromosomes. The intriguing observation of multiple rearrangements would be consistent with the presence of multiple neoplastic clones, or the evolution of a single clone through serial transformation. Finally, the study raises the possibility that clonal rearrangements might occur in the absence of clinical evidence of neoplasia. This is exemplified by the TCR-γ rearrangement documented in the dog with ehrlichiosis.

Comment

This is a highly significant and clinically relevant paper. The methodology described will potentially revolutionize our ability to confirm a diagnosis of lymphoid malignancy in situations where standard cytological or histopathological examination provides an unequivocal result. Such testing already has an important place in human medicine, and is part of the molecular revolution through which veterinary laboratory diagnosis is now proceeding. Molecular diagnosis is now commonplace for the identification of infectious disease (see above) and genetic defects (see below), and will soon become important for determining the genetic predisposition to disease (see below).

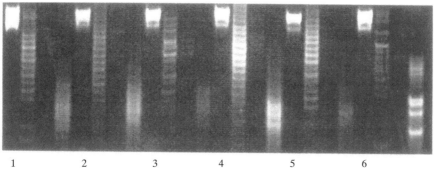

Sample number

Fig. 2.3 Examples of positive and negative PCR results obtained with a variety of sample types. Source: Burnett *et al.* (2003).

In clinical terms, molecular testing of clonality is likely to have a greater impact than immunophenotypic characterization of lymphoma. Although numerous studies have now been performed to determine whether canine and feline lymphomas are of T- or B-cell origin, this information still appears to provide little prognostic benefit. Only a single, relatively early, study clearly shows that immunophenotype correlates with outcome for canine lymphoma |**15**|, but such correlation has proven more problematic to demonstrate for the cat |**16**|.

Like all laboratory tests, the sensitivity and specificity of this molecular methodology will require further evaluation in a clinical setting as the authors of this paper are quick to point out. The 'false positive' result obtained in this study with the TCR-γ rearrangement identified in a dog with ehrlichiosis appears a not uncommon finding in this disease (unpublished data cited by the authors) and might be consistent with the fact that dogs with monocytic ehrlichiosis do sometimes develop monoclonal gammopathy and therefore presumptive clonal expansion of B lymphocytes |**17**|. It would be interesting to examine clonality in dogs infected by *Leishmania* where similar massive expansion of lymphoid populations and monoclonal gammopathy may occur |**18**|.

Susceptibility to visceral leishmaniasis in the domestic dog is associated with MHC class II polymorphism

Quinnell RJ, Kennedy LJ, Barnes A, et al. Immunogenetics 2003; **55**: 23–8

BACKGROUND. All mammalian species have a cluster of genes that encode molecules that are intrinsically involved in the initiation and regulation of immune responses. This gene cluster is known as the major histocompatibility complex (MHC) and is named differently in each species—the canine MHC being termed the 'dog leucocyte antigen' (DLA) system. The so-called 'class II' genes of the MHC encode surface membrane proteins expressed by antigen-presenting cells that carry out the 'presentation' of peptide fragments of antigen to antigen-specific TCR molecules. Genes of the MHC are among the most polymorphic in the entire genome and numerous allotypes are recognized at each locus. The expression of particular allelic variants of these loci has been clearly associated with disease susceptibility or resistance in a number of species.

Recent studies have characterized the canine MHC and breed variation in allotypes of selected loci |19|. Canine class II loci are extensively polymorphic, with 67 DLA-DRB1, 18 DLA-DQA1 and 47 DLA-DQB1 alleles reported to date. In this study, DLA class II allotype expression was examined in a cohort of Brazilian dogs naturally infected with the protozoan parasite *Leishmania infantum* and the hypothesis tested that expression of particular alleles may be associated with the nature of the immune response to the infection, and thus clinical outcome.

INTERPRETATION. The investigation described here is part of a long-term study of the kinetics of canine leishmaniasis in an endemic area of Brazil. The study involved 126 cross-bred dogs, 99 of which were obtained as naïve pups from a non-endemic area and 27 of which were born within the study area but were confirmed seronegative. The dogs were placed in cohorts with households in the endemic area and serially monitored over the period April 1993 to July 1995. Blood and bone marrow were collected at each sampling point and clinical signs of the disease scored. Infection was determined by PCR, parasite culture or serology, and 86 of the 126 dogs became infected. Levels of *Leishmania*-specific IgG and IgG subclasses |12|, blood lymphocyte proliferative responses and bone marrow cytokine production |20| were also tested. DNA extracted from bone marrow was used to genotype the dogs for their DLA-DRB1, DLA-DQA1 and DLA-DQB1 alleles by sequence-based typing. The most important finding of the study was a clear association between expression of the allele DLA-DRB1*01502 and high levels of serum antigen-specific IgG and PCR positivity for infection (odds ratio 37). Carriage of this allele also appeared to be higher in dogs with greater mean clinical scores, but this was not significant. Dogs are phenotypically either susceptible or resistant to leishmaniasis, and the disease outcome is determined by the nature of the immune response to the pathogen. Susceptibility is clearly linked to a serological response that dominates cell-mediated immunity (the 'Th2 phenotype'), whereas resistance correlates with a strong cell-mediated immune response with low antibody production (the 'Th1 phenotype'). The results of the present study suggest either that DLA-DRB1*01502 is directly associated with susceptibility, or is in 'linkage disequilibrium' with another susceptibility allele at another locus. Such information may have practical relevance in terms of more effective vaccine design for this devastating zoonotic disease.

Comment

This study provides new insight into our understanding of the immune response to *Leishmania* infection in the dog. There is now clear evidence for susceptible (Th2) and resistant (Th1) phenotypes within this species, and a recent study shows that resistance is a particular characteristic of one breed within an endemic area |21|. A second genetic association between susceptibility and expression of an allele of the NRAMP1 gene has also recently been reported in the dog |22|. This knowledge will become important in vaccine design. Vaccination of the canine population is one possible means of control in this zoonotic infection, and current vaccine studies have begun to utilize antigenic fractions of the causative organism |23|.

Outwith the specific field of *Leishmania* research, this study is also important proof of concept for the investigation of genetic linkage with aspects of the canine immune response and canine disease. MHC–disease association is a significant area of research in human medicine, where the expression of particular MHC alleles (generally alleles of several loci in combination) is strongly associated with the development of a range of autoimmune and immune-mediated diseases (e.g. rheumatoid arthritis, lymphocytic thyroiditis, multiple sclerosis). Early studies predicted that similar linkage would be found for canine disease |24| and the present investigation would support that hypothesis.

Molecular typing methods for the canine MHC are now perfected, and we have baseline knowledge of the range of alleles that are found among different dog breeds. The way is now open for studies of MHC associations in a wide range of canine disease states. Indeed, this is the purpose of the multicentre collaborative Companion Animal DNA Archive that was established in the United Kingdom during 2003. There are likely to be rapid advances in this field over the coming years.

Advances in immunomodulatory therapy

The third theme of this chapter is immunomodulatory therapy. In this section, one paper re-evaluates our use of a 'traditional' immunosuppressive agent and one describes studies leading up to the licensing of a new immunosuppressive. A further paper examines the potential for therapy of primary immunodeficiency disease in the dog. Although this is now theoretically possible, the most ready application is in experimental model studies for human disease. Finally, we now understand that immunomodulation does not only imply immunosuppression in diseased animals, but includes the concept of 'immunological health' that is now widely discussed—in particular how we might enhance this by dietary manipulation.

Cyclophosphamide exerts no beneficial effect over prednisone alone in the initial treatment of acute immune-mediated hemolytic anemia in dogs: a randomized controlled clinical trial

Mason N, Duval D, Shofer FS, Giger U. *J Vet Intern Med* 2003; **17**: 206–12

BACKGROUND. IMHA is one of the most commonly recognized immune-mediated diseases in companion animal practice. The mainstay of therapy is immuno-suppression, but as no single study has sufficiently addressed what might be the optimum immunosuppressive protocol, a variety of such regimens are in common

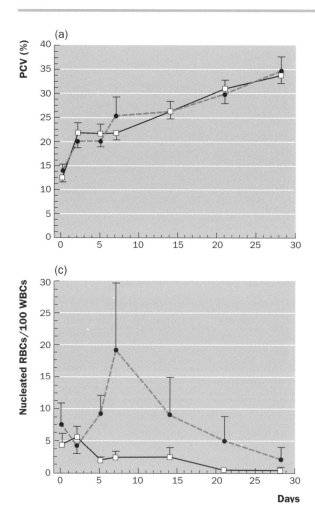

use. Most commonly, affected dogs would be treated with an immunosuppressive dose of prednisolone, but in more severe disease prednisolone is used in combination with azathioprine or cyclophosphamide. Although other agents (e.g. intravenous immunoglobulin or cyclosporin) have been successfully used to treat canine IMHA, their application is often precluded by expense. The present study compares whether the use of prednisolone and cyclophosphamide is of greater benefit than treatment with prednisolone alone.

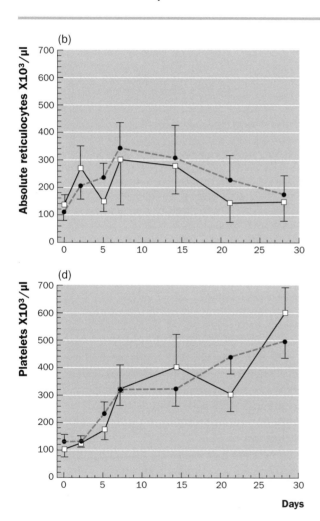

Fig. 2.4 (a) PCV, (b) absolute reticulocyte count, (c) nucleated red blood cell count, and (d) platelet count of dogs with acute, severe idiopathic immune-mediated haemolytic anaemia randomly assigned to the P group (*closed circles*) or the PC group (*open squares*). Sequential mean and SD values for each treatment group are joined by a solid line (P group) or a dotted line (PC group). Source: Mason *et al.* (2003).

INTERPRETATION. The study involved 18 dogs with primary, idiopathic IMHA characterized by compatible history (of less than 1 week) and clinical signs, haemolytic anaemia (with packed cell volume less than 20%) and either positive in-saline agglutination or Coombs' test. Additionally, the dogs had not received immunosuppressive drugs for a period of greater than 3 days before referral. The dogs were randomly assigned to one of two treatment groups. Ten dogs received oral prednisolone alone (1–2 mg/kg every 12 h), or in the event of failure to tolerate oral medication, dogs were administered intravenous dexamethasone sodium succinate (0.5–1 mg/kg every 24 h) (P group). Eight dogs received prednisolone (or dexamethasone) as described above, in addition to cyclophosphamide given either orally or intravenously at 50 mg/m^2 every 24 h for four consecutive days each week for 4 weeks (PC group). Other treatments, including packed red blood cell transfusion, were given as required. A range of parameters (physical examination, haematological examination including reticulocyte and platelet counts, urinalysis) was assessed on days 2, 3, 5, 7 and then weekly for 4 weeks. Coombs' testing was performed on days 3 and 7, and then weekly for 4 weeks.

Two of 10 dogs in the P group, and three of eight dogs in the PC group died during the first 8 days of the trial. These deaths were generally related to pulmonary thromboembolism or disseminated intravascular coagulation, which are well-documented complications of canine IMHA. Haematologically, there were few differences between the dogs in each group but reticulocytosis occurred earlier in the P group and spherocytosis resolved more rapidly in these dogs (Fig. 2.4). There was no difference between groups with respect to time taken to achieve a negative Coombs' test. Dogs in the PC group required a second blood transfusion more frequently (87.5%) than dogs in the P group (40%). Similarly, 37.5% of dogs in the PC group required a third transfusion compared with 20% of dogs in the P group. Overall, the results of this trial indicate that the concurrent use of cyclophosphamide and prednisolone offers no benefit over the use of prednisolone alone. More importantly, the use of cyclophosphamide was associated with a greater incidence of deleterious effects and should be contraindicated for the treatment of canine IMHA.

Comment

This is a simple, but very important, investigation with major practical relevance for first opinion companion animal practice. The study provides clear evidence that the use of prednisolone in combination with cyclophosphamide for the treatment of canine IMHA should be discontinued. Although the study included only 18 dogs and was performed in a single referral centre, it was prospective and randomized and is therefore an advance on the majority of reported series of canine IMHA. What is ideally required for this (and other) immune-mediated diseases is a much larger, multicentre, controlled prospective study to optimize the treatment protocol.

The second most commonly utilized combination therapy for canine IMHA is the use of prednisolone and azathioprine. This regimen would also benefit from such critical analysis. In at least one country, even the use of this protocol is discouraged in favour of prednisolone monotherapy—the reason relating to the perceived danger to humans of administration of cytotoxic agents to pet animals.

This investigation also provides insight into the monitoring of patients undergoing therapy for IMHA. The reticulocyte count is clearly a useful parameter for monitoring purposes, but the authors also describe sequential reduction in the number of circulating spherocytes, the presence of autoagglutination and the titre of the direct Coombs' test. This is in contrast to a study performed by our laboratory which showed long-term persistence of autoantibody in the majority of dogs undergoing therapy |25|. The discrepancy might relate to differences in the population of dogs studied, or methodological differences in the Coombs' test itself.

Comparison of cyclosporine A with methylprednisolone for treatment of canine atopic dermatitis: a parallel, blinded, randomized controlled trial

Steffan J, Alexander D, Brovedani F, Fisch R. *Vet Dermatol* 2003; **14**: 11–22

BACKGROUND. Atopic dermatitis is a disease of major importance in companion animal practice. Although there have been recent advances in diagnosis and management of this disease, the mainstay of initial therapy remains oral glucocorticoid administration. The adverse side effects of prolonged glucocorticoid therapy have led to studies of alternative anti-inflammatory agents such as cyclosporin A (CsA). First developed for use in human transplantation surgery, this drug has potent effects that primarily inhibit T-lymphocyte function via inhibiting transcription of the gene encoding the cytokine IL-2. Several studies have previously shown that administration of CsA has beneficial effects in dogs with atopic dermatitis, and one trial has compared the use of CsA with oral prednisolone for management of affected dogs during the first 6 weeks of therapy.

The present study is the most extensive evaluation of CsA for treatment of canine atopic dermatitis. This is a multicentre, parallel, blinded, randomized controlled study involving 117 dogs treated with CsA and 59 dogs treated with methylprednisolone over a 4-month period. The aims of the study were to compare the two treatment regimens, to investigate tapering of the dose of CsA into a maintenance phase of therapy, and to evaluate the safety of long-term administration of CsA.

INTERPRETATION. The study was conducted to the standard of Good Clinical Practice (GCP) in 30 dermatology referral centres in five European countries. The dogs with atopic dermatitis were selected on the basis of defined clinical criteria for this disease and were scored on the severity of cutaneous lesions using a Canine Atopic Dermatitis Extent and Severity Index (CADESI score). All dogs entering the trial had a baseline CADESI score of at least 25 and a defined washout period was set for various medications that may have been previously administered to the patients. The cases were randomized by computer, and the attending clinicians were unaware of the treatment administered, which was dispensed by a third party. CsA was administered at 5 mg/kg every 24 h for 4 weeks then gradually tapered on the basis of CADESI score. Methylprednisolone was administered at 0.5–1 mg/kg (mean dose 0.75 mg/kg) every 24 h for 1 week, then on alternate days for 3 weeks, following which it was also tapered in response to improving CADESI score. In addition to monitoring the patients by CADESI score, owners recorded pruritus on a visual analogue scale and the investigators also assessed pruritus at each revisit. Blood concentration of CsA was measured at 4 weeks, and haematological and biochemical parameters were checked at the initial and final visits. Eleven dogs in each group did not complete the trial.

At the conclusion of the trial, dogs treated with CsA had a mean 52% reduction in CADESI score and 36% reduction in pruritus score. Methylprednisolone-treated dogs had a mean 45% reduction in CADESI score and 33% reduction in pruritus score (Fig. 2.5). The differences between the treatment groups were not statistically significant. In addition to these scores, at the end of the trial both owners and investigators rated the response to treatment on a four-point scale. Using this index, 76% of dogs treated with CsA were said to show 'good' or 'excellent' overall response, compared with 63% of dogs treated with methylprednisolone. Neither group displayed changes in haematological or biochemical parameters when samples from initial and final visit were compared.

Adverse effects were recorded in 80% of dogs treated with methylprednisolone and 81% of dogs given CsA, but these were generally considered mild or moderate in severity. The most common side effects of CsA therapy were vomiting, diarrhoea or soft stools. In seven of 117 dogs, this was sufficiently severe to interrupt therapy, following which there was spontaneous resolution of the signs. The most common side effects of methylprednisolone therapy were bacterial or fungal dermatitis, otitis or conjunctivitis. Although these reactions occurred with similar frequency in CsA-treated dogs, they were more severe in the methylprednisolone group. Polyuria, polydipsia, increased appetite and weight gain was more frequently recorded in the methylprednisolone-treated dogs, whereas occasional CsA-treated dogs developed gingivitis (probably gingival hyperplasia) or reduced appetite.

Overall, the objective study has shown equal efficacy between the two treatments, but a subjective perception among owners and investigators that CsA produced better efficacy. The recorded adverse effects to either therapy are compatible with what is already known about these drugs.

Comment

This paper presents an excellent example of a well-designed clinical trial based on significant numbers of subjects. Trials of this magnitude and complexity are difficult to undertake in companion animal medicine without the resource afforded by commercial sponsorship. Perhaps the most surprising aspect of the study design was the choice of methylprednisolone, rather than the more commonly used prednisolone, as the comparator therapy. Overall, the study shows that CsA and methylprednisolone have equivalent efficacy when used as primary therapy for the induction and maintenance of dogs with severe atopic dermatitis. As pointed out by the authors in the discussion, it was not their intention to prove the superiority of CsA over methylprednisolone, although the subjective overall assessment measure would suggest this interpretation.

This paper is published against the background of the recent licensing of CsA for the treatment of canine atopic dermatitis. The licensing of a new immunomodulatory agent is an uncommon event in companion animal clinical immunology, which was one reason for my including this paper in this annual selection. CsA clearly has numerous other applications for the treatment of small animal immune-mediated disease for which it does not yet have a license—indeed in the same issue of the journal, there is a useful review article that summarizes the application of this drug to treatment of cutaneous lupus erythematosus, pseudopelade, pemphigus, anal furunculosis and sebaceous adenitis |26|. Moreover, there are limited studies of the application of CsA to other immune-mediated disorders such as IMHA and IMTP

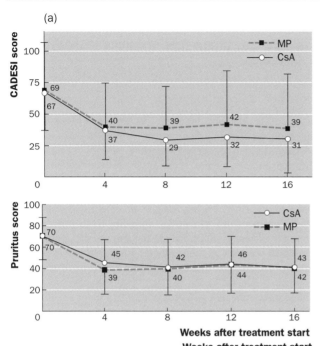

Fig. 2.5 Evolution of (a) mean Canine Atopic Dermatitis Extent and Severity Index (CADESI) lesional scores and (b) mean owner pruritus scores (visual analogue scale), during the course of the study. The dogs received cyclosporine (CsA, 5 mg/kg daily) or methylprednisolone (MP, 0.5–1 mg/kg daily for 1 week then every other day for 3 weeks) for a month. The dose was then tapered according to the clinical response. Means for all dogs included in the study (n = 117 in the CsA group and 59 in the MP group, intent-to-treat analysis). Source: Steffan et al. (2003).

(immune-mediated thrombocytopenia) |**27**|, and of course its application to the field of transplantation surgery |**28**| and the topical treatment of canine keratoconjunctivitis sicca |**29**|.

Although CsA therapy represents an advance in immunomodulatory treatment due to its relatively selective effect on T lymphocytes, in immunological terms this remains quite 'crude' immunosuppression, which has blanket effects on all T cells, not just those that mediate the disease under question. What will be particularly interesting, is to see whether the novel immunomodulatory products now available and under development for human use eventually translate into companion animal medicine. The example of monoclonal antibodies that neutralize specific cytokines has been discussed above, but of equal interest are approaches that seek to inhibit lymphocytes of particular antigen specificity—for example, the mucosal delivery of peptides derived from particular autoantigens or allergens |**7**|.

Mixed chimeric haematopoietic stem cell transplant reverses the disease phenotype in canine leukocyte adhesion deficiency

Creevy KE, Bauer Jr TR, Tuschong LM, et al. Vet Immunol Immunopathol 2003; **95**: 113–21

BACKGROUND. Canine leucocyte adhesion deficiency (CLAD) is one of the best understood of the primary immunodeficiency disorders of the dog. The disease has been recognized for many years in Irish red, or red and white, setters in a number of countries. These dogs develop multiple, severe, recurrent bacterial infections that lead to death or euthanasia by about 6 months of age. Affected dogs have marked leucocytosis, but these cells cannot migrate from the blood to infected tissue, so infection continues unchecked. Recently, the precise genetic defect underlying this disease has been identified. This is a single nucleotide mutation in the gene encoding the leucocyte integrin molecule CD18. Failure to generate CD18 prevents the formation of the CD11/CD18 complex on the leucocyte surface. It is this complex that interacts with ligands on vascular endothelium to initiate migration of white cells into infected tissue.

Humans also develop leucocyte adhesion deficiency but with a wider spectrum of mutations in the CD18 gene. The disease has a spectrum of clinical severity in humans, but can lead to lethal infection early in life. Human patients have been treated with myeloablative haematopoietic stem cell transplantation. This procedure involves complete destruction of the patient bone marrow, and reconstitution of the marrow compartment by transfer of stem cells from a donor individual. The patient essentially becomes a 'chimera' as the haemopoietic cells within them are entirely of donor origin (termed '100% donor chimerism'). As myeloablation is clearly a very severe process, this therapy is restricted in its application.

The spontaneously arising canine disease provides a useful experimental model for investigation of therapeutic options for human patients. In this study, the authors have established an experimental breeding colony of CLAD dogs for this purpose. They investigate whether a less severe (non-myeloablative) conditioning of a canine patient would lead to successful establishment of tissue matched (histocompatible) donor stem cells and reverse the disease phenotype.

INTERPRETATION. The study involved a 4-month-old CLAD dog bred from heterozygous Irish setter parents. The dog had characteristic features of CLAD, including hypertrophic osteodystrophy (Fig. 2.6). The donor dog was a histocompatible, clinically normal littermate. Two hours before the bone marrow transplant, the recipient dog received a dose of total body irradiation at a sublethal dose of 200 cGy. Marrow was collected from the donor dog and filtered before a total of 1.95×10^8 nucleated cells per kg were infused into the recipient intravenously over 15 min. A sample of marrow was tested to show that 1.3% of the transferred cells were stem cells expressing the marker CD34. Post-transplantation, the recipient dog received immunosuppression with CsA (tapered over 60 days) and mycophenolic acid mofetil for 28 days.

The response of the recipient dog to transplantation was remarkable. There was clinical improvement by 2 weeks post-transplant, with a single episode of pyrexia, anorexia and lethargy at 12 weeks, which responded rapidly to antimicrobials and non-steroidal anti-inflammatory drugs. The dog has shown no further signs of CLAD for over 12 months post-transplantation and the initial hypertrophic osteodystrophy lesions resolved completely (Fig. 2.6). The elevated leucocyte count that characterizes CLAD was stably reversed following transplantation (Fig. 2.7) and leucocytes expressing CD18 were readily identified in the blood. The mixed chimeric state of the recipient was assessed by testing for a genetic marker that differed between the recipient and donor. The proportion of donor DNA within

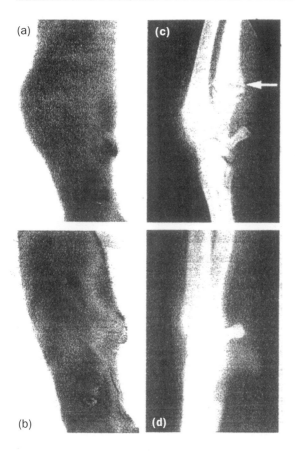

Fig. 2.6 Hypertrophic osteodystrophy (HOD) of the right carpus of the CLAD dog before and 1 year after bone marrow transplant. (a) Photograph demonstrating metaphyseal soft tissue swelling at 2 months of age, taken during a period of lameness. (b) Radiographic metaphyseal lucency in the right radius and ulna, with increased density immediately adjacent to the physis (double physis sign) typical of HOD. (c) Normal carpus from the same dog at 16 months of age, 1 year following transplant. (d) Radiographic resolution of metaphyseal lucency, along with closed physes in the CLAD dog at 16 months of age. Source: Creevy *et al.* (2003).

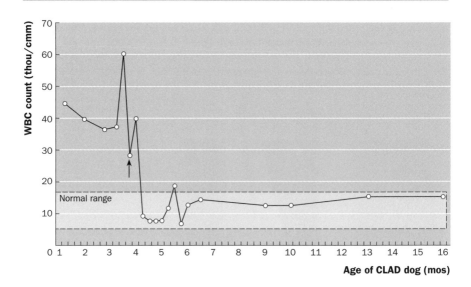

Fig. 2.7 Total WBC counts prior to and following matched littermate bone marrow transplant. The WBC count (y axis) was measured at the designated time intervals (x axis). The time of matched littermate bone marrow transplant is designated by the arrow. The lighter area represents the normal WBC count range. Source: Creevy *et al.* (2003).

DNA extracted from leucocytes correlated with the proportion of CD18 expressing leucocytes in the blood. The results of this experiment suggest that complete replacement of recipient haemopoietic tissue by donor cells may not be required to successfully treat leucocyte adhesion deficiency in humans.

Comment

This is an important and exciting paper that very clearly demonstrates the contribution that companion animal immunology can make to human disease. While the prime concern of veterinarians is for the health and welfare of their animal patients, it should also be recognized that our companion animals do develop spontaneously arising diseases that are excellent models for human counterparts. The study of naturally occurring disease, in an outbred, large animal that shares an environment with humans, can often be a more powerful model than an investigation conducted into induced disease in inbred laboratory rodents.

The CLAD story is one of the great successes in the field of companion animal immunology. First identified in 1975 |**30**|, the immunological abnormality was identified at the protein |**31**| and subsequently the molecular level |**32**|. The widespread availability of a genetic test for this mutation has now enabled the Irish setter breed group to work towards the elimination of this trait in the breed, via the identification of carriers and modified breeding programmes |33|. The present study demonstrates the further benefit that these studies have provided for human medicine.

Effects of dietary n-6 and n-3 fatty acids and vitamin E on the immune response of healthy geriatric dogs

Hall JA, Tooley KA, Gradin JL, Jewell DE, Wander RC. *Am J Vet Res* 2003; **64**: 762–72

BACKGROUND. This study is based upon two background strands of information: (i) the recognition of age-related changes in the canine immune system, and (ii) the ability to modulate the systemic immune system by the incorporation of a range of dietary components. The immunological changes that occur in elderly dogs include decreased total leucocyte count and lymphocyte proliferative responses, and altered ratios of T-cell subsets with a reduction in CD4+ cells. The overall aim of this study was to determine whether these immunological parameters could be altered in older dogs by dietary manipulation.

The dietary factors under consideration were the n-3 polyunsaturated fatty acids (PUFAs) and α-tocopheryl acetate. n-3 PUFAs, such as those derived from fish oil, are associated with dampening of a wide range of inflammatory and immune parameters, and dietary supplementation has previously been shown to reduce the cutaneous delayed hypersensitivity (DTH) response in aged beagle dogs. By contrast, α-tocopheryl acetate is inhibitory of lipid peroxidation, and it has been suggested that when diets are enriched for n-3 PUFAs there should be accompanying increased intake of α-tocopheryl acetate. Therefore, a specific aim of this study was to determine whether the concentration of α-tocopheryl acetate added to food supplemented with n-3 PUFAs was related to the immunological effects of this diet in elderly dogs.

INTERPRETATION. The study involved 32 beagle dogs aged between 7 and 10 years that were initially acclimatized to a commercial diet with low n-3 PUFA content (n-6 to n-3 ratio of 18:1). The dogs were divided into six groups, each fed a different diet for a 17-week period. Three groups were fed a low n-3 PUFA diet (n-6 to n-3 ratio of 40:1), and three groups received a high n-3 PUFA diet (n-6 to n-3 ratio of 1.4:1). Within each of these two types of diet, there were three subtypes characterized by the content of α-tocopheryl acetate (low, medium and high).

Blood samples were taken before the trial and at 12, 13 and 15 weeks for routine haematological examination and determination of T-lymphocyte subsets by flow cytometry. Dogs were injected with a novel antigen (keyhole limpet haemocyanin; KLH) at weeks 13 and 15 and blood taken at week 17 to determine antibody response. One day after the second injection, a DTH skin test was performed with KLH.

Dogs fed the high n-3 PUFA diet had similar DTH test reactions at 48–96 h for all three concentrations of α-tocopheryl acetate. By contrast, dogs fed a low n-3 PUFA diet had significantly greater DTH reaction at 72 and 96 h when they received the medium concentration of α-tocopherol acetate (Fig. 2.8). These findings suggest that vitamin E supplementation of a low n-3 PUFA diet can enhance the DTH response, but that this effect is inhibited when the optimum vitamin E supplementation is given with a high n-3 PUFA diet. There was no significant difference in the KLH antibody response at week 17 between dogs in any group.

Dogs receiving high α-tocopheryl acetate had more blood lymphocytes on weeks 13 and 15 compared with week 12, and dogs fed the high n-3 PUFA diet had more blood lymphocytes on week 13 compared with week 12. The percentage of blood CD8+ T lymphocytes and the CD4 to CD8 ratio was lower at week 12 in dogs consuming the low α-tocopheryl acetate diets. Although there was no significant difference in these parameters between groups at week 13, the ratio of CD4 to CD8 cells was significantly greater at week 15 only for dogs on the high n-3 PUFA and low α-tocopheryl acetate diet. Overall, these observations suggest that vitamin E supplementation enhances the CD8+ T-lymphocyte count regardless of the n-3 to n-6 ratio of the diet. The authors speculate that there may be

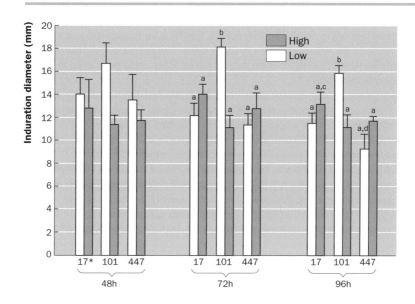

Fig. 2.8 Effect of feeding dogs six foods containing high (*grey bars*) or low (*white bars*) amounts of n-3 fatty acids and three differing concentrations of α-tocopheryl acetate (low = 17 mg of α-tocopheryl acetate/kg of food; medium = 101 mg/kg; high = 447 mg/kg) on the delayed-type hypersensitivity skin test at 48, 72, and 96 hours. Dogs were challenged with an intradermal injection of keyhole limpet haemocyanin (KLH) to which they had been previously sensitized. Each bar represents the mean (± SEM) induration diameter after dogs had consumed their respective food for 15 weeks. A significant ($P < 0.05$) interaction was found between concentration of dietary α-tocopheryl acetate and n-3 fatty acids at 72 and 96 hours; therefore, effects of α-tocopheryl acetate at each amount of n-3 fatty acids were compared separately. a, b, c, d, Different letters above bars at each time indicate values that differed significantly ($P < 0.05$). Source: Hall *et al.* (2003).

a relationship between the ability of vitamin E supplementation to enhance the numbers of blood CD8+ T cells and the cutaneous DTH response.

Comment

This is a relatively complex experimental protocol that has resulted in a detailed and lengthy manuscript. Regardless of the finer points of the experimental data, the overall conclusion of the study is important. It is widely recognized that older animals have weakened immune defences that predispose them to disease. This study is just one of a growing number of publications that clearly demonstrate that systemic immune function can be enhanced by the inclusion of optimum concentrations of particular dietary supplements. Although it might be argued that some effects observed in a controlled experimental study might not readily translate to animals in the field (i.e. a 7-year-old laboratory beagle may be quite different to a 14-year-old German shepherd dog living on a farm), the basic premise is sound and must be to the benefit of the companion animal population. The wide range of commercially available diets designed for various disease states is now an important part of patient management for these disorders. This next phase of dietary manipulation aims to optimize the health of animals without overt disease, particularly at-risk groups such as geriatrics. These studies will eventually have enormous practical significance for clinical practice.

Advances in vaccinology

The final theme of this chapter covers vaccination. So much emphasis is now placed on the adverse effects of vaccination that I have selected one paper on the most investigated of such reactions—the feline vaccine-associated sarcoma. The second paper in this section investigates whether vaccination has different effects in young and old dogs, and the final study is a taste of the future of vaccination, demonstrating the efficacy of so-called 'naked DNA' vaccines in the dog.

Multicenter case-control study of risk factors associated with development of vaccine-associated sarcomas in cats

Kass PH, Spangler WL, Hendrick MJ, et al. J Am Vet Med Assoc 2003; **223**: 1283–92

BACKGROUND. The association between the development of aggressive fibrosarcoma and prior injection of vaccine at the tumour site was first reported in 1991, but continues to exercise much interest and debate within the veterinary profession. Numerous aspects of the epidemiology and pathogenesis of this lesion have been studied since the inception of the US Vaccine Associated Feline Sarcoma

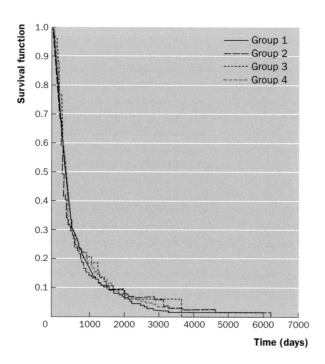

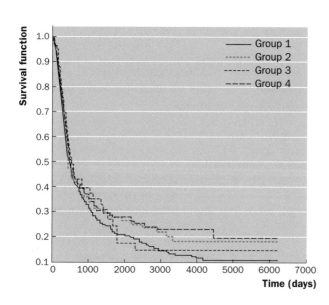

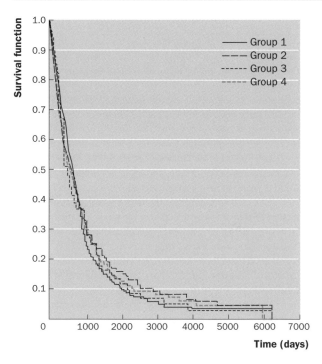

Fig. 2.9 Distribution of time between the last administration of a (a) feline viral rhinotracheitis-calicivirus-panleukopenia vaccine; (b) FeLV vaccine; and (c) rabies vaccine, and diagnosis of a tumour in various groups of cats. Group 1 ($n = 643$) consisted of cats with a soft tissue sarcoma at a site where vaccines are frequently administered (e.g. interscapular and femoral regions). Group 2 ($n = 131$) consisted of cats with a sarcoma at a site where vaccines are infrequently given (e.g. thoracic, shoulder, lumbar, gluteal, and flank regions). Group 3 ($n = 72$) consisted of cats with a sarcoma at a site where vaccines are not given (e.g. ears, head, toes, and tail). Group 4 ($n = 217$) consisted of cats with a basal cell tumour. Source: Kass *et al.* (2003).

Taskforce, but there is still much to be understood about this entity and even the true prevalence of these sarcomas is not clear.

Early US studies suggested an increased risk among cats receiving vaccination for feline leukaemia virus (FeLV) or rabies, and an association with the use of adjuvant, and these findings have been replicated in European investigations |34|. The simple avoidance of vaccination is not a viable answer to this problem, as maintaining protection among the feline population is crucial to the control of serious infectious diseases, and there are legal and zoonotic implications to rabies vaccination. The present paper reports a prospective, multicentre, case–control study that aims to identify risk factors for the occurrence of feline vaccine-associated sarcoma. Specific factors examined included brand of vaccine, use of other injectables, vaccination practice and host factors.

INTERPRETATION. Case material for the study was generated through seven university or laboratory centres, including the US Pharmacopeia to which there is voluntary reporting of feline vaccine-associated sarcoma. Inclusion criteria were that a cat should have developed a histologically confirmed soft tissue sarcoma at a site commonly used for vaccination over the period January 1998 to June 1999. Veterinarians and owners were contacted to obtain relevant history. The sarcomas recorded covered the full histopathological spectrum of these lesions that has been previously documented.

Control cats were of two sources and were identified over the same time frame. The first control group comprised cats from the same centres (except the US Pharmacopeia) that had been diagnosed with histologically confirmed basal cell tumour. The second control group consisted of cats with histologically confirmed soft tissue sarcomas arising at sites not generally used for vaccination (e.g. head, digits, ventral abdomen, ears or tail). Data were analysed using different definitions of case and control cats, and using five different 'time windows' (3 and 6 months, 1, 2 and 3 years) to take into account whether vaccines had actually been administered into the site of the sarcoma, and the time interval between onset of sarcoma and vaccination. A total of 1598 cats were included in the study, of which further information was obtained on 1347 cats, but not all animals were included in all analyses. The range of vaccines used in this population included 17 rabies vaccines from eight manufacturers, 14 FeLV vaccines from 10 manufacturers and 26 FVRCP (feline viral rhinotracheitis, calicivirus and parvovirus) vaccines from 11 manufacturers. Almost all rabies and FeLV vaccines were adjuvanted.

These analyses failed to document clear associations between feline vaccine-associated sarcoma and factors such as: (i) whether cats lived in multicat households; (ii) whether cats were seropositive for FeLV or feline immunodeficiency virus; (iii) previous trauma at the site of the sarcoma; (iv) specific types of vaccine within a class of antigen; or (v) specific brands of vaccine. There was no association with vaccination practice, with the possible exception of vaccine temperature prior to injection where administration of cold vaccine was associated with a greater risk of sarcoma. Other vaccine practices assessed included: mixing vaccines in a single syringe, reusing syringes after sterilization, type of syringe, gauge of needle, whether multidose vials were shaken before use and whether the vaccine site was massaged. Of most interest was the finding that the administration of injectable long-acting penicillin or methylprednisolone acetate may be associated with sarcoma formation.

The interval between the diagnosis of tumour and the most recent administration of rabies, FeLV or FVRCP vaccine was analysed when cats were grouped by tumour location (sarcomas at sites used for vaccination, sites less commonly used for vaccination, sites generally not used for vaccination and basal cell tumours). No significant difference was found even when cats were excluded from the analysis when the vaccination to diagnosis interval was up to 120 days (Fig. 2.9).

Comment

This is a complex epidemiological study that is significant for the numbers of animals included and the strict attention to case definition utilized. The authors were relatively conservative concerning the interpretation of their findings, and suggest that any potential for association between sarcoma and administration of other injectables or the temperature at which vaccines are administered, should be corroborated by others. It is pointed out in discussion that this study was performed at a time when newer vaccine products (e.g. non-adjuvanted recombinant products) had been only recently introduced and did not account for a sizeable proportion of the vaccines administered in the study. It might be expected that the prevalence of adverse reactions might change over time with the availability of such products.

The authors also comment as to the amount and quality of data available for assessment. This is an international problem, and reflects the fact that reporting of adverse reactions occurs on a voluntary basis and the recording of the detail of administration of vaccines to individual animals by veterinarians is limited.

The debate concerning the frequency of adverse reactions to vaccination in companion animal species has now continued for several years, and in North America at least has led to significant changes in vaccine practice based on recommendations produced by the American Association of Feline Practitioners (AAFP) |**35**|, American Veterinary Medical Association (AVMA) |**36**| and American Animal Hospital Association |**37**|. There is no more tangible area of veterinary immunology for the veterinarian in first opinion practice than vaccination and the issues surrounding it.

Effect of age on immune parameters and the immune response of dogs to vaccines: a cross-sectional study

HogenEsch H, Thompson S, Dunham A, Ceddia M, Hayek M. *Vet Immunol Immunopathol* 2004; **97**: 77–85

BACKGROUND. The background to this paper is not dissimilar to the study of Hall *et al.* discussed above. It is recognized that there are changes in the immune system of older dogs, and one aim of the present paper was to further define these differences in immune function of elderly animals. The more interesting purpose of the investigation was to determine whether older dogs responded less effectively to vaccination than younger animals. This is an important question, addressed against the current background of discussions about duration of immunity for companion animal vaccines and the wisdom of extending revaccination intervals for these animals.

INTERPRETATION. The study involved 65 pet dogs recruited through a university first opinion practice. There were 32 young dogs (mean age 3.15 ± 0.8 years) of 10 different breeds, the greatest number being crossbred ($n = 14$). There were 19 females (17 neutered) and 13 males (11 neutered). There were 33 old dogs (mean age 12.1 ± 1.3 years) of 15 different breeds (including 10 crossbred). This group included 20 females (19 neutered) and 13 males (11 neutered). On the day of recruitment, the dogs were blood sampled and given a killed rabies vaccine plus standard multivalent vaccine. A second blood sample was collected 2 weeks after vaccination. Saliva was collected using cotton swabs.

A range of immunological tests was performed on each sample. A whole-blood lymphocyte proliferation assay was performed, whereby blood lymphocytes were stimulated with the mitogens concanavalin A, pokeweed mitogen, phytohaemagglutinin and staphylococcal enterotoxin B. Lymphocyte phenotyping was performed by flow cytometry using antibodies to detect the markers CD3, CD21, CD4, CD8, CD45R and CD29. Serum antibody titres to canine distemper virus, canine parvovirus-2 and rabies virus were determined, and the total

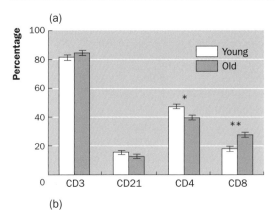

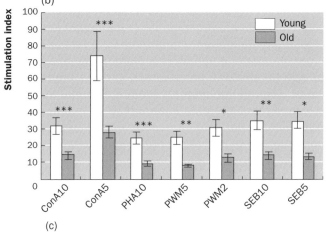

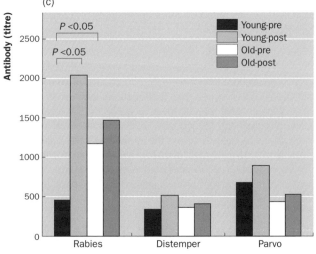

Fig. 2.10 The effect of age on (a) the percentage of lymphocyte subpopulations in the peripheral blood of dogs. The bars indicate the SEM. *$P = 0.005$; **$P = 0.001$; (b) lymphocyte proliferation. Whole blood cultures were stimulated with the indicated mitogens at 2.5 or 10 μm/ml. The stimulation index was calculated and presented as mean $\pm$ SEM. There were significant differences between the young and old dogs for all mitogens. *$P < 0.01$; **$P = 0.001$; ***$P < 0.001$; (c) the antibody response to vaccines in dogs. Serum collected pre- and 2 weeks post-vaccination was tested for antibodies against rabies virus (fluorescence focus inhibition assay), canine distemper virus (virus neutralization) and canine parvovirus-2 (haemagglutination inhibition). The bars represent the geometric means. There was a significant difference of anti-rabies titre between the young and old pre-vaccination titres and a significant increase of titre in young dogs following rabies vaccination ($P < 0.05$). Source: HogenEsch et al. (2004).

concentrations of serum IgG, IgM and IgA were assessed. The concentration of salivary IgA was also measured.

Old dogs had significantly reduced lymphocyte proliferative responses to all mitogens tested. Although there was no significant difference in the percentage of CD3+ T lymphocytes or CD21+ B lymphocytes between the groups, the older dogs had lower CD4 and higher CD8 percentages resulting in a lower CD4/CD8 ratio. Older dogs also had significantly fewer CD45+/CD4+ T cells than younger dogs.

Old dogs had significantly more IgA in the serum than young dogs, but there were no differences in IgG or IgM concentration. Salivary IgA concentration was greater in older dogs, but when this parameter was adjusted for salivary flow rate by relating concentration to total protein, there was no significant difference between the groups.

All dogs had antibody titres to each of the three viruses that were above the 'minimum protective titre' before vaccination. When pre- and postvaccinal titres were compared, vaccination did not induce a significant rise in antibodies to distemper or parvovirus in either group. By contrast, older dogs had a higher prevaccinal rabies titre than younger dogs, but vaccination induced a significantly greater response to this antigen in the younger dogs. The findings of the study suggest that there are immunological changes in older dogs, but in terms of the serological response to vaccination, the protocol of annual vaccination used in these animals was sufficient to maintain protective immunity.

Comment

This paper makes a significant contribution to our understanding of the age-related changes in the canine immune system. Many previous studies of elderly canines have involved relatively homogeneous populations of dogs housed in experimental facilities (for example the study of Hall et al. described above). The major advance in the present work is that an outbred, mixed population of pet animals living in a natural environment was utilized. The findings confirm and extend previous observations. Of all the observations, those that were most conclusive and might serve as useful biomarkers for ageing were the proliferative response to concanavalin A and phyto-haemagglutinin, the CD4/CD8 ratio and the percentage of CD45R+/CD4+ T cells in the blood. This latter finding may be interpreted to mean that older dogs have reduced numbers of 'naive' (cells not stimulated by antigen) T cells, although the canine CD45R molecule has not yet definitively been shown to mark a naive T-cell subset. The elevated serum IgA concentration in older dogs is consistent with find-ings in humans, and leakage of serum IgA into saliva might explain the raised salivary IgA concentration in the same group of dogs |38|.

Of equal importance are the observations made on the vaccinal immune responses in these dogs. The dogs in this study were annually revaccinated with both rabies and standard multivalent canine vaccine. This protocol had clearly induced antibody titres to all tested components that were considered protective. The greater baseline antibody titre to rabies in the older dogs was interpreted to associate with the longer usage of this product in this population over time. As the authors point out, it would be interesting to compare the results of this study to a similar investigation con-ducted on a group of dogs that had received a triennial revaccination schedule.

There is mounting evidence to suggest that many companion animal vaccines induce prolonged seropositivity and therefore likely have a longer duration of immun-ity than there is currently evidence to support |39|. A number of studies have now shown that animals that do not receive annual revaccination (sometimes for many years) retain protective antibody titres |40|. This does not, however, necessarily mean that each individual within a population will respond in the same way to less frequent revaccination, so tailor-made vaccination schedules based on serological testing may be required. A further argument concerns the validity of serological testing as a measure of protection. Although there is evidence to support the presence of anti-body to some viruses as indicating protection, this is less clear for others. In fact, measurement of T-cell responsiveness would be an immunologically more sensible means of assessing the immune response to viral antigens, but in practical terms this is very difficult to achieve. The debate over companion animal revaccination sched-ules is likely to continue, until such time as there is increased availability of licensed products with a claim for extended duration of immunity.

Canine rabies DNA vaccination: a single-dose intradermal injection into ear pinnae elicits elevated and persistent levels of neutralizing antibody

Lodmell DL, Parnell MJ, Weyhrich JT, Ewalt LC. *Vaccine* 2003; **21**: 3998–4002

BACKGROUND. This investigation concerns the development of improved canine rabies vaccines. In rabies endemic areas it is difficult to achieve more than 30–50% vaccination coverage of the canine population, particularly when dogs require booster vaccinations to maintain immunity. The availability of a vaccine that gave long-term protective immunity after a single vaccination would go some way towards addressing this problem. A good candidate to achieve this aim would be a DNA vaccine. A single DNA vaccination has been shown to confer lifetime protection of experimental mice, and preliminary studies have shown that rabies DNA vaccination can induce protection in dogs. A further advantage of molecular vaccines is that such products may be administered to young animals, as their action is less likely to be inhibited by maternally derived antibody.

INTERPRETATION. The studies described here used a DNA vaccine comprising a plasmid containing the gene encoding the glycoprotein of the rabies virus. The study used 13–15-month-old beagle dogs that had not previously been vaccinated for rabies. Four groups of three dogs each received the DNA vaccine via a different route. Group 1 received a total of 10 μg of DNA delivered into each ear pinna by a 'gene gun'. Group 2 received a total of 200 μg of DNA given by intradermal injection to the skin on each side of the neck. Group 3 received a total of 200 μg of DNA given by intradermal injection to the inner surface of each ear pinna. Group 4 received a total of 100 μg of DNA by intramuscular injection into the quadriceps muscle. Blood samples for determination of antibody titre were collected on days 0, 10, 30, 60, 90, 120 and 150. On day 150, all dogs received a booster vaccination of 100 μg of DNA by intradermal injection into the ear pinnae. In the final part of the study, a group of mice was injected intraperitoneally with 1 ml of dog serum (previously determined to contain 5 IU of rabies virus neutralizing antibody). Seven days later the mice were challenged with virulent rabies virus and at the same time given a further 5 IU of canine antibody. Canine antibody was also given to the mice 7, 14 and 21 days after viral challenge. A control group of mice received non-immune canine serum, and both groups were monitored for 60 days after rabies challenge.

In the canine experiment, serum collected 10 days post-vaccination showed rabies antibody only in Group 3 dogs. At day 30, the titres of antibody in these dogs had increased and one dog from Group 2 had a low titred antibody response. There was no change in this pattern through to 150 days, suggesting that only the Group 3 dogs had made a successful and long-term response to vaccination. Ten days after the booster vaccine at day 150, the Group 2 dogs had a greater than 100-fold increase in rabies antibody titre, and an increase of similar magnitude was detected in two of the three dogs in Group 2. Additionally, two dogs of Group 1 and one dog of Group 4 now had detectable antibody. Thirty days after the booster, all dogs (except one animal in Group 1) had serum antibody to rabies of >0.5 IU/ml. In the murine experiment, all eight mice receiving canine serum were protected from rabies, whereas all controls developed rabies.

The results of the study show that dogs receiving intradermal rabies DNA vaccination into the pinnae respond by developing long-term seropositivity. The superiority of this route of administration likely relates the ready transfection of dendritic cells that migrate to the regional lymph node to activate T cells.

Comment

The studies described in this paper give a glimpse into the future of companion animal vaccinology. Already we have licensed molecular vaccines that rely on the use of a vector virus to carry the genes of interest from organisms such as rabies, canine distemper or FeLV |41|. The next stage of such development is the use of 'naked DNA' such as the plasmids described here. Such plasmids are capable of not only carrying genes for structural components of microbes, but also an array of 'molecular adjuvants', such as bacterial CpG motifs or cytokine genes derived from the target animal species. These molecular vaccines are exceptionally potent and appear to provide long-lasting immunity of both humoral and cell-mediated type.

The attraction for use in companion animal practice is obvious. These are non-adjuvanted products that could be given with an extended duration of immunity, and molecular vaccines might also be effective in young pups or kittens in the face of maternal immunity |**42**|. Of course, these products will not appear in the market-place in the near future. The lead-in time for production and licensing of new immunological products is long, and there are particular issues with respect to the use of 'genetically modified' products, but the future of vaccinology is an exciting place.

Conclusion

The preceding 12 papers provide a snapshot of veterinary immunology relating to companion animal practice in the year 2003–2004. The breadth of the topics covered is a good reflection of the many areas of small animal practice that involve aspects of the immune system. The papers have shown how recent advances in understanding the canine and feline immune systems are based in the application of molecular technology, and how this same technology has carried through into laboratory diagnosis and heralds the development of a new era in vaccine production and therapeutics. Vaccination and therapy may in future go hand-in-hand with genetic testing (such as described for susceptibility to leishmaniasis), so that vaccines and drugs are designed for the requirements of individual patients (or breeds of animal) on the basis of their genotype. Designer therapy may be accompanied by designer pet foods—manu-factured to enhance specifically the immune system of different patient groups, for example the elderly, or breeds of dog where immune defects are documented.

The selection of papers also makes the point that even in the short term there is room for continued re-evaluation of paradigms in immunology. For many years we have accepted that immune-mediated diseases are best treated with a limited reper-toire of immunosuppressive agents, but it would now seem that at least one of these (cyclophosphamide) does not lead to the clinical benefits ascribed to it. The adoption of new immunomodulatory drugs (for example CsA) by the veterinary profession need not be based solely on their having a more potent effect, but such decisions might be a result of the less severe side effects that might be associated with them. A further example of fundamental rethinking in immunology relates to the example given of the interaction between arthropod-borne infectious agents and the immune system. There is increasing evidence that many of the 'primary, idiopathic immune-mediated' diseases with which we deal in veterinary practice, might actually have an infectious aetiology.

This is an exciting time to work in companion animal practice, and to be able to witness the practical application of breakthroughs in molecular technology to the health and welfare of our patients.

References

1. Nuttall TJ, Knight PA, McAleese SM, Lamb JR, Hill PB. Expression of Th1, Th2 and immunosuppressive cytokine gene transcripts in canine atopic dermatitis. *Clin Exp Allergy* 2002; **32**: 789–95.

2. Peters IR, Helps CR, Calvert EL, Hall EJ, Day MJ. Cytokine mRNA quantification in canine duodenal mucosa by real-time RT–PCR. *Vet Immunol Immunopathol* 2004; in press.

3. Taglinger K, Nguyen Van N, Helps CR, Day MJ, Foster AP. Quantitative real-time RT–PCR for the measurement of feline cytokine mRNA expression in skin of normal cats and cats with allergic skin disease. *World Congress Vet Dermatol*, Vienna, 2004. Published in *Vet Dermatol* 2004; **15**(Suppl 1): 31.

4. Adorini L. Cytokine-based immunointervention in the treatment of autoimmune diseases. *Clin Exp Immunol* 2003; **132**: 185–92.

5. Day MJ. Antigen specificity in canine autoimmune haemolytic anaemia. *Vet Immunol Immunopathol* 1999; **69**: 215–24.

6. Lewis DC, Myers KM. Studies of platelet-bound and serum platelet-bindable immunoglobulins in dogs with idiopathic thrombocytopenia purpura. *Exp Haematol* 1996; **24**: 696–701.

7. Wraith DC. Antigen-specific immunotherapy of autoimmune disease: a commentary. *Clin Exp Immunol* 1996; **103**: 349–52.

8. Murphy KM, Reiner SL. The lineage decisions of helper T cells. *Nat Rev Immunol* 2002; **2**: 933–44.

9. Mazza G, Whiting AH, Day MJ, Duffus WPH. The preparation of monoclonal antibodies specific for the subclasses of canine immunoglobulin G. *Res Vet Sci* 1994; **57**: 140–5.

10. Deplazes P, Smith NC, Arnold P, Lutz H, Eckert J. Specific IgG1 and IgG2 antibody response of dogs to *Leishmania infantum* and other parasites. *Parasite Immunol* 1995; **17**: 451–8.

11. McBride JW, Corstvet RE, Gaunt SD, Boudreaux C, Guedry T, Walker DH. Kinetics of antibody response to *Ehrlichia canis* immunoreactive proteins. *Infect Immun* 2003; **71**: 2516–24.

12. Quinnell RJ, Courtenay O, Garcez L, Kaye PM, Shaw M-A, Dye C, Day MJ. IgG subclass responses in a longitudinal study of canine visceral leishmaniasis. *Vet Immunol Immunopathol* 2003; **91**: 161–8.

13. Shaw SE, Day MJ, Birtles RJ, Breitschwerdt EB. Tick-borne infectious diseases of dogs. *Trends Parasitol* 2001; **17**: 74–80.

14. Shaw SE, Lerga AI, Williams S, Beugnet F, Birtles RJ, Day MJ, Kenny MJ. Review of exotic infectious diseases in small animals entering the United Kingdom from abroad diagnosed by PCR. *Vet Rec* 2003; **152**: 176–7.

15. Teske E, van Heerde P, Rutteman GR, Kurzman ID, Moore PF, MacEwan G. Prognostic factors for treatment of malignant lymphoma in dogs. *J Am Vet Med Assoc* 1994; **205**: 1722–8.

16. Vail DM, Moore AS, Ogilvie GK, Volk LM. Feline lymphoma (145 cases): proliferation indicies, cluster of differentiation 3 immunoreactivity, and their association with prognosis in 90 cats. *J Vet Intern Med* 1998; **12**: 349–54.

17. Giraudel JM, Pages J-P, Guelfi J-F. Monoclonal gammopathies in the dog: a retrospective study of 18 cases (1986–1999) and literature review. *J Am Anim Hosp Assoc* 2002; **38**: 135–47.

18. Ciaramella P, Corona M. Canine leishmaniasis: clinical and diagnostic aspects. *Comp Cont Educ Pract Vet* 2003; **25**: 358–68.

19. Kennedy LJ, Barnes A, Happ GM, Quinnell RJ, Bennett D, Angles JM, Day MJ, Carmichael N, Innes JF, Isherwood D, Carter SD, Thomson W, Ollier WER. Extensive interbreed, but minimal intrabreed, variation of DLA class II alleles and haplotypes in dogs. *Tissue Antigens* 2002; **59**: 194–204.

20. Quinnell RJ, Courtenay O, Shaw M-A, Day MJ, Garcez L, Kaye PM, Dye C. Tissue cytokine response in canine visceral leishmaniasis. *J Infect Dis* 2001; **183**: 1421–4.

21. Solano-Gallego L, Llull J, Ramos G, Riera C, Arboix M, Alberola J, Ferrer L. The Ibizian hound presents a predominantly cellular immune response against natural *Leishmania* infection. *Vet Parasitol* 2000; **90**: 37–45.

22. Altet L, Francino O, Solano-Gallego L, Renier C, Sanchez A. Mapping and sequencing of the canine NRAMP1 gene and identification of mutations in leishmaniasis-susceptible dogs. *Infect Immun* 2002; **70**: 2763–71.

23. Molano I, Garcia Alonso M, Miron C, Redondo E, Requena JM, Soto M, Gomez Nieto C, Alonso C. A *Leishmania infantum* multi-component antigenic protein mixed with live BCG confers protection to dogs experimentally infected with *L. infantum. Vet Immunol Immunopathol* 2003; **92**: 1–13.

24. Day MJ, Penhale WJ. A review of major histocompatibility disease associations in man and dog. *Vet Res Comm* 1987; **11**: 119–32.

25. Day MJ. Serial monitoring of clinical, haematological and immunological parameters in canine autoimmune haemolytic anaemia. *J Small Anim Pract* 1996; **37**: 523–34.

26. Robson DC, Burton GC. Cyclosporin: applications in small animal dermatology. *Vet Dermatol* 2003; **14**: 1–9.

27. Grundy SA, Barton C. Influence of drug treatment on survival of dogs with immune-mediated hemolytic anemia: 88 cases (1989–1999). *J Am Vet Med Assoc* 2001; **218**: 543–6.

28. Mathews KG, Gregory CR. Renal transplants in cats: 66 cases (1987–1996). *J Am Vet Med Assoc* 1997; **211**: 1432–6.

29. Izci C, Celik I, Alkan F, Ogurtan Z, Ceylan C, Sur E, Ozkan Y. Histologic characteristics and local cellular immunity of the gland of the third eyelid after topical ophthalmic administration of 2% cyclosporine for treatment of dogs with keratoconjunctivitis sicca. *Am J Vet Res* 2002; **63**: 688–94.

30. Renshaw HW, Chatburn C, Bryan GM, Bartsch RC, Davis WC. Canine granulocytopathy syndrome: neutrophil dysfunction in a dog with recurrent infections. *J Am Vet Med Assoc* 1975; **166**: 443–7.

31. Giger U, Boxer LA, Simpson PJ, Lucchesi BR, Todd III RF. Deficiency of leukocyte surface glycoproteins Mo1, LFA-1 and Leu M5 in a dog with recurrent bacterial infections: an animal model. *Blood* 1987; **69**: 1622–30.

32. Kijas JM, Bauer Jr TR, Gafvert S, Marklund S, Trowald-Wigh G, Johannisson A, Hedham-mar A, Binns M, Juneja RK, Hickstein DD, Andersson L. A missense mutation in the β-2 integrin gene (ITGB2) causes canine leukocyte adhesion deficiency. *Genomics* 1999; **61**: 101–7.

33. Jobling AI, Ryan J, Augusteyn RC. The frequency of the canine leukocyte adhesion deficiency (CLAD) allele within the Irish Setter population of Australia. *Aust Vet J* 2003; **81**: 763–5.

34. Gaskell R, Gettinby G, Graham S, Skilton D. *Veterinary Products Committee (VPC) Working Group on feline and canine vaccination.* London: DEFRA, 2001.

35. Elston T, Rodan H, Flemming D, Ford RB, Hustead DR, Richards JR, Rosen DK, Scherk-Nixon MA, Scott PW. 1998 report of the American Association of Feline Practitioners and Academy of Feline Medicine Advisory Panel on Feline Vaccines. *J Am Vet Med Assoc* 1998; **212**: 227–41.

36. Klingborg DJ, Hustead DR, Curry-Galvin EA, Gumley NR, Henry SC, Bain FT, Paul MA, Boothe DM, Blood KS, Huxsoll DL, Reynolds DL, Riddell Jr MG, Reid JS, Short CR. AVMA Council on Biologic and Therapeutic Agents' report on cat and dog vaccines. *J Am Vet Med Assoc* 2002; **221**: 1401–7.

37. Paul MA, Appel M, Barrett R, Carmichael LE, Childers H, Cotter S, Davidson A, Ford R, Keil D, Lappin M, Schultz RD, Thacker E, Trumpeter JL, Welborn L. Report of the American Animal Hospital Association (AAHA) Canine Vaccine Task Force: executive summary and 2003 canine vaccine guidelines and recommendations. *J Am Anim Hosp Assoc* 2003; **39**: 119–31.

38. German AJ, Hall EJ, Day MJ. Measurement of IgG, IgM and IgA concentrations in canine serum, saliva, tears and bile. *Vet Immunol Immunopathol* 1998; **64**: 107–21.

39. Scott FW, Geissinger CM. Long-term immunity in cats vaccinated with an inactivated trivalent vaccine. *Am J Vet Res* 1999; **60**: 652–8.

40. Twark L, Dodds WJ. Clinical use of serum parvovirus and distemper virus antibody titers for determining revaccination strategies in healthy dogs. *J Am Vet Med Assoc* 2000; **217**: 1021–4.

41. Pardo MC, Bauman JE, Mackowiak M. Protection of dogs against canine distemper by vaccination with a canarypox virus recombinant expressing canine distemper virus fusion and hemagglutinin glycoproteins. *Am J Vet Res* 1997; **58**: 833–6.

42. Fischer L, Tronel J-P, Pardo-David C, Tanner P, Colombet G, Minke J, Audonnet J-C. Vaccination of puppies born to immune dams with a canine adenovirus-based vaccine protects against a canine distemper virus challenge. *Vaccine* 2002; **20**: 3485–97.

3

Oncology

ANN HOHENHAUS

Introduction

This chapter will focus on recent publications in three main subdisciplines of clinical oncology: biological behaviour of tumours, diagnostic testing for cancer and clinical evaluation of cancer treatments. The papers were chosen for a variety of reasons and in an attempt to present information about clinically important tumours. Mast cell tumours, lymphoma and osteosarcoma are commonly treated tumours; consequently, one publication on each tumour is included in this chapter written by Geiger *et al.*, Charney *et al.* and Bailey *et al.* Several studies included involve a large number of patients. Larger studies provide information that is more applicable to the general patient population than are single case reports or small case series. Data from studies using a control group allow stronger conclusions to be made than can be made from studies lacking a control group. The studies by Charney *et al.*, Henry *et al.* and Penninck *et al.* include a control group. Two studies provide 'new' information; one is a description of a new use for computed tomography (CT) scanning by Johnson *et al.*, and the other, a previously described tumour in a new species by Vascellari *et al.* Finally, the tables of contents of several non-American veterinary journals published in English were reviewed to widen the scope of information included in this chapter.

Diagnostic procedures

In humans, early detection of cancer has translated into the potential to cure some cancers. Few screening tests for cancer, other than a thorough physical examination, are available for veterinary patients. The diagnostic kit for transitional cell carcinoma described by Henry *et al.*, is a screening test, which appears to be useful in the differentiation of lower urinary tract disorders. Abdominal ultrasonography has been widely utilized in the diagnostic evaluation of intestinal diseases. In this paper, Penninck *et al.* use ultrasonography to differentiate inflammation from neoplasia. Finally, the diagnosis of pulmonary metastasis may be difficult in some cases based on standard radiographic techniques and Johnson *et al.* use CT to diagnose pulmonary metastasis.

Diagnostic value of ultrasonography in differentiating enteritis from intestinal neoplasia in dogs

Pennick D, Smyers B, Webster CRL, et al. Vet Radiol Ultrasound 2003; **44**: 570–5

BACKGROUND. Ultrasonography is commonly used in the diagnostic evaluation of dogs with clinical signs of gastrointestinal disease. This retrospective study compares ultrasonographic findings in dogs with histologically confirmed enteritis and neoplasia to quantify the features typical of each disorder. Main parameters measured during the ultrasound included wall thickness, wall layering, lymph node thickness, regional motility and lesion distribution, either diffuse or focal.

INTERPRETATION. Sixty-one dogs with enteritis and 89 dogs with neoplasia were evaluated using standard abdominal ultrasonography techniques. A statistically significant difference was found between all parameters evaluated in the enteritis and neoplasia groups (Table 3.1). Wall and lymph node thickness were greater in the neoplasia group. Layering and regional motility were reduced or lost more commonly in the neoplasia group. Neoplasia was more commonly a focal lesion and enteritis was more commonly diffuse.

Comment

The diagnosis of enteritis versus neoplasia can only be made based on cytological or histological samples. This study is useful in identifying parameters found on ultrasound, a non-invasive test which may assist the veterinarian predict the findings

Table 3.1 Main ultrasonographic features in dogs with enteritis and dogs with intestinal tumour

Parameter	Enteritis (61 dogs)	Neoplasia (89 dogs)
Wall thickness (cm) P <0.001	Median: 0.6 Range: 0.2–2.9	Median: 1.5 Range: 0.5–7.9
Wall layering P <0.001	Normal: 16 (26%) Reduced: 38 (62%) Lost: 7 (11%)	Normal: 1 (1%) Reduced: 0 (0%) Lost: 88 (99%)
Distribution of lesion P <0.001	Diffuse: 44 (72%) Not diffuse: 17 (28%)	Diffuse: 2 (2%) Not diffuse: 87 (98%)
Lymph node thickness (cm) P =0.001	Median: 1.0 Range: 0.6–2.6 Dogs tested 24/61	Median: 1.9 Range: 0.3–9.0 Dogs tested 56/89
Regional motility P =0.055	Normal: 4 (22%) Increased: 3 (17%) Decreased: 11 (61%) Dogs tested 18/61	Normal: 3 (7%) Increased: 3 (7%) Decreased: 39 (87%) Dogs tested 45/89

Source: Penninck et al. (2003).

from a biopsy. The findings will help direct the pre-biopsy testing, including the need to obtain thoracic radiographs to identify pulmonary metastasis. The feature most commonly found in dogs with intestinal neoplasia was a loss of normal intestinal layering. Ultrasound has also been used to describe abnormalities in gastric neoplasia where loss of normal layering is a common finding |**1,2**|. Dogs found to have lost normal layering were 51 times more likely to have an intestinal tumour; although, some dogs with enteritis also had loss of normal intestinal layering. There was also significant overlap in the wall thickness between the two groups. Therefore, a biopsy is still required for the diagnosis of intestinal disease even if abnormal layering is found.

Evaluation of a bladder tumor antigen test as screening test for transitional cell carcinoma of the lower urinary tract in dog

Henry CJ, Tyler JW, McEntee MC, et al. Am J Vet Res 2003; **64**: 1017–20

BACKGROUND. Histologically, 50–75% of canine bladder tumours are transitional cell carcinoma. An early detection method for canine transitional cell carcinoma is needed because the diagnosis of transitional cell carcinoma of the urinary bladder is typically made when the disease is too advanced for complete surgical resection. The disease is also poorly responsive to chemotherapy, and survival time is short following diagnosis. The bladder tumour antigen test is designed to be performed in the veterinarian's office. It is a rapid latex agglutination dipstick test for the identification of glycoproteins in the urine associated with transitional cell carcinoma.

INTERPRETATION. This study evaluated four groups of dogs: 48 with transitional cell carcinoma, 82 healthy control dogs, 71 sick dogs with urinary tract disease and 28 sick dogs without urinary tract disease. Overall, the sensitivity of the test was 90%. Specificity was low, with false-positive results occurring in dogs with non-neoplastic urinary tract abnormalities such as proteinuria or haematuria. Centrifugation of the urine sample prior to performing the test improved accuracy of the test. The negative predictive value of this test is 0.999.

Comment

A perfect test would have high sensitivity and high specificity. A patient with a positive test would have the disease being tested for, and a patient with a negative test would not have the disease. As there are no perfect tests, a good screening test is defined as one with high sensitivity; in other words, it misses few cases of the disease. It may have a low specificity and a high rate of false-positive tests. The bladder tumour antigen test meets the criteria for a good screening test. Dogs with transitional cell carcinoma have a positive bladder tumour antigen test, but so do some dogs with other lower urinary diseases. Dogs with a negative bladder tumour antigen test would not be expected to have a transitional cell carcinoma.

This test should be useful to help the general practitioner differentiate between the various causes of recurrent lower urinary tract signs in dogs. If the test is negative, there is a 99.9% chance that the dog does not have transitional cell carcinoma. That information helps to remove some of the urgency from the diagnostic evaluation, although further testing is indicated to determine if the cause of the lower urinary tract signs is a chronic infection, urolithiasis or a tumour other than transitional cell carcinoma. A positive test requires a more immediate diagnostic evaluation, including a urine culture, abdominal radiographs, abdominal ultrasonography, and contrast cystourethrogram. If a mass lesion is identified, cystoscopy or cystotomy should be performed to obtain a biopsy for confirmation of a malignancy.

Thoracic high-resolution computed tomography in the diagnosis of metastatic carcinoma

Johnson VS, Ramsey IK, Thompson H, *et al*. *J Small Anim Pract* 2004; **45**: 134–43

BACKGROUND. Thoracic radiography is considered essential in the diagnostic evaluation of patients with neoplastic disease. Identification of pulmonary metastasis can be made using two-view thoracic radiographs, but more recently, it has become the standard to obtain three-view thoracic radiographs (right lateral, left lateral, dorsoventral or ventrodorsal) to increase sensitivity and specificity for the diagnosis of metastasis. Despite the improvement in diagnostic accuracy with three-view radiographs, limitations still exist. CT is becoming more widely available to veterinary practitioners and will likely improve diagnostic ability in dogs with suspected pulmonary metastasis. This small study demonstrates the utility of CT scanning in the diagnosis of metastatic carcinoma.

INTERPRETATION. Three dogs with suspected pulmonary metastasis based on routine thoracic radiography underwent thoracic CT scanning immediately following radiography. Owing to the poor prognosis and progression of clinical signs, the dogs were euthanized and underwent post mortem examination. Multiple radiologists reviewed radiographs from the three study dogs and from five other dogs. The same radiologists also reviewed CT scans. Radiographic, CT scan and pathological findings were compared. Despite minimal changes on the thoracic radiographs, abnormalities were identified in the subpleural region on CT scan. There were regions of ground glass opacity and parenchymal bands, which were identified as metastatic carcinoma based on the pathological findings. Wedge-shaped areas were found to be infarcts caused by blockage of tumour vessels by neoplastic cells (Fig. 3.1).

Comment

The new generation of CT scanners is fast and has a greater resolution than previous ones. This makes them ideal for rapid diagnosis of pulmonary metastasis in cases where the results of standard radiography are inconclusive. Although the authors do not report the total time per scan, each 'slice' of the CT scan took 1 s to complete

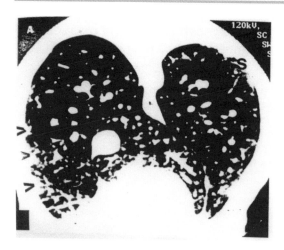

Fig. 3.1 Lung high resolution computed tomography (HRCT) and histopathological findings in dog 2. A marked band of subpleural interstitial infiltrate (S) is present in zone 2 of the dorsal part of the left caudal lobe. Wedge-shaped regions (*arrowheads*) of ground glass opacity and subpleural interstitial thickening lie along the ventral half of the right caudal lobe. Diffuse ground glass opacity is present throughout all lobes visualized.
Source: Johnson *et al.* (2004).

making the entire scan a very rapid process. Even if high resolution scanning is not available, the older generation of CT scanners has demonstrated utility in the diagnosis of pulmonary metastasis, and should be considered when the diagnosis of pulmonary metastasis using standard radiography is uncertain.

Biological behaviour of tumours

A complete understanding of a tumour's behaviour is an essential component of developing prevention and treatment strategies for a particular tumour. Once the diagnosis of a tumour is made, a treatment plan must be developed. Treatment is based on the typical behaviour of a tumour. Tumours, which are likely to recur locally, need surgical excision and/or radiation therapy. Those tumours with a high metastatic potential may benefit from systemic therapy such as chemotherapy. Williams *et al.* describe the behaviour of apocrine gland adenocarcinoma and Geiger *et al.* describe the behaviour of mast cell tumours occurring on the muzzle. Both are frequently metastatic, but dogs with metastatic apocrine gland tumours have a short survival while metastatic muzzle mast cell tumours do not always result in rapidly progressive disease. The description of injection site sarcomas in dogs by Vascellari *et al.* will spur further investigation into the behaviour of this newly described tumour.

Biologic behavior and prognostic factors for mast cell tumors of the canine muzzle: 24 cases (1990–2001)

Gieger TL, Theon AP, Werner JK, et al. J Vet Intern Med 2003; **17**: 687–92

BACKGROUND. The location of a tumour on the body can affect its biological behaviour. Melanomas of the haired skin are considered benign, while melanomas in the oral cavity have a highly malignant behaviour |3|. Mast cell tumours, which are the most common malignant skin tumour in the dog, have previously been shown to behave in a more malignant manner if located on the trunk when compared with the appendages |4|. This study describes the behaviour of mast cell tumours occurring on the muzzle of dogs.

INTERPRETATION. This retrospective multicentre study reviews the outcome of treatment in 24 dogs with muzzle mast cell tumours. All tumours were graded according to the Patnaik histological grading scale for mast cell tumours. This scale defines grade I tumours as the least malignant and grade III tumours as the most malignant. Tumour recurrence and survival are linked to the grade of tumour. Grade I tumours have the longest survival and the lowest rate of tumour recurrence, and grade III tumours have a high rate of recurrence with a shorter survival. There appeared to be a greater number of grade II and III tumours in this group of dogs than has typically been seen in other mast cell tumour studies |4|. There were two grade I, 15 grade II and seven grade III tumours. In this study, high-grade tumours were associated with a greater risk of metastasis and a shorter survival time. Fifty-eight per cent of dogs had lymph node metastasis, but systemic metastasis was rare (Fig. 3.2). The presence of lymph node metastasis was not uniformly associated with rapidly progressive disease because five dogs in this study with lymph node metastasis did not show any disease progression. However, dogs with metastasis were almost eight times more likely to die of mast cell disease.

Comment

Results of this study should be interpreted with some caution due to its retrospective nature and lack of a control group. Retrospective studies can under- or overestimate the occurrence and severity of a tumour as not every case of tumour is identified, and the comparison group is not concurrent, but historical. Historical control groups are not necessarily treated equivalently to the treatment group due to changes in medical practice over time. All patients in a retrospective study do not receive identical treatment, making the data more difficult to interpret.

Even with the imperfections of a retrospective study, this article has important implications for the management of dogs with muzzle mast cell tumours. This group of dogs studied is similar to other groups of dogs with mast cell tumours reported in the literature; all but one dog was purebred and the median age was 8 years |5|. Higher-grade tumours tended to recur locally; therefore, if a high-grade tumour is not completely resected, additional surgery or follow-up radiation therapy should be considered for the dog. The presence of lymph node metastasis indicated that a dog was more likely to die of mast cell tumour, but not all dogs with lymph node meta-

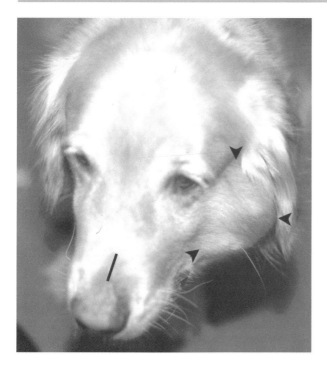

Fig. 3.2 The black bar represents the excision site of a muzzle mast cell tumour. The arrowheads demarcate the massively enlarged lymph node from metastatic mast cell tumour.

stasis experienced disease progression. Therefore, treatment should be considered even in the presence of metastasis.

Because of the wide variety of treatments given to this group of dogs, no conclusions about the efficacy of treatment could be made. Several other published studies on the treatment of canine mast cell tumours clearly indicate prolonged survival can be attained with radiation therapy following incomplete surgical excision of grade II mast cell tumours |**5,6**|.

Carcinoma of the apocrine glands of the anal sac in dogs: 113 cases (1985–1995)
Williams LE, Gliato JM, Dodge RK, et al. J Am Vet Med Assoc 2003: **223**: 825–31

BACKGROUND. Two histologically distinct tumours of the anal sac occur: the anal sac adenocarcinoma (hepatoid tumour) and the apocrine gland carcinoma of the anal

sac. The apocrine gland carcinoma comprises 16.5% of perianal tumours. Dogs with
the tumour have been reported to be older, female dogs |7|. Prognosis for dogs with
apocrine gland carcinoma has previously been reported to be poor, as metastasis
and hypercalcaemia are common |7|.

INTERPRETATION. One hundred and thirteen dogs were entered into this study. An equal
number of male and female dogs with apocrine gland carcinoma are reported, which differs
from the previous reports. The presence of hypercalcaemia carried a worse prognosis
confirming data from previous reports. Treatment of any type (surgery, chemotherapy or
radiation therapy) increased survival over dogs that did not receive treatment (median survival
with treatment 544 days (without treatment median survival time not reported). Treatment
with a single modality of therapy (chemotherapy or surgery or radiation therapy) did not
improve survival, although dogs receiving surgery as part of their treatment protocol did have
longer survival times (receiving surgery median survival 548 days, not receiving surgery
median survival 402 days). Dogs with tumours <10 cm^2 had longer survival times (median
584 days) than those with tumours >10 cm^2 (median 292 days) (Fig. 3.3).

Comment

This study contains the largest case series of apocrine gland carcinoma reported to
date. The large number of cases and the multiple institutions contributing to the
study make it a significant contribution to the literature. It confirms the findings of
previous studies where approximately 25% of dogs were hypercalcaemic and hypercalcaemia conferred a poor prognosis.

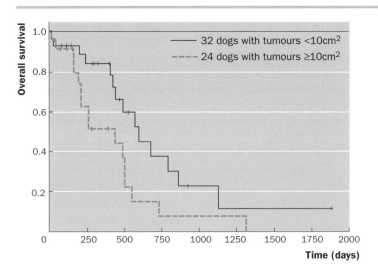

Fig. 3.3 Kaplan–Meier survival curves for 56 dogs with carcinoma of the apocrine glands of
the anal sac, grouped according to tumour size. The solid line represents 32 dogs with
tumours <10cm^2, and the dashed line represents 24 dogs with tumours ≥10cm^2. Vertical
lines denote dogs that were censored from analysis. Source: Williams et al. (2003).

Because dogs with smaller tumours have a better prognosis, and because half of the dogs had a palpable mass at the time of diagnosis, rectal examination and careful assessment of the history given by the owner will help to identify these tumours early and result in an improved prognosis for dogs with apocrine gland carcinoma. The results of this study indicate survival time may be long in dogs with this tumour. Previous studies report only a 6–8-month median survival time [7]. A treatment protocol, which includes surgery, appears to give the best survival; although, because of the retrospective nature of this study, it is unknown if dogs able to undergo surgery may have had smaller tumours and thus a better prognosis than those dogs who did not undergo surgery.

Fibrosarcomas at presumed sites of injection in dogs: characteristics and comparison with non-vaccination site fibrosarcomas and feline post vaccinal fibrosarcomas

Vascellari M, Melchiotti E, Bozza MA, Mutinelli F. *J Vet Med A* 2003; **50**: 286–91

BACKGROUND. Since they were first described in 1991, injection site sarcomas in the cat have received a significant amount of attention in the veterinary literature because of their aggressive biological behaviour and their association with treatments given to protect the patient from infectious diseases. Because vaccination and other injections cause inflammation in dogs as well as cats, veterinarians have been concerned injection site sarcomas could develop in dogs. This paper seeks to determine if there are similarities between feline post-vaccinal fibrosarcomas, fibrosarcomas at presumed sites of injections in dogs, and fibrosarcomas at non-injection sites in dogs.

INTERPRETATION. Based on the information presented in this paper, it appears that dogs may develop a similar tumour to feline injection site sarcomas, although the tumour is rare. This study reviews biopsies of three tumour types: injection site sarcomas in cats, and injection site fibrosarcomas and non-injection site fibrosarcomas in dogs. Fibrosarcomas at injection sites in dogs have a similar histological appearance to those in cats. The tumours have inflammatory cell infiltrates consisting of lymphocytic follicle-like aggregates in the tumour periphery and myofibroblasts. Aluminium, a component of some vaccine adjuvants was detected in canine injection site sarcomas as has been previously described in feline vaccinal fibrosarcomas [8] (Fig. 3.4).

Comment

Although designated vaccine-associated sarcomas in cats, it is believed sarcomas can arise from any type of injection that causes irritation and inflammation at the injection site. This paper confirms that a similar tumour occurs in the dog. The designation, injection site sarcoma is a more appropriate descriptive term for these

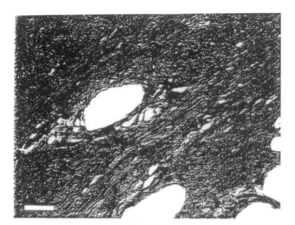

Fig. 3.4 Canine fibrosarcoma from presumed injection site. Aluminium deposits revealed by the aurintricarboxylic acid method in the fibrous stroma of the excised tumours. Bar = 25 μm. Source: Vascellari *et al.* (2003).

tumours as the histology is not limited to fibrosarcoma, but can be any soft tissue sarcoma, including chondrosarcoma, malignant fibrous histiocytoma, extraskeletal osteosarcoma, myofibrosarcoma and undifferentiated sarcoma. In this study, the authors describe the histological appearance of the tumours based on morphology and a limited panel of immunohistochemical stains. All tumours were confirmed to be of mesenchymal origin based on positive staining for vimentin and negative staining for desmin. Further immunohistochemical staining of these tumours would likely reclassify some as other types of soft tissue sarcomas

The biological behaviour of the injection site sarcomas in this group of dogs was not described and further work will be necessary to describe the tumour's behaviour and determine the optimal course of treatment. Until this information is known, wide surgical resection of an injection site sarcoma should be recommended. Following surgical resection, careful monitoring of the surgery site will be necessary, as recurrence is likely based on the behaviour of this tumour in cats.

Therapeutic interventions

The first two sections of this chapter focus on the diagnosis of a tumour and understanding the biological behaviour of a tumour, leading up to development of a treatment strategy. This section describes three publications regarding treatment strategies for three different tumours: a retrospective study of several different radiation therapy protocols for the treatment of oral melanoma by Proulx *et al.*, a prospective, but uncontrolled study of doxorubicin and carboplatin for the treatment of osteosarcoma by Bailey *et al.*, and a case–control study of the use of furosemide as an adjunct to chemotherapy for lymphoma in an attempt to prevent cyclophosphamide cystitis by Charney *et al.*

A retrospective analysis of 140 dogs with oral melanoma treated with external beam radiation

Proulx DR, Ruslander DM, Dodge RK, *et al*. *J Vet Radiol Ultrasound* 2003; **44**: 352–9

BACKGROUND. **Oral melanoma is the most common oral tumour in dogs. It is locally invasive and highly metastatic. Reported median survival with radical surgical resection alone is 9–10 months |3|. A previous report indicates oral melanoma is responsive to large doses of radiation therapy given less frequently than traditional fractionation schemes |9|. Radiation therapy addresses control of local disease, but not systemic spread of tumour. This large retrospective study evaluates several radiation therapy fractionation schemes, evaluates factors influencing prognosis and determines the influence of chemotherapy on outcome in 140 dogs with oral melanoma.**

INTERPRETATION. Three dose fractionation schemes were studied. The first group included 69 dogs treated with three 10-Gy fractions given on days 1, 7 and 21. The second group included 54 dogs treated with four 9-Gy fractions on days 1, 7, 14 and 21. The third group included 17 dogs treated with 12–19 2–4-Gy fractions. In addition to the radiation therapy, 80 dogs received chemotherapy. The most commonly used drug was carboplatin, which was given to 60 dogs. Time to first event was analysed. First event was categorized five ways: development of new metastasis, tumour recurrence, death, progression of metastasis, or local recurrence and metastasis. Overall, median time to first event was 5 months. Overall median survival was 7 months. The occurrence of the first event and survival were predicted by tumour volume, sublocation, and presence of bone lysis at the tumour site. Median survival was longest, 21 months, in dogs with small, rostral tumours without bone lysis. Median survival of dogs with one of the three risk factors was 11 months, two risk factors 5 months, and three risk factors 3 months (Fig. 3.5). There was no difference in outcome based on radiation therapy dose fractionation scheme. Chemotherapy treatment did not impact on time to first event or survival.

Comment

The biological behaviour of oral melanoma is similar to the other common oral tumours, squamous cell carcinoma and fibrosarcoma, because of its highly invasive nature and frequent recurrence. Oral melanoma differs from the other two tumours as it has a high metastatic rate and metastasis occurs even if the primary tumour is controlled with surgery or radiation therapy. The tumours in this study were highly metastatic as expected. Forty-six per cent first events were metastasis. Radiation therapy was effective in controlling local tumour and 51% of dogs with measurable disease underwent a complete remission, corroborating the data from other studies.

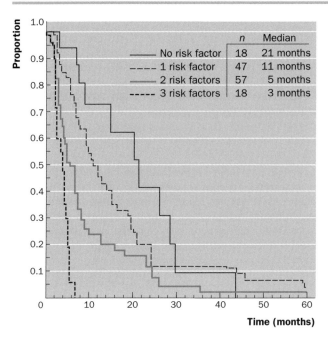

Fig. 3.5 Kaplan–Meier survival curves for dogs grouped according to number of risk factors present (tumour volume, tumour sublocation, bone lysis). Source: Proulx *et al.* (2003).

Similar to other studies, tumour volume inversely correlated with survival. At first glance, it is surprising chemotherapy did not have a greater impact on survival; however, the median dose of carboplatin given in this study was 7.8 mg/kg. The dose given to responding dogs in a previous study was 15.1 mg/kg |10|. The lack of response seen in this study may be attributable to inadequate dosing. Because of the retrospective nature of the study, it may also be attributable to chemotherapy treatment of dogs with a higher tumour burden compared with the dogs not receiving chemotherapy. As the fractionation scheme does not impact on survival, the most convenient scheme can be used. If chemotherapy is prescribed, adequate dosing is essential.

Carboplatin and doxorubicin combination chemotherapy for the treatment of appendicular osteosarcoma in the dog

Bailey D, Erb H, Williams L, *et al. J Vet Intern Med* 2003; **17**: 199–205

BACKGROUND. Osteosarcoma is the most common skeletal tumour of the dog. Current standard of care is control of local tumour by amputation or limb-sparing surgery followed by chemotherapy. Chemotherapy, with doxorubicin, carboplatin and cisplatin, has been described and results in roughly equivalent survival |11–13|. This study reports the outcome of dogs treated with a combination of carboplatin and doxorubicin.

INTERPRETATION. Following amputation or a limb-sparing procedure, 24 dogs received chemotherapy. Day 1, 175 mg/m^2 of carboplatin was administered and on day 2, 15 mg/m^2 of doxorubicin was administered. Treatment was administered every 21 days for up to four cycles of treatment. The treatment protocol had acceptable toxicity and only one chemotherapy cycle resulted in hospitalization of a dog for gastrointestinal signs. Median disease-free interval was 195 days and median survival time 235 days.

Comment

Although this study seems to indicate that treatment with the described protocol offers no advantage over previously reported chemotherapy protocols, the comparison should be made with caution. Studies comparing two contemporaneous treatment groups, which have been randomly allocated to the different treatment arms, are required to state, with certainty, whether two treatments are or are not equivalent. Until such a study is performed, no chemotherapy protocol for osteosarcoma should be considered optimal. Following amputation, chemotherapy has

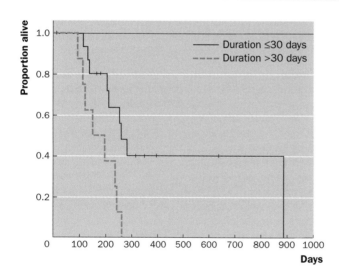

Fig. 3.6 Kaplan–Meier curves comparing survival for patients whose duration of clinical signs was 30 days or less before surgery ($n = 15$) with those whose duration of clinical signs was more than 30 days ($n = 9$). Vertical tick marks represent censored observations. Cox proportional hazard ratio for patients with a longer duration of clinical signs was 3.7 (95% confidence interval 1.8–7.1, $P = 0.2$). Source: Bailey *et al.* (2003).

been shown to improve survival over amputation alone |**14**|. Chemotherapy with single agent doxorubicin, cisplatin or carboplatin or combinations of those agents is a reasonable choice for the treatment of osteosarcoma. Another interesting finding in this study was the duration of clinical signs prior to diagnosis and surgery was inversely correlated with survival time indicating that early diagnosis and timely treatment improve prognosis in dogs with osteosarcoma (Fig. 3.6).

Risk factors for sterile hemorrhagic cystitis in dogs with lymphoma receiving cyclophosphamide with or without concurrent administration of furosemide: 216 cases (1990–1996)

Charney SC, Bergman PJ, Hohenhaus AE, McKnight JA. *J Am Vet Med Assoc* 2003; **222**: 1388–93

BACKGROUND. Administration of cyclophosphamide is known to cause sterile haemorrhagic cystitis because a metabolite of cyclophosphamide, arcolein, excreted in the urine, is an irritant to the urothelium (Fig. 3.7). Frequent and uncontrolled urinations result in a poor quality of life for both the owner and the dog. Cyclophosphamide administration has also been linked to the development of transitional cell carcinoma of the bladder. This case–control retrospective study investigated the frequency of occurrence of sterile haemorrhagic cystitis in dogs receiving chemotherapy for lymphoma with two similar but not identical protocols containing cyclophosphamide. In one protocol, cyclophosphamide was administered concurrently with furosemide to promote urination in an attempt to prevent cyclophosphamide cystitis.

INTERPRETATION. A total of 216 dogs' medical records were reviewed. In both protocols, the dogs received cyclophosphamide at a dosage of 200 mg/m^2 i.v. In one protocol, the dogs received 2.2 mg/kg i.v. of furosemide at the time of cyclophosphamide administration. The two groups were compared to identify risk factors for the development of sterile haemorrhagic cystitis. Nine per cent of dogs not receiving furosemide developed sterile haemorrhagic cystitis and only 1% of those receiving furosemide did. The median number of treatments of cyclophosphamide prior to the development of sterile haemorrhagic cystitis was 2. Age, sex, breed, body weight, prior urinary tract disease, neutropenia and chemotherapy agent administered prior to the dose of cyclophosphamide causing sterile haemorrhagic cystitis did not correlate with the development of cystitis. This study also describes the course of cyclophosphamide cystitis. Its duration ranged from 21 to 136 days. Cyclophosphamide was successfully and safely administered to dogs following an episode of cyclophosphamide cystitis when furosemide was concurrently administered.

Comment

The results of this study allow several strong recommendations about the management of dogs receiving cyclophosphamide for the treatment of lymphoma to be made. The recommendations are strong because the groups of dogs studied are typical for

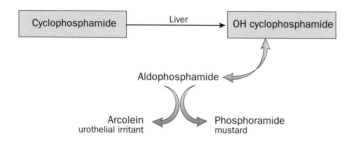

Fig. 3.7 The metabolic pathway of cyclophosphamide to arcolein, which is believed to be the cause of cyclophosphamide cystitis.

dogs reported with lymphoma, they received drugs commonly used for the treatment of lymphoma and were closely monitored to identify the occurrence of cyclophosphamide cystitis. The incidence of cyclophosphamide cystitis was similar to previously reported studies (approximately 10%) and occurred early in the course of treatment |15,16|. The incidence of cyclophosphamide cystitis was statistically significantly decreased ($P = 0.047$) in dogs receiving furosemide. Administration of furosemide is simple and inexpensive and appears to decrease the incidence of sterile haemorrhagic cystitis. Its use should be considered routinely in dogs receiving a lymphoma chemotherapy protocol containing cyclophosphamide.

Conclusion

The overall unifying theme of these selected publications focuses on improving the survival of patients with cancer. First, the diagnostic procedures concentrated on early and accurate detection of tumours. Early diagnosis is important as the papers presented here also demonstrate that early detection translates to improved survival. When it comes to tumours, the 'wait and watch' approach is detrimental to the patient. Allowing clinical signs to persist or the tumour to enlarge worsens the patient's prognosis. In dogs with apocrine gland carcinoma and oral melanoma, smaller tumour volume translated into longer survival. In dogs with osteosarcoma, longer duration of clinical signs prior to treatment shortened survival. The goal for the future is to diagnose tumours such as transitional cell carcinoma earlier using tests like the bladder tumour antigen test in order to improve survival. Although the rapid diagnosis of pulmonary metastasis using CT does not prolong survival, it allows for an accurate prognosis to be given, thus preventing treatment from being administered for a condition unlikely to respond.

New information presented here indicates that the prognosis in some tumours may be different than previously published. Survival in apocrine gland carcinoma appears to be more favourable than previously believed and treatment is not futile; conversely, the prognosis of muzzle mast cell tumours may be less favourable than for mast cell tumours occurring at other locations. These data also suggest multimodality therapy may be indicated in dogs with muzzle mast cell tumours and apocrine gland carcinoma.

Another facet of the publications presented is how different therapeutic modalities are combined to control tumours and extend survival. Local tumour control is achieved by surgery or radiation therapy and disseminated tumours are treated with chemotherapy as described in dogs with osteosarcoma and apocrine gland carcinoma. Multimodality therapy is becoming increasingly common as more is learned about the biological behaviour of tumours and the effect that surgery, chemotherapy and radiation therapy have on patient survival.

References

1. Rivers BJ, Walter PA, Johnston GR, Feeney DA, Hardy RM. Canine gastric neoplasia: utility of ultrasonography in diagnosis. *J Am Anim Hosp Assoc* 1997; **33**: 144–55.
2. Penninck D, Moore A, Gliatto J. Ultrasonography of canine gastric epithelial neoplasia. *Vet Rad Ultrasound* 1998; **39**(4): 342–8.
3. Harvey HJ, MacEwen EG, Braun D, Patnaik AK, Withrow SJ, Jongeward S. Prognostic criteria for dogs with oral melanoma. *J Am Vet Med Assoc* 1981; **178**(6): 580–2.
4. Turrel J, Kitchell B, Miller L, Theon A. Prognostic factors for radiation treatment of mast cell tumor in 85 dogs. *J Am Vet Med Assoc* 1988; **193**(8): 936–40.
5. LaDue T, Price GS, Dodge R, Page RL, Thrall DE. Radiation therapy for incompletely resected canine mast cell tumors. *Vet Radiol Ultrasound* 1998; **39**: 57–62.
6. Frimberger AE, Moore AS, LaRue SM, Gliatto JM, Bengtson AE. Radiotherapy of incompletely resected, moderately differentiated mast cell tumors in the dog: 37 cases (1989–1993). *J Am Anim Hosp Assoc* 1997; **33**: 320–4.
7. Ross J, Scavelli T, Matthiesen D, Patnaik A. Adenocarcinoma of the apocrine glands of the anal sac in dogs: a review of 32 cases. *J Am Anim Hosp Assoc* 1991; **27**: 349–55.
8. Hendrick MJ, Goldschmidt MH, Shofer FS, Wang YY, Somlyo AP. Postvaccinal sarcomas in the cat: epidemiology and electron probe microanalytical identification of aluminum. *Cancer Res* 1992; **52**: 5391–4.
9. Bateman KE, Catton PA, Pennock PW, Kruth SA. 0–7–21 radiation therapy for the treatment of canine oral melanoma. *J Vet Intern Med* 1994; **8**: 267–72.
10. Rassnick KM, Ruslander DM, Cotter SM, Al-Sarraf R, Bruyette DS, Gamblin RM, Meleo KA, Moore AS. Use of carboplatin for treatment of dogs with malignant melanoma: 27 cases (1989–2000). *J Am Vet Med Assoc* 2001; **218**: 1444–8.

11. Straw RC, Withrow SJ, Richter SL, Powers BE, Klein MK, Postorino NC, LaRue SM, Ogilvie GK, Vail DM, Morrison WB. Amputation and cisplatin for treatment of canine osteosarcoma. *J Vet Intern Med* 1991; 5: 205–10.

12. Chun R, Kurzman ID, Couto CG, Klausner J, Henry C, MacEwen EG. Cisplatin and doxorubicin combination chemotherapy for the treatment of canine osteosarcoma: a pilot study. *J Vet Intern Med* 2000; 14: 495–8.

13. Bergman PJ, MacEwen EG, Kurzman ID, Henry CJ, Hammer AS, Knapp DW, Hale A, Kruth SA, Klein MK, Klausner J, Norris AM, McCaw D, Straw RC, Withrow SJ. Amputation and carboplatin for treatment of dogs with osteosarcoma: 48 cases (1991 to 1993). *J Vet Intern Med* 1996; 10(2): 76–81.

14. Spodnick GJ, Berg J, Rand WM, Schelling SH, Couto G, Harvey HJ, Henderson RA, MacEwen G, Mauldin N, McCaw DL. Prognosis for dogs with appendicular osteosarcoma treated by amputation alone: 162 cases (1978–1988). *J Am Vet Med Assoc* 1992; 200(7): 995–8.

15. Henness AM. Treatment of cyclophosphamide induced cystitis. *J Am Vet Med Assoc* 1985; 187: 4–5.

16. Crow SE, Theilen GH, Madewell BR, Weller RE, Henness AM. Cyclophosphamide-induced cystitis in the dog and cat. *J Am Vet Med Assoc* 1977; 171: 259–62.

4

Critical care

LINDA BARTON

Introduction

Emergency and critical care practitioners treat patients presenting with a wide variety of medical and surgical disease processes. These patients are often presented in an unstable and/or rapidly changing clinical condition and must be treated before complete diagnostic information is available. Clinicians must rely on their clinical experience and thorough knowledge of the underlying disease process to successfully treat unstable, severely affected patients. New information presented in the current literature can add to this body of knowledge and aid practitioners in patient management. The articles selected for inclusion in this review reflect the variety of disease processes encountered by the emergency/critical care practitioner and can be placed into two broad categories: studies designed to generate new evidence to support or refute common clinical procedures, and articles offering new solutions to difficult problems.

Re-examining current procedures

Many common practices are based on sound physiological principles, clinical experience or borrowed from human medicine, but have not been rigorously evaluated in veterinary patients. The need to critically examine new diagnostic and therapeutic procedures is highlighted by the first article in this category. Despite increased availability of advanced diagnostics, no significant change in discordance between the ante mortem and post mortem diagnosis was demonstrated in dogs autopsied at a veterinary teaching hospital in 1989 compared with 1999. Each of the other articles included in this category provide additional evidence about procedures commonly used in veterinary practice; enteral nutritional support, furosemide delivered by constant rate infusion (CRI), and prophylactic fenestration for the prevention of recurrent thoracolumbar disk extrusion.

Concurrence between clinical and pathologic diagnosis in a veterinary medical teaching hospital: 623 cases (1989 and 1999)

Kent MS, Lucroy MD, Gillian D, Lehenbauer TW, Madewell BR. *J Am Vet Med Assoc* 2004; **224**: 403–6

BACKGROUND. In the past 15 years, there have been a number of advances in the diagnostic methods available to veterinary practitioners, including endoscopic and advanced imaging capacities, and increased availability of clinical laboratory services. It is reasonable to assume that these technological advances have improved our ability to make an accurate clinical ante mortem diagnosis. However, this assumption has not been critically evaluated. The purpose of this retrospective study was to determine the rate of discordance between the ante mortem clinical diagnosis and post mortem pathological diagnosis in dogs undergoing autopsy at a veterinary teaching hospital in 1989 compared with 1999.

INTERPRETATION. The medical records of all dogs autopsied following death or euthanasia at a veterinary medical teaching hospital in 1989 and 1999 were reviewed. The records were reviewed for the clinical diagnosis recorded by the attending clinician and for the pathological diagnosis determined at autopsy. Table 4.1 lists the number of in-hospital deaths, percentage of dogs autopsied and agreement between clinical and pathological diagnosis in each of the years evaluated. The percentage of hospitalized dogs that died was not significantly different between 1989 and 1999. There was a significant decline in the rate of autopsy from 58.9% of in-hospital deaths in 1989 compared with 48.3% in 1999. The emergency/critical care service was the only hospital service found to increase the percentage of cases autopsied in 1999 compared with 1989. There was no significant change in the discordance between the ante mortem and post mortem diagnosis over the time periods examined. In both 1989 and 1999, the clinical services with the highest rates of discrepancies between clinical and pathological diagnosis were dermatology, emergency/critical care and internal medicine.

Comment

Similar to the trend reported in human medicine, this study demonstrates a decline in the autopsy rate between 1989 and 1999. The cause for the decline reported in this

Table 4.1 The number of in-hospital deaths, percentage of dogs autopsied and agreement between clinical and pathological diagnosis in 1989 and 1999

Year	Dogs/visits	Deaths	Autopsy	Agree Yes	Agree No
1989	6822/14 496	576 (8.4%)	339 (58.9%)	204 (60.2%)	135 (39.8%)
1999	7654/16 266	588 (7.7%)	284 (48.3%)	179 (63.0%)	105 (37.0%)

Source: Kent *et al.* (2004).

study was not determined. Suggested possibilities include cost of the procedure, reluctance to ask for owner permission, overconfidence that clinical diagnosis is correct, and fear that autopsy will disclose errors and possibility lead to litigation.

Despite marked advancements in diagnostic technology over the time period evaluated, no improvement in the accuracy of ante mortem diagnosis was demonstrated. The approximate 40% rate of discordance reported in this study is comparable with a discrepancy rate of 6–65% reported in human medicine. In a study of 41 human patients from a medical intensive care unit (ICU), Blosser *et al.* reported agreement between clinical and pathological diagnosis in 37 of 41 patients |1|. However, in 27 of 41 patients the pathological cause of death differed from the suspected cause of death. A new active diagnosis was demonstrated in the post mortem exam that had not been detected premortem in 37 of 41 patients. The new diagnosis was most often infectious or thromboembolic. Perhaps most important, the authors concluded that the autopsy findings would have changed therapy in the ICU in 11 patients.

The study highlights the importance of autopsy. Post mortem examination serves as an important quality assurance indicator of our clinical acumen and a measure of the efficacy and appropriateness of our diagnostic and therapeutic interventions.

Effect of early enteral nutrition on intestinal permeability, intestinal protein loss, and outcome in dogs with severe parvoviral enteritis

Mohr AJ, Leisewitz AL, Jacobson LS, Steiner JM, Ruaux CG, Williams DA. *J Vet Intern Med* 2003; **17**: 791–8

BACKGROUND. Early enteral nutritional (EEN) support is recommended to reduce morbidity and mortality in critically ill veterinary patients. In critically ill humans, enteral nutrition has been shown to reduce intestinal mucosal permeability, reduce the incidence of bacteraemia, endotoxaemia and septic morbidity, attenuate the acute-phase response, reduce the incidence of multiple organ failure, improve immunological status, reduce catabolism and preserve positive nitrogen balance, and improve clinical outcome. In a 2002 retrospective study of partial parenteral nutrition, Chan *et al.* reported a significant increase in survival in dogs and cats that received some enteral nutrition during partial parenteral nutrition compared with animals not receiving any enteral nutrition |2|. The clinical effects of enteral nutrition in critically ill veterinary patients has not previously been critically evaluated. The objective of this prospective, randomized study was to evaluate the effect of EEN on intestinal permeability, intestinal protein loss and clinical outcome in naturally occurring severe canine parvovirus (CPV) enteritis.

INTERPRETATION. Puppies diagnosed with severe CPV and hospitalized for intensive supportive care were prospectively randomized to receive no food until vomiting had stopped (NPO group) or to receive EEN via a nasoesophageal feeding tube starting 12 h after hospital admission. A clinical score was assigned daily to semiquantify the clinical condition in each patient. The clinical score was applied by the scheme outlined in Table 4.2. In addition, body

Table 4.2 Daily clinical scoring system used to semiquantify clinical disease in dogs with parvoviral enteritis

	0	1	2	3
General attitude	Normal	Mild to moderate depression	Severe depression	Collapsed or moribund
Appetite	Normal	Voluntarily eats small amounts	No interest in food	N/A
Vomiting	Absent	Mild; 1 × /12 h	Moderate; 2–5 × /12 h	Severe; >6 × /12 h
Faeces	Well-formed	Soft or pasty faeces	Watery diarrhoea, non-bloody	Watery; bloody diarrhoea

Source: Mohr et al. (2003).

weight was measured daily and serum albumin concentrations were measured on days 1, 2, 4 and 6. Thirty dogs were enrolled in the study (15 NPO group, 15 EEN group). Body weight significantly increased ($P = 0.003$) from admission on all days in the EEN group, but not in the NPO group. There was no significant difference in serum albumin levels between the two groups. There was significant improvement in composite clinical score from admission values on day 2 in EEN versus day 3 in NPO. The median time taken to the normalization of general attitude and appetite and the resolution of vomiting and diarrhoea were consistently 1 day shorter for the EEN group. There was no significant difference in survival between the groups.

Comment

This is the first prospective study to demonstrate a reduction in morbidity associated with early enteral feeding. This study and its conclusions can be questioned for several reasons. The finding of reduced morbidity was based primarily on the more rapid improvement in clinical score and could be affected by observer bias in assignment of the scores. Total hospital days were not reported for the dogs in the study. However, a difference in total hospitalization time between the groups would support the conclusion of the study. Additionally, tolerance of the enteral feeding was assumed based on the increase in body weight and more rapid resolution of vomiting and diarrhoea seen in the EEN group. Placement of a nasogastric tube rather than a nasoesophageal tube would have allowed measurement of gastric residuals and better evaluation of feeding tolerance. The authors do not describe any tube dislodgement during the course of the study, which is always a concern in vomiting patients.

Traditionally, patients with diseases such as CPV enteritis associated with vomiting and gut dysfunction have been managed by complete gut rest. This study demonstrates that EEN can be safely administered to patients with CPV enteritis and, noting the limitations discussed above, can reduce morbidity in this patient population. More studies designed to evaluate the clinical effects of EEN in critically ill veterinary patients need to be conducted.

Intermittent bolus injection versus continuous infusion of furosemide in normal adult greyhound dogs

Adin DA, Taylor AW, Hill RC, Scott KC, Martin FG. *J Vet Intern Med* 2003; **17**: 632–6

BACKGROUND. Furosemide is a diuretic frequently used in veterinary patients. Furosemide, a loop diuretic is secreted into the proximal tubule and exerts its effect from the luminal side of the renal tubule by blocking the active transport of chloride and sodium in the thick ascending loop of Henle. Furosemide is administered orally, by intermittent intravenous (i.v.) bolus and more recently by i.v. CRI. The recommendation to administer furosemide by CRI is based on sound pharmacodynamic principles. In addition to the absolute amount of drug delivered to the site of action, the time course of delivery to the site of action is also an important determinant of the overall diuretic response. Fig. 4.1 illustrates the rate of urinary furosemide excretion, a measure of drug availability at the active site, in normal human volunteers following either an i.v. bolus or a CRI of furosemide |3|. When administered as a CRI, there is a constant rate of urinary furosemide excretion throughout the study period. By contrast, after bolus injection a peak value of urinary furosemide excretion is seen during the first hour followed by a dramatic decrease during the subsequent hours. Sodium and water retention in the 'drug-free' interval between i.v. boluses is thought to be one cause of diuretic resistance that may develop in patients. CRI administration of furosemide has been advocated to avoid diuretic resistance, improve efficacy and reduce toxic side effects.

Clinical studies designed to evaluate the efficacy of i.v. bolus versus CRI administration of furosemide have produced conflicting results. Differing results may be attributed to different patient populations (reason for diuretic administration), doses administered and presence or absence of concurrent fluid therapy. CRI administration of furosemide has been shown to produce more diuresis in normal horses and normal dogs given i.v. fluid replacement, but has not previously been examined in normal dogs in the absence of i.v. fluid replacement, a situation analogous to the clinical use of the drug in the treatment of congestive heart failure. The purpose of this prospective study was to compare the diuretic efficacy of furosemide administered by intermittent bolus (IB) and CRI to normal greyhound dogs in the absence of i.v. fluid replacement.

INTERPRETATION. In a randomized crossover design, six healthy adult greyhound dogs received equal doses of furosemide by either IBs (3 mg/kg at 0 and 4 h) or CRI (0.66 mg/kg i.v., then 0.66 mg/kg per h $\times$ 8 h). Water was offered hourly during the period of measurement. Urine, water and serum chemistry values significantly different between the two methods of administration are listed in Tables 4.3 and 4.4. Urine production and water intake were significantly greater for the CRI compared with the IB group. Packed cell volume (PCV), TS (total solids—measured by refractometer) and serum creatinine were significantly higher in the CRI group. Subjectively, five of six dogs became anxious and restless during the CRI.

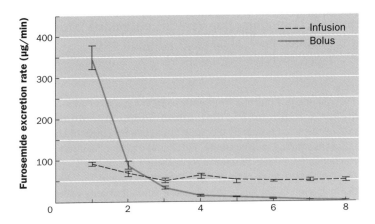

Fig. 4.1 Furosemide excretion rate in healthy human volunteers after bolus injection and continuous infusion of 40 mg furosemide. Source: Van Meyel *et al.* (1992) |**3**|.

Table 4.3 Mean ± SD for urine and water variables for CRI furosemide and IB furosemide. The *P* value represents the difference between methods of administration when averaged over all time periods (except baseline)

	CRI	IB	*P*
Mean urine production/h	7.5 ± 1.0	5.4 ± 0.9	0.003
Total urine production	59.9 ± 8.1	43.2 ± 6.8	0.003
Mean water intake/h	4.3 ± 0.7	2.9 ± 1.5	0.05
Total water intake	34.4 ± 6.0	23.1 ± 7.6	0.05
Total urinary K^+ loss	5.1 ± 0.7	6.6 ± 1.0	0.03
Total urinary Ca^{2+} loss	146.1 ± 37.9	90.7 ± 25.6	0.01
Total urine sodium loss	8.5 ± 0.6	7.4 ± 1.0	0.04

Source: Adin *et al.* (2003).

Table 4.4 Mean ± SD for blood and serum variables for CRI furosemide and IB furosemide. The *P* value represents the difference between methods of administration when averaged over all time periods (except baseline)

	CRI	IB	*P*
PCV	69 ± 4	59 ± 4	0.003
Total protein	8.1 ± 0.4	6.6 ± 0.5	0.01
Serum creatinine	1.5 ± 0.1	1.3 ± 0.1	0.04
Serum chloride	104 ± 2	109 ± 2	0.003

Source: Adin *et al.* (2003).

Comment

In this group of healthy dogs, CRI administration of furosemide compared with IB dosing resulted in a significantly increased diuresis, natriuresis and calciuresis with statistically significant, but clinically insignificant changes in PCV, total protein, serum creatinine and serum chloride. However, the study does not determine if this difference would translate to a change in clinical outcome. In human medicine, furosemide CRI is recommended in patients thought most likely to demonstrate diuretic tolerance with standard i.v. administration. This includes patients likely to experience rebound sodium and water retention during the drug-free interval between i.v. bolus doses because of neurohumeral activation.

Owing to the constant hourly urine production it may be easier to titrate the diuresis in patients receiving CRI furosemide. However, furosemide administration by CRI may complicate patient management because furosemide is incompatible with many other intravenously administered drugs. Further studies are required to determine the population of veterinary patients most likely to benefit from CRI furosemide administration.

Recurrence of thoracolumbar intervertebral disk extrusion in chondrodystrophic dogs after surgical decompression with or without prophylactic fenestration: 265 cases (1995–1999)

Brisson BA, Moffatt SL, Swayne SL, Parent JM. *J Am Vet Med Assoc* 2004; **224**(11): 1808–14

BACKGROUND. Acute neurological dysfunction secondary to thoracolumbar intervertebral disk extrusion is a common emergency presentation. Surgical decompression with fenestration at the site of intervertebral disk extrusion is the recommended treatment for dogs with severe or progressive clinical signs. Controversy exists, however, about the efficacy of prophylactic fenestration of the remaining disk spaces in the thoracolumbar region to prevent recurrent episodes of intervertebral disk extrusion. In their 1982 retrospective study, Levine *et al.* reported on recurrent thoracolumbar disk disease in 130 dogs. The recurrence rate for dogs treated with decompressive surgery alone was 26.5% compared with 16.6% for dogs treated with decompression and fenestration |4|. In 1999, Dhupa *et al.* reported on 30 dogs that underwent a second decompressive thoracolumbar surgery for recurrent intervertebral disc extrusion |5|. They found dachshunds to be at increased risk for recurrence. Additionally, they reported that the recurrence occurred at a site remote from the previously operated site in more than 80% of the cases. They did not include data about prophylactic fenestration but noted that in >70% of the cases the disk responsible for reoperation was within the T11–12 to L2–3 region and could have been easily fenestrated at the time of the first surgery. The objective of this retrospective study was to evaluate the rate and location of recurrence of intervertebral disk extrusion in a large population of chrondystrophic dogs treated for

thoracolumbar Hansen type 1 disk disease by use of surgical decompression with or without prophylactic fenestration.

INTERPRETATION. Chondrodystrophic dogs with Hansen type 1 thoracolumbar intervertebral disk disease confirmed at surgery were included in the study. A total of 265 cases were identified. Recurrence was defined by compatible clinical signs and removal of extruded disk material during a second decompressive surgery. Follow-up phone calls were made to owners and referring veterinarians to identify possible recurrence; defined as clinical signs compatible with intervertebral disk extrusion. Dogs exhibiting back pain without any neurological deficits were not included. In 37 of 252 (15%) of dogs, fenestration was performed at the site of decompression only at the time of the first surgery. In the remaining 215 dogs (85%) prophylactic fenestration was performed in three to six disk spaces in the thoracolumbar region. The recurrence rate was 4.4% (CI 2.3–7.7%). Twelve instances of recurrence (in 11 dogs) were confirmed at surgery. Table 4.5 lists the sites of first and second disk extrusion and the sites fenestrated in the dogs identified with a recurrent episode of intervertebral disk extrusion. Dachshunds were shown to have an increased incidence of recurrence (OR 9.7; CI 2.0–64.2). There was no significant difference in the rate of recurrence in dogs with single fenestration and the dogs with prophylactic fenestration of three to six disk spaces ($P = 0.67$). Recurrence was 5.86 times more likely to occur at a non-fenestrated disk space. Recurrence often occurred at a site immediately adjacent to a series of fenestrated disk spaces. Eighteen cases of possible recurrence were identified. There was no significant difference in the rate of possible recurrence in the dogs with or without prophylactic fenestration.

Comment

Recurrent intervertebral disk extrusion is a serious problem and strategies to prevent recurrence should be actively pursued. Many owners are reluctant or financially unable to undergo a second surgical procedure. The euthanasia rate for dogs with a

Table 4.5 Summary of twelve recurrences of intervertebral disk extrusion and sites of fenestration in eleven dogs

Dog	1st surgery	Fenestration	2nd surgery
1	T11–12	T11–12 to L2–3	T13–L1
2	T12–13	T11–12 to L3–4	T13–L1
3	T12–13	T11–12 to L2–3	L4–5
4	L1–2	T11–12 to L3–4	L4–5*
5	L3–4	T12–13 to L3–4	L4–5*
6	T12–13	T12–13 only	L2–3
6	NA	T13–L1 to L3–4	L4–5*
7	T12–13	T11–12 to T13–L1 and L2–3	L3–4*
8	T13–L1	T11–12 to L3–4	L4–5*
9	L1–2	L1–2 only	T12–13
10	L1–2	T12–13 to L3–4	T 11–12*
11	L3–4	T12–13 to L3–4	T 11–12*

*Recurrence at a non-fenestrated site adjacent to a fenestrated disk space. Source: Brisson et al. (2004).

possible recurrence without repeat decompressive surgery in this study was 44%. The use of prophylactic fenestration remains controversial. Although recurrent disk extrusion was more likely to occur at a non-fenestrated site, a significant reduction in recurrence following prophylactic fenestration has not been demonstrated. Prophylactic fenestration at the time of decompressive surgery increases the length of anaesthesia and surgery and cost to the client. Additionally, the frequent recurrence at sites immediately adjacent to a series of fenestrated disks is worrisome, suggests that abnormal biomechanical forces may be exerted on disks adjacent to fenestrated sites and requires further investigation.

New solutions to old problems

The remaining articles selected for inclusion in this review offer new solutions to common clinical problems encountered by emergency and critical care practitioners; chylothorax, collapsing trachea and predicting the severity of canine pancreatitis. In keeping with the trend of more rigorous examination of new diagnostic and therapeutic interventions, the new therapy is critically compared with the current clinical practice standard.

Management of advanced tracheal collapse in dogs using intraluminal self-expanding biliary wallstents

Moritz A, Schneider M, Bauer N. *J Vet Intern Med* 2004; **18**: 31–42

BACKGROUND. Collapsing trachea is a common problem in middle-aged to older small breed dogs. Patients presented on emergency for episodes of dyspnoea are treated with sedation, oxygen, ± corticosteroids and cage rest. Long-term medical management includes weight control, exercise restriction, cough suppressants and bronchodilators. Extraluminal stabilization of the trachea with polypropylene prosthetic rings is the preferred procedure for the dogs that fail medical management. Clinical signs are improved in the majority of patients following external stabilization; however, the procedure is invasive and associated with severe complications, including laryngeal paralysis, tracheal necrosis and loosening or failure of the implant. Additionally, the procedure is not recommended for patients with collapse of the intrathoracic portion of the trachea. Stabilization of the trachea with intraluminal endoprostheses has been reported. Initial experience with intraluminal stabilization suggests that this may be an effective method of managing small dogs with severe collapsing trachea. The objective of this retrospective study was to evaluate the efficacy of intraluminal stents for the management of severe collapsing trachea in 24 dogs. Immediate and long-term outcomes were compared with extraluminal stabilization.

INTERPRETATION. The study group included dogs with collapsing trachea diagnosed by physical examination, thoracic radiography and bronchoscopy and presenting with severe clinical signs despite medical management. Yorkshire terriers were over-represented. Twenty-two dogs survived the immediate post-implant period and showed immediate improvement in clinical signs. Eighteen dogs were available for re-evaluation at a median interval of 68 days (range 21–880 days). At the time of re-evaluation, six of 18 (33.3%) dogs were asymptomatic, 11 of 18 (61.1%) showed marked improvement and only one of 18 (5.6%) remained symptomatic. Several dogs presented with recurrence of clinical signs. Recurrent signs were often associated with the development of excessive granulation tissue at the ends of the prosthesis. In these dogs, signs resolved following therapy with corticosteroids.

Comment

Both initial survival and long-term outcome reported in this study were comparable with the rates reported for surgical methods of extraluminal stabilization. Compared with extraluminal methods of fixation, intraluminal stent placement is atraumatic, faster and technically easier than surgery. Intraluminal stabilization can be performed over the entire length of the trachea, while extraluminal prosthetic ring placement is limited to collapse of the cervical trachea. Patients receiving intraluminal stents required minimal post-procedure care. The size of stents commercially available limits the procedure to small to medium dogs. Stent migration following placement has previously been reported, but did not occur in this study population. This study demonstrated that intraluminal stabilization with a Wallstent appears to be an effective method of managing small dogs with severe collapsing trachea.

Thoracic duct ligation and pericardectomy for treatment of idiopathic chylothorax

Fossum TW, Mertens MM, Miller MW, et al. J Vet Intern Med 2004; **18**: 307–10

BACKGROUND. Idiopathic chylothorax is the accumulation of chyle in the pleural space in the absence of an underlying cause (heart disease, cranial mediastinal mass lesions). Affected patients often present with mild to severe respiratory distress. Thoracocentesis and oxygen therapy are needed for emergency stabilization of severely affected patients. Long-term medical management consisting of feeding a low fat diet, intermittent needle thoracocentesis and administration of a benzopyrone such as rutin fails in many cases. Surgery is recommended for patients failing medical therapy. Surgical intervention, most commonly thoracic duct ligation is reported to eliminate pleural fluid accumulation in only about 50% of cases. Based on the observation of thickened pericardial tissue in some patients requiring thoracotomy for treatment of chylothorax, the authors of this study hypothesized that a thickened pericardium could increase venous pressures and impede drainage of chyle via lymphaticovenous channels and that these effects could be reversed by removal of the pericardium. This study reports the treatment of 20 patients presented with idiopathic chylothorax treated with thoracic duct ligation plus pericardectomy or pericardectomy alone.

INTERPRETATION. The study population consisted of 20 patients (10 dogs, 10 cats) treated for idiopathic chylothorax with thoracic duct ligation plus pericardectomy or pericardectomy alone. The surgery was considered successful if the animal had radiographic evidence of minimal or no pleural fluid accumulation or no clinical signs associated with pleural effusion at least 60 days post-operatively. The patients were followed for a mean of 20.6 months (range, 0.65–63 months). There was resolution of pleural fluid accumulation in 90% of the patients (10 of 10 dogs, eight of 10 cats).

Comment

The 90% success rate reported in this study is higher than that previously reported for thoracic duct ligation without pericardectomy. Although increased expertise of the surgeon performing all of the procedures in this study cannot be ruled out as a factor contributing to the improved surgical success, removal of the pericardium appears to be an important factor in the resolution of effusion in the patients in this study. Removal of the abnormal pericardium is thought to reduce right-sided venous pressures and allow increased drainage of pleural fluid via normal lymphaticovenous channels. Pericardectomy performed in conjunction with thoracic duct ligation does not require an additional thoracotomy incision, adds minimal morbidity to the procedure and based on the results of this study is recommended for patients with idiopathic chylous effusion.

Assessing the severity of canine pancreatitis
Mansfield CS, Jones BR, Spillman T. *Res Vet Sci* 2003; **74**: 137–44

BACKGROUND. Pancreatitis is a commonly diagnosed disease in dogs. Diagnosis of pancreatitis can be difficult and is generally based on a combination of compatible clinical signs (anorexia, vomiting, abdominal pain) and abdominal ultrasound findings (enlarged, hypoechoic pancreas with hyperechoic, peripancreatic fat). The clinical presentation of the disease can vary from mild and self-limiting to the development of severe and sometimes fatal systemic complications. Differentiating severe from mild disease would be useful in communicating with clients about appropriate therapy and prognosis, but is difficult based on initial presentation and/or traditional laboratory tests. Ruaux and Atwell did not find any difference in mean trypsin-like immunoreactivity (TLI) or α-macroglobulin concentrations in dogs with mild pancreatitis compared with those with severe forms of the disease |6|. In human patients C-reactive protein and trypsinogen activation peptides (TAP) have been shown to correlate with severity of pancreatitis. The objective of this prospective study was to determine the usefulness of currently available laboratory tests to provide prognostic information in canine pancreatitis.

INTERPRETATION. Twenty-one dogs with pancreatitis were included in the study. The clinical diagnosis of pancreatitis was confirmed by pancreatic biopsy obtained during exploratory coeliotomy, laparoscopy or at post mortem. Blood was collected for routine biochemical profile, lipase and amylase, and serum TLI. Additionally, blood and urine samples were collected for measurement of TAP. Twelve dogs were classified as having severe disease based on the criteria published by Bradley |7|. The remaining dogs were classified as having mild disease. There was no significant difference in plasma TAP and serum TLI concentrations in dogs with mild pancreatitis compared with dogs with severe disease. The urinary TAP-to-

Table 4.6 Statistical analysis of differences between dogs with mild and severe pancreatitis

Criteria	P value	Diagnostic cut-off value	AUC	Sensitivity (%)	Specificity (%)
Plasma TAP	>0.10	≥6.9 nmol/l	0.659	54.5	90.0
Urinary TAP	>0.10	≥308.0 nmol/l	0.562	37.5	100.0
UTCR	<0.01	≥3.78	0.929	85.7	100.0
TLI	>0.10	≥4010 μg/l	0.500	30.0	100.0
Lipase	<0.01	≥4010 U/l	0.873	63.6	100.0
Amylase	>0.10	≥1165 U/l	0.545	90.9	30.0
Phosphate	<0.02	≥1.14 mmol/l	0.875	87.5	62.5
Creatinine	<0.05	≥106.0 μmol/l	0.812	75.0	87.5
Urine specific gravity	<0.05	≥1.018	0.835	71.4	50.0

TAP, trypsinogen activation peptide; UTCR, urinary TAP-to-creatinine ratio; TLI, trypsin-like immunoreactivity; AUC, area under the curve. A significant difference using Mann-Whitney analysis was taken when $P = 0.05$. Receiver operating curve characteristics were used to determine the AUC, optimal diagnostic cut-off value and relative specificities and sensitivities.
Source: Mansfield et al. (2003).

creatinine ratio (UTCR) was significantly higher in the severe group compared with the dogs with mild pancreatitis. A summary of the sensitivities and specificities for the tests evaluated for the ability to differentiate mild from severe pancreatitis is included in Table 4.6.

Comment

In this study, the UTCR was the most sensitive and specific pancreas-specific marker for differentiating severe pancreatitis from milder forms of the disease. TAP measurements are not widely commercially available, but can be obtained from specialized veterinary laboratories. The UTCR is the first laboratory marker shown to correlate with the severity of pancreatic inflammation in dogs and can be recommended to veterinary practitioners in predicting the severity of disease in dogs diagnosed with pancreatitis.

Conclusion

The information presented in these recently published articles is very useful to veterinarians treating emergency and critically ill patients. Prevalent ideas regarding improved diagnostic acumen, the beneficial effects of early enteral nutrition, methods of furosemide administration and prophylactic fenestration to prevent recurrent intervertebral disk extrusion, are subjected to more rigorous evaluation. Additionally, practitioners are offered good alternatives to current standards of care for idiopathic chylothorax, severe collapsing trachea, and for predicting the severity of canine pancreatitis.

References

1. Blosser SA, Zimmerman HE, Stauffer JL. Do autopsies of critically ill patients reveal important findings that were clinically undetected? *Crit Care Med* 1998; **26**: 1332–6.

2. Chan DL, Freeman LM, Labato MA, Rush JE. Retrospective evaluation of partial parenteral nutrition in dogs and cats. *J Vet Intern Med* 2002; **16**: 440–5.

3. van Meyel JJM, Smits P, Russel FGM, Gerlag PG, Tan Y, Gribnau FW. Diuretic efficiency of furosemide during continuous administration versus bolus injection in healthy volunteers. *Clin Pharmacol Ther* 1992; **51**: 440–4.

4. Levine SH, Caywood DD. Recurrence of neurological defects in dogs treated for thoracolumbar disk disease. *J Am Anim Hosp Assoc* 1984; **20**: 889–94.

5. Dhupha S, Glickman N, Waters DJ. Reoperative neurosurgery in dogs with thoracolumbar disk disease. *Vet Surg* 1999; **28**: 421–8.

6. Ruaux CG, Atwell RB. Levels of total α-macroglobulin and trypsin-like immunoreactivity are poor indicators of clinical severity in spontaneous canine acute pancreatitis. *Res Vet Sci* 1999; **67**: 83–7.

7. Bradley EL. A clinically based classification system for acute pancreatitis; summary of the international symposium on acute pancreatitis. Atlanta, Georgia, September 11–13, 1992. *Arch Surg* 1993; **128**: 586–90.

5

Upper and lower respiratory diseases in dogs and cats

CECILE CLERCX

Introduction

Chronic nasal disorders are very commonly encountered in veterinary practice, in both dogs and cats. Specific conditions, such as canine aspergillosis and nasal tumours, are quite easy to diagnose but very challenging to treat. A large number of studies report the relative efficacy of numerous therapeutic regimens, including systemic, invasive or non-invasive topical application of antifungal medication, with increasing success rates. Despite this, treatment failure or recurrence may still occur. Therefore, new treatment strategies continue to be investigated (Hotston Moore, 2003).

In many chronic nasal diseases in both dogs and cats, no aetiology can be clearly demonstrated: therapeutic regimens are often empirical and rarely curative. A retrospective study in cats reports the histopathology and cytology findings in these cases (Michiels *et al.*, 2003), and another retrospective study is devoted to so-called 'idiopathic lymphoplasmacytic rhinitis' (LPR) in dogs (Windsor *et al.*, 2004).

Laryngeal paralysis is a condition that can be inherited or acquired. The acquired form is common in large and giant breed dogs. Diagnosis is usually made during laryngoscopy under a light plane of anaesthesia, as a too deep plane of anaesthesia causes changes in active laryngeal motion, altering the diagnostic possibilities. The influence of some anaesthetic agents on laryngeal motion has been investigated (Jackson *et al.*, 2004).

Tracheal collapse is a common disorder in middle-aged toy and miniature dogs. The most effective management of this condition is still controversial. Placement of external prostheses has become the preferred technique for surgical treatment, although the procedure is difficult, invasive and associated with severe complications. An innovative successful therapy, which consists of stabilization of the trachea with intraluminal self-expanding endoprostheses, has been reported in dogs (Moritz *et al.*, 2004).

Lower airways disorders of infectious origin in cats are uncommon and documented reports of these disorders are rare. However, two recent retrospective studies deal with lower respiratory tract infections (LRTIs) in cats (Macdonald *et al.*, 2003; Foster *et al.*, 2004a). Inflammatory airways disease with no identified aetiology is quite common: these cases have been termed feline bronchitis, feline asthma or asthmatic bronchitis, as the distinction between chronic bronchitis and feline asthma is not clear-cut and not easy to make. Foster *et al.* (2004b) also reported in a retrospective study a series of 25 cats with feline bronchial disease (FBD), and also a retrospective analysis of bronchoalveolar lavage (BAL) in the same species. Several interesting studies aim at a better understanding of the immunopathogenesis in allergic asthma using feline experimental models (Norris *et al.*, 2003). Such studies will help in the future to characterize better the different forms of FBD and possibly give rise to some new therapeutic considerations.

The clinical significance and implication of *structural pulmonary changes in dogs*, such as blebs, bullae or development of bronchiectasis, are yet to be fully elucidated. The rupture of blebs and bullae is the most common cause of spontaneous pneumo-thorax, and management of pneumothorax is challenging. One comprehensive retrospective study analyses such cases in dogs (Lipscomb *et al.*, 2003) and another study related to canine cases of bronchiectasis (Hawkins *et al.*, 2003) are then reviewed.

An interesting and hence still poorly understood syndrome is *acute dyspnoea*, which is described in Swedish hunting dogs by Egenvall *et al.* (2003).

Finally, the last paper relates to a condition of uncertain origin, leading to pro-gressive rhinitis and bronchopneumonia, which resembles the hereditary disease primary ciliary dyskinesia (PCD) in the Irish wolfhound (Clercx *et al.*, 2003).

Use of topical povidone-iodine dressings in the management of mycotic rhinitis in three dogs
Moore AH. *J Small Anim Pract* 2003; **44**: 326–9

BACKGROUND. This paper describes the treatment of three dogs with mycotic rhinitis with a proprietary wound dressing product intended to produce a sustained release of povidone-iodine. The dogs had been refractory to several treatments, including clotrimazole infusion on five occasions, followed by enilconazole treatment through frontal sinus catheters in case 1, terbinafine (a systemic antifungal drug) given for 8 weeks in case 2, and oral itraconazole given for 3 weeks in case 3. This treatment was designed because there is some evidence that topical povidone-iodine used as a 'paint' after open rhinotomy can be considered as an alternative treatment |1|. The use of a slow release form of dressing was expected to maintain adequate levels of active iodine locally, and to reduce the frequency of handling the animal.

INTERPRETATION. The affected nasal cavity and/or frontal sinus was exposed via a dorsal approach and partial turbinectomy was performed. The wound dressing was applied and retained with a 'tie-over' dressing. The dressing was replaced every 48–72 h mostly under general anaesthesia, and sometimes under sedation, according to the patient's temperament, until all exposed tissue was covered by healthy granulation tissue, at which time the rhinotomy was closed by soft tissue reconstruction. The duration of topical povidone-iodine therapy was 18 days (six changes), 21 days (seven changes) and 15 days (five changes) in the three patients, respectively. There was no evidence of recurrence of the fungal infection at a follow-up of 14, 18 and 20 months post-surgery, respectively.

Comment

The diagnosis of canine aspergillosis is based on clinical, radiological and rhinoscopic findings. A large number of studies report the relative efficacy of numerous therapeutic regimens, including systemic or invasive topical application of antifungal medication, but none has been satisfactory |2,3|. More recent treatments propose rhinoscopic debridement combined with repeated topical non-invasive antifungal therapy with an increasing success rate |4,5|, but it is likely that no treatment method is expected to be successful in all cases. The topical povidone-iodine pack used in the present study was more invasive than any other alternative option. Cases 2 and 3 did not get a chance to undergo potentially adequate and less invasive treatments, as they had been refractory only to oral terbinafine and oral itraconazole, respectively, as the efficacy of terbinafine is not well established, and the success rate of oral administration of itraconazole is rather poor. Besides, and as underlined by the authors, the local absorption of the agent from this site is unknown and, although no toxic effects were noted, systemic levels of iodine should be investigated if the treatment was to be used widely. As the authors conclude, the invasiveness of this technique makes it unsuitable for use in routine cases, but could represent a useful option in complicated cases.

Fungal rhinitis and sinusitis is quite rarely encountered in cats. Three cases are reported in a recent publication |6|, which presents an interesting discussion about some questionable aspects of the disease, among others a comparison with similar conditions in human beings.

A retrospective study of non-specific rhinitis in 22 cats and the value of nasal cytology and histopathology

Michiels L, Day MJ, Snaps F, Hansen P, Clercx C. *J Fel Med Surg* 2003; **5**: 279–85

BACKGROUND. Feline chronic rhinitis is a diagnostic and therapeutic challenge. Despite a complete diagnostic investigation, aetiology is not often defined. Treatment is rarely curative, particularly in cats with chronic, non-specific disease. Moreover, treatment regimens are often empirical and are generally not based on the cytological and histopathological assessment of the lesions. The aim of this retrospective study was to review the clinical, radiographic and rhinoscopic findings in a series of cats with chronic rhinitis for which no underlying cause could be found, and to analyse the cytological and histological results in those cases. The agreement between cytology and histopathology was also assessed.

INTERPRETATION. Case records from 22 cats subjected to rhinoscopic examination for investigation of chronic nasal disease, and in which no specific underlying cause was detected, were reviewed. The radiographic and rhinoscopic findings were variable and non-specific. Cultures were positive in 15 of 21 cats, and more than one type of bacteria was isolated in nine of these. Mucosal biopsy specimens were obtained in 20 cases. Histopathology indicated acute inflammation in four, chronic lymphoplasmacytic inflammation in two and mixed (lymphoplasmacytic and neutrophilic) inflammation in 14 cats. Four of the 17 cytological specimens, obtained by brush sampling, were not diagnostic; acute inflammation was diagnosed ($n = 11$) more commonly than chronic ($n = 1$) or mixed inflammation ($n = 1$). Concurrent samples, of quality suitable for both histopathological and cytological interpretation, were collected from 12 cases only. Cytological results were in agreement with the histological results in 25% of these cases, the main discrepancy being the nature of the dominant inflammatory cell type.

Comment

In the present study, clinical signs, radiographic and rhinoscopic findings were comparable with those commonly described in upper respiratory diseases in general. As expected, blood work was not specific. In agreement with previous data from the literature, there is a low prevalence of feline leukaemia virus and feline immunodeficiency virus infection in those cats with non-specific nasal chronic disease. The study failed to investigate possible involvement of feline herpesvirus and calicivirus. The bacteria isolated (cultures were positive in 15 of 21 cats, and more than one type of bacteria was isolated in nine of them) was variable and non-specific; however, the presence of *Mycoplasma* was not examined. *Bordetella bronchiseptica*, which has been reported to act as the primary pathogen in cats with respiratory tract disease, particularly in kittens and in cats living in a stressful environment, was not identified in this study.

In the present study, all tissue specimens were of suitable quality for histopathological interpretation to be made; this is higher than in other studies of dogs |7|, where approximately a quarter of tissue specimens, obtained using perendoscopic biopsy forceps, were unevaluable. By contrast, the proportion of diagnostic cytological samples was lower (13 of 17 cases, or 76%).

Despite clinical signs of more than 4 weeks' duration, histopathology indicated acute inflammation in four cases; acute inflammation was diagnosed by cytology ($n = 11$) more commonly than chronic ($n = 1$) or mixed inflammation ($n = 1$). This finding might simply reflect the random choice of site for mucosal biopsies, but could also indicate that even in cats that exhibit clinical signs for more than 4 weeks, chronic histopathological modifications of the nasal mucosa are not yet present. Another explanation would be that the presence of a deep mucosal chronic infiltrate can be hidden by a superficial neutrophilic inflammatory process. It would be interesting to determine whether such cases of acute inflammation are more responsive to treatment than others. Cytological results were in agreement with the histological results in 25% of these cases, the main discrepancy being the nature of the dominant inflammatory cell type. Therefore, cytology does not appear to be a reliable means for the detection of chronic inflammation. In the future, it would be interesting to investigate whether a correlation exists between the nature of mucosal inflammation as defined by both histological and cytological evaluation, and prognosis and therapy in feline chronic rhinitis.

Idiopathic lymphoplasmacytic rhinitis in dogs: 37 cases (1997–2002)

Windsor RC, Johnson LR, Herrgesell EJ, De Cock HE. *J Am Vet Med Assoc* 2004; **224**: 1952–7

BACKGROUND. Idiopathic LPR in dogs refers to chronic rhinitis in which the underlying cause is not apparent. Two previous reports of this condition involved five dogs each |8,9|, but specific characteristics of the disease have not been fully described. The purpose of this retrospective study was to determine clinical signs, effectiveness of past treatment, rhinoscopic findings, computed tomograph abnormalities, and histological abnormalities in dogs with idiopathic LPR. Dogs in which a histological diagnosis of LPR had been made and no underlying cause of the lesions (e.g. neoplasia, aspergillosis, nasal foreign body, oronasal fistula) could be identified were eligible for inclusion in the study. Dogs were included only if a biopsy specimen had been obtained from both nasal passages.

INTERPRETATION. The 37 selected dogs ranged from 1.5 to 14 years old (mean: 8 years) and most were large breed dogs. Nasal discharge was unilateral in 11 of 26 dogs (42%) and bilateral in 58%. In dogs with unilateral disease, duration of clinical signs ranged from 1.5 to 36 months (mean 8.25 months), and in dogs with bilateral disease, from 1.25 to 30 (mean 6.5 months). Computed tomography (CT; $n = 33$) most often revealed fluid accumulation (82%), turbinate destruction (70%) and frontal sinus opacification (42%). Rhinoscopy ($n = 37$) commonly demonstrated increased mucus and epithelial inflammation; turbinate destruction was detected in 22% of the dogs. Bilateral biopsy specimens from the 37 dogs were examined. Four dogs had only unilateral changes, the remaining 33 dogs had bilateral lesions; in 20, lesions were more severe on one side than the other. These findings suggest that idiopathic LPR is most often a bilateral disease even among dogs with unilateral nasal discharge.

Comment

This condition mainly affects middle-aged to older dogs. Common clinical signs of chronic nasal inflammation (discharge, sneezing, stertor, ocular discharge, and regional lymph node lymphadenopathy related to moderate lymph node reactivity) were variably present; moreover, several had experienced episodes of epistaxis and some demonstrated cough. This study also collected information on previous treatments used and their relative efficacy. Oral antimicrobials, antihistamines and glucocorticoids had not been very effective in eliminating clinical signs in the present study. Radiography has some sensitivity in differentiating inflammatory rhinitis from neoplasia or aspergillosis; however, CT provides better definition of the extent and severity of the lesions |**10,11**|. In the present study, CT demonstrated that in idiopathic LPR: (i) turbinate destruction can be present; (ii) frontal sinus can be involved (in 42% of the cases); and (iii) a bilateral and diffuse distribution of the lesions is seen in many dogs with unilateral signs. Rhinoscopic findings were related to non-specific chronic inflammation. Such findings are difficult to interpret especially in the hands of inexperienced rhinoscopists; they include hyperaemia, inflammation, excessive mucus, plaque-like or mass-like lesions and excessive friability of tissue.

The authors then discuss some potential causes for idiopathic LPR, which include unidentified foreign body, undiagnosed neoplastic or mycotic process; hypotheses of immune dysregulation, allergy or high microbial load are also evoked. In fact, a lymphoplasmacytic infiltration is the most common histological finding in nasal mucosal biopsy specimens in most dogs with chronic clinical signs of nasal disease, whatever the origin, e.g. in association with canine aspergillosis |12|, and this is also true in cats with chronic nasal disease (Michiels *et al.*, 2003). Therefore, LPR could be viewed as a common type of infiltration resulting from a variety of possible causes responsible for chronic disease, during the insult or after appropriate therapy, rather than to a specific idiopathic disease. Therefore, it is likely that no treatment, used orally or systemically, exists that will cure the disease and eliminate clinical signs. Better results may be possible with the use of intranasal or nebulized therapies, but this needs to be investigated in future prospective studies.

Effects of various anesthetic agents on laryngeal motion during laryngoscopy in normal dogs

Jackson AM, Tobias K, Long C, Bartges J, Harvey R. *Vet Surg* 2004; **33**: 102–6

BACKGROUND. Laryngeal paralysis is a common upper airways disease, which can be congenital in young Siberian huskies and Bouvier des Flandres or acquired. A recent paper describes the disease in three young Siberian huskies crossbreeds, and discusses the pathogenesis of the disease |13|. Diagnosis is usually made during laryngoscopy under a light plane of anaesthesia, as a too deep plane of anaesthesia causes changes in active laryngeal motion, altering the diagnostic possibilities. This study was designed to evaluate the effects of various anaesthetics and anaesthetic protocols conventionally used for anaesthesia on arytenoid cartilage motion during laryngoscopy in normal dogs. Therefore, six large breed healthy dogs were randomly assigned to different injectable anaesthetic protocols and to isoflurane protocol, once a week for 7 weeks. Videolaryngoscopy was performed and recorded immediately after induction until dogs could no longer be safely restrained for endoscopy. Images for maximal inspiration and expiration were imported into an image analysis software program.

INTERPRETATION. Within each protocol, laryngeal motion, defined as change in normalized glottal gap area (NGGA = area of the laryngeal ostium normalized for its height), was not significantly different at induction from laryngeal motion measured at recovery. Additionally, no significant differences were found in arytenoid motion immediately after induction when anaesthetic protocols were compared. Arytenoid motion before recovery was significantly greater with thiopental when compared with protocol, ketamine + diazepam, acepromazine + thiopental, and acepromazine + propofol. No significant difference in arytenoid motion was seen immediately after induction or before recovery when acepromazine + butorphanol + isoflurane and thiopental were compared (Table 5.1).

Comment

Mean change in NGGA was significantly reduced with the following protocols: acepromazine i.m. + propofol i.v., propofol i.v., ketamine i.v. and diazepam i.v., because at least half of the dogs had no arytenoid abduction on inspiration while arytenoid motion was normal using other protocols. Therefore, the authors recommend against the use of those three protocols, which can lead to a false diagnosis; laryngeal function in normal dogs seems best assessed with i.v. thiopental. As acepromazine reduces the amount of anaesthetic required for induction, premedication can be useful, but in this case, the authors advise mask induction with isoflurane if further anaesthetic administration is needed.

It is indeed desirable for the examiner to be able to observe laryngeal motion during several deep breaths while noting the stage of respiration to verify that the larynx is abducting effectively during inspiration. Duration of the examination is limited by return of jaw tone and risk of trauma to the equipment or examiner. In the present paper, the authors evaluated laryngeal function by measuring NGGA, implying the use of expensive equipment, a videoendoscope, which needs to be inserted far enough into the mouth and over the tip of the epiglottis in order to make the entire laryngeal ostium visible on the monitor, and to further allow analysis by the software program. Hence, laryngeal function can indeed better be evaluated under a minimal plane of anaesthesia, just enough to permit minimal retraction of the jaws. Then, if laryngeal abduction was evaluated by direct examination (visualization) rather than

Table 5.1 Mean (±SD) dosages of anaesthetic drugs and mean (±SD) duration of anaesthetic examination used for evaluation of laryngeal function in six normal dogs

Anaesthesia protocol (route of administration)	Dosage (mg/kg)	Examination duration (min:s)
Acepromazine (i.m.)	0.05	12:53 ± 8:13
Oxymorphone (i.v.)	0.05 ± 0.019	
Acepromazine (i.m.)	0.05	2:27 ± 1:41
Thiopental (i.v.)	9.82 ± 2.09	
Thiopental (i.v.)	14 ± 2.26	3:07 ± 1:04
Acepromazine (i.m.)	0.05	7:47 ± 5:01
Propofol (i.v.)	3.7 ± 1.31	
Propofol (i.v.)	5.6 ± 1.14	5:01 ± 2:31
Ketamine (i.v.)	8.5 ± 2.91	3:25 ± 1:33
Diazepam (i.v.)	0.4 ± 0.15	
Acepromazine (i.m.)	0.2	9:58 ± 8:35
Butorphanol (i.m.)	0.4	
Isoflurane	Mask induction	

Source: Jackson et al. (2004).

by the use of expensive material, the acceptable plane of anaesthesia would probably be lighter and the corresponding dosage lower. Therefore, the procedure could be less dependent on the agent use for induction.

The authors quote that they currently use doxapram hydrochloride (2–5 mg/kg, i.v.) to stimulate vigorous respiratory motion during laryngoscopy when propofol had been used as an induction agent. The effect of dopram on intrinsic laryngeal motion in dogs has already previously been described and advocated for routine use in the diagnosis of suspected laryngeal disease |14|. Another recent paper refers to the use of transnasal laryngoscopy for the diagnosis of laryngeal paralysis in dogs under sedation and local anaesthesia. This technique, which is used in human medicine, is not routinely used in dogs |15|.

Management of advanced tracheal collapse in dogs using intraluminal self-expanding biliary Wallstents™
Moritz AM, Schneider M, Bauer N. *J Vet Intern Med* 2004; **18**: 31–42

BACKGROUND. Tracheal collapse is a common disorder in middle-aged toy and miniature and dogs. The most effective management of this condition is still controversial. Placement of external prostheses has become the preferred technique for surgical treatment, but the procedure is difficult, invasive and associated with severe complications. The purpose of this retrospective study was to evaluate the efficacy of endoscopic placement of an intraluminal self-expanding stainless steel endoprosthesis (Wallstent) and to report the results of the follow-up after stent implantation. Twenty-four client-owned dogs with tracheal collapse refractory to conventional treatment underwent management with this technique.

INTERPRETATION. Initial improvement of clinical signs was observed in 95.8% of the dogs. Two dogs (8.3%) died within days after stent implantation. Of the dogs treated, 30.4% were reported to be asymptomatic after stent implantation, 60.9% markedly improved, and 4.3% remained symptomatic. Endoscopy rechecks, performed in 18 dogs, showed that the Wallstents were almost completely covered with tracheal epithelium, a consequent shortening of the endoprosthesis was frequently noted (in 15 dogs) and steroid-responsive granuloma formation resulted in a severe reduction of the tracheal lumen in three patients. The results suggest that implantation of Wallstents was minimally invasive and provided stabilization of collapsed thoracic tracheal portions in addition to the cervical part of the trachea.

Comment

Tracheal collapse is a common disorder in middle-aged toy and miniature dogs. The most effective management is still controversial. Retrospective studies have shown that many dogs respond to symptomatic medical therapy together with management of initiating or aggravating causes. Therefore, many clinicians are still in favour of conservative medical treatment and advise it in most cases, rather than surgical procedures. However, the management of tracheal collapse using endoscopic placement of intraluminal self-expanding stents, as described in the present paper, appears extremely attractive, and such methods could become a therapy of choice in the future. Indeed, in contrast with surgical methods of extraluminal stabilization, the implantation of stents is atraumatic and comparatively quicker. Furthermore, stabilization is performed along the entire length of the trachea rather than along the extrathoracic portion. However, there are potentially severe complications associated with the procedure, such as risk of perforation by the terminal sharp ends of the stent leading to emphysema and pneumomediastinum, severe tracheal collapse cranial to the stented area due to the progressive shortening and concurrent increase in diameter and the formation of steroid-responsive granulomas. Potential supplementary technical problems arise from the choice of the length and diameter of the stent and from bad positioning (once expanded, the stent cannot be removed or repositioned) and these can be overcome in the hands of experienced clinicians. Therefore it is important to select patients the same way they did in the present study. Selected patients should evidence a marked reduction of the dog's quality of life due to persistence of one or more severe clinical signs such as dyspnoea, cyanosis, severe paroxysmal coughing, and syncope due to hypoxaemia, despite conservative management. Patients with mild clinical signs and dogs in which most clinical signs are caused by diseases other than severe tracheal collapse (i.e. cardiac disease, chronic bronchopulmonary disease) are not good candidates.

Clinicopathologic and radiographic features and etiologic agents in cats with histologically confirmed infectious pneumonia: 39 cases (1991–2000)

Macdonald ES, Norris CR, Berghaus RB, Griffey SM. *J Am Vet Med Assoc* 2003; **223**: 1142–50

BACKGROUND. Infectious pneumonia is uncommon in cats, and there are few documented reports of this disorder. The objectives of this retrospective study were to evaluate clinicopathological and radiographic features and aetiological agents in cats with infectious pneumonia in which the diagnosis was confirmed during histological examination. Medical records of 31 323 cats that underwent autopsy were reviewed. Of these, 110 cats with pneumonia were identified, but only 39 were selected for the study. Inclusion criteria required a histological diagnosis of pneumonia and identification of an infectious (bacterial, viral, fungal, protozoal or parasitic) agent.

INTERPRETATION. Clinical signs referable to the respiratory tract were detected in 25 (64%) of the selected cats, and included, essentially, tachypnoea or dyspnoea (19 cats), nasal discharge (eight) and coughing (three). Clinical signs of systemic illness (lethargy, anorexia, fever) were recorded in 23 cats (59%). Results of complete blood count (CBC) and radiography were unremarkable in four of 18 and three of 13 cats, respectively. Aetiological agents included more frequently bacteria (n = 22) and viruses (n = 11), including coronavirus (n = 9) and feline herpesvirus (n = 1). Most bacterial infections were attributable to anaerobes (17 of 21) and eight of 13 were single isolates; the majority (12 of

20) resulted from haematogenous spread. In 11 cats, histological lesions were limited to the respiratory tract and the 28 others had evidence of systemic disease.

Comment

The findings in this retrospective study confirm that the ante mortem diagnosis of infectious pneumonia in cats is very challenging in cases that lack clinical signs, haematological or radiographic abnormalities that support the diagnosis. This is true in dogs as well, as the diagnosis of pneumonia can also be difficult to confirm |16|. In both species, lack of coughing is frequent. As noted in this study, clinicians should use respiratory signs as a clinical indicator of potential advanced respiratory tract disease, because cats that had respiratory signs were shown to be more likely to have severe histological changes. On the other hand, this study failed to demonstrate any correlation between the severity of histological lesions and evidence of signs of systemic illness. Besides, clinical signs of respiratory disease were not helpful in predicting the cause as signs were not significantly associated with the aetiological agents.

Therefore, a major conclusion of this paper is indeed that clinicians should maintain a high index of suspicion for pneumonia and evaluate the respiratory tract when infection is detected in other organ systems.

As in dogs, lack of abnormalities on a CBC and on thoracic radiographs are not adequate to rule out infectious pneumonia.

Other diagnostic techniques traditionally considered helpful in the diagnosis of infectious pneumonia are culture and cytology of airways lavage and fine-needle aspiration of the pulmonary parenchyma; however, all these techniques have several inherent limitations. Indeed, bacteria cultured from lavage fluid could be a contaminant, a positive result of a lavage sample can be secondary to a non-infectious lung disease or to another infectious disease such as a viral disease. Also, an organism could fail to grow for many reasons. Cytological examination of specimens obtained by lavage or by the use of fine-needle aspiration is a successfully used diagnostic tool for the detection of infectious or non-infectious pneumonia, and results of examination of fine-needle aspirates correlate well with results of histological examination. However, cytology can be inadequate to obtain a definitive diagnosis as well. Histological examination remains the gold standard for definitive confirmation of a diagnosis of infectious pneumonia and is helpful in identifying the aetiological agent. However, it is not a recommended procedure for ante mortem diagnosis!

This study confirmed that bacterial pneumonia is the most common cause of infectious pneumonia, aerobic infection being the most common. Viral infection was identified in 11 cats, and feline infectious peritonitis was associated with nine of them, with a higher risk for juvenile and purebred cats. However, it is unusual for those cats to be examined primarily because of clinical signs associated with pulmonary involvement. Pneumonia can indeed rarely be attributable to herpesvirus (one cat in this study). It is more common for calicivirus to cause interstitial pneumonia in cats, although no cats with calicivirus-induced pneumonia were found in this study. The frequency of fungal pneumonia (15% in this study) certainly depends on geographical area, and is probably much less in most European countries.

Lower respiratory tract infections in cats: 21 cases (1995–2000)

Foster SF, Martin P, Allan GS, Barrs VR, Malik R. *J Fel Med Surg* 2004a; **6**: 167–80

BACKGROUND. Twenty-one LRTIs diagnosed in cats at the University of Sydney Veterinary Centre between 1995 and 2000 were identified from a retrospective study of BAL cytology and microbiology |17|. The diagnosis required a significant pure culture of bacterium and fungus (moderate to heavy growth of any microbe with minimal growth of oral contaminant), together with supportive historical, clinical, radiographic and cytological findings, and unambiguous response to appropriate antimicrobial therapy. Patient records were analysed to determine historical, clinical, clinicopathological and radiographic features of non-viral LRTIs. Response to therapy was also assessed.

INTERPRETATION. The median age was 10 years; males were 2.4 times more likely to have LRTIs than females. Serological testing for feline immunodeficiency virus antibody was positive in four of 12 cats. Serological testing for feline leukaemia virus antigen in seven cases was negative in each. Infectious agents identified were essentially *Mycoplasma* spp. as a single agent (11 cases) or in combination (two cases), but also *Pasteurella* spp. (three cases), *Salmonella typhimurium* (two cases), *Aelurostrongylus abstrusus* (two cases), and *Pseudomonas* sp., *Bordetella bronchiseptica*, *Mycobacterium thermoresistible*, *Cryptococcus neoformans*, *Toxoplasma gondii*, and *Eucoleus aerophilus* (one case of each). Cough or dyspnoea were present in all but two cases. Neutrophilic leucocytosis was detected in 11 of 12 cases tested. BAL cytology revealed neutrophilic inflammation in all but two of 19 cases.

Comment

In this study, diagnosis was based on ante mortem findings, rather than on autopsy findings, as in the previous paper (Macdonald *et al.*, 2003) and the inclusion criteria were different. This probably accounts for the differences in clinical findings with regard to clinical signs, haematological and radiographic abnormalities between both retrospective studies. Differences in the nature and frequency of causative infectious agents described in both studies probably also partly relies on geographic differences. In the present study, *Mycoplasma* appears as the more common infectious agent of feline LRTIs. Mycoplasmal LRTIs are often considered to be a consequence of pre-existing pulmonary diseases. The authors hypothesize that the mycoplasmal LRTIs, while of clinical significance, were possibly secondary to FBD. The role of *Mycoplasma* is being increasingly examined in human asthma, but so far the exact role of *Mycoplasma* in asthmatic and/or bronchial disease in humans and animals is still poorly defined. In the present study, oral doxycycline, 5 mg/kg twice daily, appeared effective in most cases and could be recommended as a first choice when *Mycoplasma* is suspected to be the aetiological agent.

Twenty-five cases of feline bronchial disease (1995–2000)

Foster SF, Allan GS, Martin P, Robertson ID, Malik R. *J Fel Med Surg* 2004b; **6**: 181–8

BACKGROUND. Bronchopulmonary disease in cats may be caused by infectious agents (viruses, bacteria, fungi, parasites), cardiac disease, neoplasia, trauma or toxins. Many cases, however, have inflammatory airways disease with no identifiable aetiology. These cases have been termed feline asthma, feline bronchitis, allergic bronchitis and FBD |18–20|. Besides, other bronchopulmonary diseases such as bacterial and parasitic infections are frequently not rigidly excluded before making a diagnosis of FBD. This retrospective study, conducted at the University of Sydney Veterinary Centre, Australia, reviews historical, clinical, clinicopathological and radiographic features in 25 cases of FBD, selected on the basis of consistent clinical signs or histopathology and no other identifiable aetiology, and after exclusion of bacterial lower respiratory tract disease.

INTERPRETATION. The cats were 2–15 years old (median 9 years), and included domestic cats (13), Siamese/oriental/Sirex/Siamese cross (four), Burmese (four), British short-hair (three), Persian (one) and Australian Mist (one). Purebred cats were no more likely to have FBD than crossbred cats; however, purebred shorthair cats (excluding Burmese and Siamese) were four times more likely to be affected than domestic cats. The main presenting complaints were coughing and dyspnoea. The most common physical finding was dyspnoea. The majority of radiographs had a bronchial pattern or a mixed bronchial pattern. BAL cytology was classified according to the predominant cell type (50% or more of the total cell count) as neutrophilic, histiocytic, lymphocytic, eosinophilic or mixed: it was neutrophilic or eosinophilic in the majority of cats. There was no association between age, breed, sex, clinical signs, BAL cytology or radiographic severity and disease severity. Twenty-three cats required oral prednisolone, bronchodilators (terbutaline, sustained-release theophylline or aminophylline), or both for improvement of clinical signs. Seventeen cats needed continuous bronchodilator and/or glucocorticoid therapy, three cats required intermittent medication, and three cats were weaned off medication.

Comment

Selected criteria of inclusion in this retrospective study are narrower than in other studies: the 25 cats selected were identified as having FBD on the basis of consistent ongoing clinical signs or histopathology and no other identified aetiology. Besides, bacterial lower respiratory tract disease had been excluded, based on the results of a retrospective study of unguided BAL cytology and microbiology |17|. Cases for which follow-up information was not available and cats that appeared to have self-limiting disease were excluded. By narrowing the selected criteria compared with previous studies, the authors hoped to identify more definitive diagnostic and prognostic features without the need for pulmonary function testing. Indeed, as the author underlines it, pulmonary function testing and immunohistochemistry in naturally occurring FBD are not used routinely. However, there is an obvious need for the use of non-invasive pulmonary function testing coupled with standardized broncho-reactivity testing, as well as of immunohistochemistry studies of feline respiratory mucosae in order to characterize the different types of bronchial diseases in cats. The mean age of the cats in the present study is older than in previous studies, which the authors attributed to the difference in selection criteria, excluding mild and self-limiting diseases. Siamese cats have been reported to be over-represented or more severely affected in earlier studies, a tendency that is not confirmed in the present study. However, the authors do not provide information about reference popula-tions of breeds of cats in Australia versus other countries or continents. In the present study, purebred short-hair cats (other than Burmese and Siamese) were four times more likely than domestic cats to have FBD. In another concurrent study from the same author |**17**|, those cats were also four times more likely to have infectious lower respiratory tract diseases, which were identified to be due to *Mycoplasma*. The authors speculate that an association between FBD and *Mycoplasma* could exist. FBD might predispose to mycoplasmal infection; however, mycoplasmal infection might cause hyperreactivity and induce FBD. However, this is a pure hypothesis as, in fact, the exact role of *Mycoplasma* remains unknown. Although this study eventually suggests that dyspnoea associated with FBD might be induced by seasonal environ-ment, the potential role of seasonal factors has not been clearly established. Changes in haematology, serum biochemistry and urinalysis are, like in previous studies, non-specific. The variability of radiographic appearance and the lack of correlation between radiographic severity and disease severity appear consistent with previous studies. Similarly, BAL cytology appeared variable in this study and does not help in predicting the severity of the disease or the response to treatment.

Allergen-specific IgG and IgA in serum and bronchoalveolar lavage fluid in a model of experimental feline asthma

Norris CR, Byerly JR, Decile KC, *et al*. *Vet Immunol Immunopathol* 2003;
96: 119–27

BACKGROUND. Allergic asthma is characterized by bronchoconstriction and airways inflammation and has classically been described as a type I hypersensitivity reaction mediated by allergen-specific IgE antibodies. Feline asthma is a naturally developing condition in pet cats and closely mimics human asthma. A model of feline asthma is useful to study the immunopathogenesis of the disease in both species. An experimental model of feline asthma using Bermuda grass allergen (BGA) has been developed, and sensitized cats develop BGA-specific IgE, airways eosinophilia, airways hyperreactivity, and have a T-helper 2 cytokine profile |**21,22**|. Because of the central role IgE plays in asthma pathogenesis, most studies evaluating the role of immunoglobulins in asthma have focused on IgE; however, other immunoglobulin classes are likely to influence the asthmatic phenotype. The objective of this study was to evaluate fluctuations in levels of serum and BAL fluid (BALF) allergen-specific IgG and IgA over the course of allergic sensitization and challenge in cats with experimentally induced asthma in order to investigate their role in the immunopathogenesis of allergic asthma.

INTERPRETATION. Levels of BGA-specific IgG and IgA, measured by an enzyme-linked immunosorbent assay (ELISA) technique, significantly increased over time in serum and BALF after allergen sensitization. Additionally, these elevated levels of BGA-specific IgG and IgA were seen in conjunction with the development of an asthmatic phenotype indicated by positive intradermal skin tests, enhanced airways hyperreactivity, and increased eosinophil percentages in the BALF. Airways hyperresponsiveness was evaluated under anaesthesia using a penumotachograph and a pressure transducer. Aerosol challenges with methacholine were used for bronchoprovocation studies. The measurement of allergen-specific IgG and IgA is likely to have important implications in both research and clinical settings. In a clinical setting, monitoring allergen-specific IgG and IgA in serum or mucosal secretions may be useful in clinical patients undergoing therapy to modulate the allergic response. In humans, subclasses of allergen-specific IgG antibodies vary in response to seasonal changes of the allergen in the environment. Much research remains to be done on the immunopathogenesis of asthma in the cat, and use of allergen-specific ELISAs for IgG and IgA in serum and BALF may help provide answers to aetiological and mechanistic questions in this and other related allergic diseases.

Comment

The feline model of experimentally induced asthma has already been used by the same author to investigate other immunopathological aspects of the disease |23|. Other experimental models of asthma have been developed in cats and several studies investigating the immunopathogenesis, potential markers of inflammation, degree of hyperresponsiveness to aerosol challenges and response to drugs have been conducted in those models |24–27|. Much research remains to be done on the immunopathogenesis and possible management of asthma in the cat, and those studies (in the present study the use of allergen-specific ELISAs for IgG and IgA in serum and BALF) may help provide answers to aetiological and mechanistic questions in this and other related allergic diseases.

For such investigations, a technique for the assessment of pulmonary function is required, as well as reactivity tests. In the present paper, lung function was evaluated under anaesthesia using a penumotachograph and a pressure transducer. Alternative non-invasive techniques, such as whole body barometric plethysmography can be used as well |26| and will be needed to investigate cats with spontaneous bronchial diseases. In the present paper, aerosols with metacholine were used for bronchoprovocation studies, although other bronchoconstrictive substances, such as carbachol or histamine, can be used as well. In order to characterize better and understand the pathogenesis of the disease in spontaneous cases of feline bronchitis, such bronchoreactivity tests will have to be used with a maximum of safety and absence of side effects in patients. The measurements of allergen-specific IgG and IgA will have to be repeated in cats with naturally occurring disease before definitive conclusions can be made regarding the mechanisms and the treatment possibilities in our feline patients

Spontaneous pneumothorax caused by pulmonary blebs and bullae in 12 dogs

Lipscomb VJ, Hardie RJ, Dubielzig RR. *J Am Vet Med Assoc* 2003; **39**: 435–45

BACKGROUND. Reported causes of spontaneous pneumothorax include bacterial pneumonia, pulmonary abscesses, neoplasia, dirofilariosis, bullous emphysema; the most common cause is the rupture of blebs or bullae. Previous reports have described the clinical findings from dogs with spontaneous pneumothorax due to pulmonary blebs, bullae/bullous emphysema; however, differences in lesion terminology (the terms bleb, bulla and bullous emphysema have been used interchangeably), lesion description and histopathological interpretation have resulted in conflicting information. The purpose of this study was to describe the clinical signs, radiographic findings, surgical treatment, post-operative complications, histopathological findings, and long-term outcome in 12 dogs with primary spontaneous pneumothorax caused by focal pulmonary blebs and bullae and to compare them with those described for humans with the same disorder.

INTERPRETATION. Radiographic evidence of blebs or bullae was seen in only one dog. Two dogs had pneumomediastinum and one had subcutaneous emphysema. None of the dogs responded to conservative treatment with thoracocentesis or thoracostomy tube drainage. A medial sternotomy was used to explore the thorax in all dogs. Blebs and bullae were resected with partial or total lobectomy. Ten of the dogs had more than one lesion, seven had bilateral lesions; the cranial lobes were more commonly affected. Histopathology results resembled lesions found in humans. None of the dogs developed recurrence of pneumothorax. The outcome following resection was excellent.

Comment

Identification of the cause of spontaneous pneumothorax in dogs is challenging as the source of air leakage can remain unclear after history taking, clinical examination and thoracic radiographs. This study confirms that spontaneous pneumothorax due to blebs or bullae is mostly found in healthy, middle-aged large-breed or deep-chested dogs with no history of respiratory disease. Respiratory signs (tachypnoea, exercise intolerance, coughing and various degrees of respiratory distress) may develop rapidly and be obvious, whereas in some dogs, non-specific signs (depression, lethargy) occur prior to the onset of respiratory signs. Lesions are usually not apparent on thoracic radiographs unless blebs or bullae become very large or develop thickened walls. The authors advise serial radiographs in order to identify eventually other potential causes of pneumothorax such as bacterial pneumonia, pulmonary abscesses, neoplasia, dirofilariosis, or tracheal, bronchial or oesophageal lesions.

In this series, thoracic CT or thoracoscopy was not used for the diagnosis. It would be very interesting to know how sensitive CT is in the detection of small pulmonary lesions. Indeed, it would be tempting to perform a lateral thoracotomy approach rather than a median sternotomy in any case where unilateral lesions are diagnosed. On the other hand, this paper shows that there is a great risk that contralateral lesions exist as well. Therefore, sternotomy should be advised in order to examine both lungs, unless the absence of lesions on one side can be accurately ascertained.

In all cases of this series, conservative treatment with thoracocentesis or thoracostomy tube drainage (together with strict rest, oxygen supplementation) was not effective. In other cases, prolonged conservative management can be effective in resolving the pneumothorax, although recurrence can occur. In contrast to dogs, conservative management in humans is generally successful. In dogs, the decisions regarding how long to pursue conservative treatment and when to undertake surgery can be difficult to make. Indeed, the results from this paper do not help to establish rules about how long the conservative management must reasonably be prolonged before deciding that it is definitely a failure, and when sternotomy should be undertaken. To this effect, thoracoscopy could be highly recommended, essentially as resection during the procedure can be performed safely with much less morbidity than during median sternotomy. The use of minimally invasive thoracoscopic techniques for detection and resection has been recently described in human beings, but also in dogs |28|, with reduced complication rates and surgical times. The recurrence rate appears to be slightly higher with this technique than with thoracotomy. Histological differentiation has been clearly demonstrated in the present paper, and bullae can be classified into three histological types, like in the human being. However, it appears that such distinctions are not directly useful for the clinician as the response to management and the prognosis is not related to the histology results. However, no new practical information about bullous emphysema is available.

Demographic, clinical, and radiographic features of bronchiectasis in dogs: 316 cases (1988–2000)

Hawkins EC, Basseches J, Berry CR, Stebbins ME, Ferris KK. *J Am Vet Med Assoc* 2003; **223**: 1628–35

BACKGROUND. Bronchiectasis refers to persistent dilatation of the bronchi resulting from chronic airways inflammation with destruction of the structural integrity of the bronchial walls. Bronchiectasis is most commonly diagnosed morphologically ante mortem through thoracic radiography. Although the condition is well known to occur in dogs, and has been described in numerous reports of lower respiratory tract diseases, few publications have primarily addressed this abnormality. Therefore, this retrospective study reviews a Veterinary Medical database (VMDB, 289 dogs) as well as the medical records of patients at a veterinary teaching hospital (VTH) (27 dogs) to determine demographic, clinical and radiographic features of bronchiectasis in dogs in the hope of identifying potential risk factors.

INTERPRETATION. The study showed that some purebred dogs such as American cocker spaniels, West Highland white terriers, miniature poodles, Siberian huskies, English springer spaniels and old dogs had an increased risk of bronchiectasis. Coughing was the most common clinical sign; a variety of bacteria were isolated, and on thoracic radiographs, cylindrical bronchiectasis, generalized disease, and right cranial lung lobe involvement were most common. There was no progression of the lesions on follow-up radiographs (seven dogs). Mean duration of clinical signs prior to the diagnosis of bronchiectasis was 9 months (range 1 day–10 years). Despite the presence of irreversible lesions, these dogs may survive for years (median survival time was 16 months; range 2 days–72 months).

Comment

Although the title mentions an analysis of bronchiectasis in 316 cases, the clinical and radiographic features relate to the 27 that were examined at the VTH. For demographic features, population statistics from the VMDB and VTH were used, respectively, for comparison.

In bronchiectasis the normal structure and function of airways are compromised. The resulting retention of secretions and decreased ability to eliminate infection perpetuates the inflammatory response. However, bronchiectasis is not a universal consequence of chronic inflammation. Therefore, the identification and understanding of risk factors for the development of bronchiectasis indeed needed to be investigated. Because of alterations of defence mechanisms at the time of diagnosis, it is difficult to identify whether infection is a consequence or an initiating cause. Infections with certain bacterial agents are thought to predispose individuals to bronchiectasis, such as *Staphylococcus aureus* and *Pseudomonas* spp. The present study does not help to document this, because, although bacterial growth was important in most dogs, a high proportion of dogs had been previously treated with antibiotics.

Most dogs with bronchiectasis in this study had a history of cough and evidence of hypersecretion of mucus and pooling of secretions. However, bronchiectasis does not appear to be the cause of haemoptysis in dogs, while it is reported in 50% of the cases in human medicine.

Dogs included in this study had clearly visible identifiable radiographic evidence of bronchiectasis. The sensitivity of thoracic radiographs in the diagnosis of bronchiectasis in people is low. Therefore, it is likely that the dogs in the present study all had advanced disease and that bronchiectasis is more common. In the present study, the incidence of bronchiectasis was quite low: 0.05% (VMDB) to 0.07% (VTH).

As suggested by the authors, the predisposition of certain purebred dogs could be the result of inherited disorders. None of the dogs in this study had obvious congenital disease, but testing for PCD was performed in only one dog. On the other hand, 70% of the dogs were older than 10, making congenital disease less probable. Focal bronchiectasis can result from endobronchial obstruction but this study shows that it is not always the case as in the three dogs of the present study with involvement of a single lobe, none had evidence of airways obstruction. Bronchiectasis has previously been shown to be associated with chronic bronchitis and eosinophilic bronchopneumopathy, but this paper is lacking consistent information about the presence of concomitant specific respiratory diseases: hence the existence of some of those concurrent diseases is probably among the most important risk factor.

An interesting feature of the study is that it tended to confirm that radiographic lesions are not reversible. Despite that and, although bronchiectasis is generally considered as an end-stage irreversible disease, clinical signs can be controlled with appropriate veterinary care.

Pulmonary oedema in Swedish hunting dogs
Egenvall A, Hansson K, Säteri H, Lord PF, Jonsson L. *J Small Anim Pract* 2003; **44**: 209–17

BACKGROUND. Since the mid-1970s, a syndrome of acute dyspnoea due to a form of neurogenic pulmonary oedema, appearing during or after hunting has been recognized; this was found mainly in Swedish hunting dogs, but also in daschunds and basset Artesien Normands |29|. Some dogs are affected almost every time they hunt, even from the first season, whereas others may be affected just once in their lifetime. Although occasionally the dogs die, they usually recover spontaneously within hours to a few days. This study aimed at characterizing the condition with respect to history, physical examination, chest radiology, echocardiography, electrocardiography, haematology, serum biochemistry, hormone analysis, and cardiac and pulmonary post mortem findings.

INTERPRETATION. The median age at which 16 hunting dogs first developed dyspnoea was 2.5 years (range 1–7), the median time between the end of run and dyspnoea was 20 min (range 0–24). The only clinical sign was dyspnoea (median respiratory rate = 60) and radiographic findings were bilateral infiltrates, predominantly dorsal, compatible with oedema; both findings were absent on re-evaluation (5–14 days after hunt). Echocardiography and electrocardiography were not remarkable and helped to rule out existing cardiac disease. There were very few statistical differences in blood haematology and serum biochemistry between dogs with pulmonary oedema and control dogs, with the exception of a higher insulin level (while cortisol was not different). Post mortem study showed no macroscopic changes in the heart, but histopathological examination showed multiple foci of subendocardial necrosis in the left ventricular myocardium.

Comment

Blood work values were adequately compared with those obtained in hunting dogs without any episodes of dyspnoea, and post mortem results were compared with those observed in hunting dogs without any attack of dyspnoea. This allowed us to see that white blood cells and neutrophil counts were elevated in all hunting dogs, which is probably a reflection of normal mobilization of cells from the marginal pool as a response to catecholamines.

The appearance of the radiographical lung lesions, the rapid progression without antibiotic treatment, the absence of trauma and bleeding, and the total disappearance of the lesions after frusemide provide evidence that the cause of dyspnoea in these dogs is transitory pulmonary oedema. Possible causes for acute transient pulmonary oedema are upper airways obstruction, epilepsy and brain trauma, all of which have been shown to be very unlikely in this study. Postictal oedema is caused by hypoglycaemia. The rapid mechanism by which the body corrects hypoglycaemia is through the release of catecholamines and glucagon, and catecholamine release is common to many causes of pulmonary oedema. Subendocardial necrosis has also been reported in conjunction with exertional cardiomyopathy, among wild animals chased by predators |**30**| and in humans with phaeochromocytoma with elevated blood levels of catecholamines. Therefore, the authors propose a pathological mechanism whereby acute sympathetic stimulation and high catecholamine release, present during hunting due to the stress of excitement and exercise, may be a factor causing myocardial and pulmonary lesions in some susceptible dogs, similar to neurogenic or postictal oedema.

This condition could possibly be encountered in all types of dogs, submitted to stress and acute huge oxygen demand, excitement and strenuous exercise, such as working, racing or sled dogs and probably also exists in hunting dogs from other countries. One should be aware of this condition and include it in the differential diagnosis whenever compatible clinical signs arise, and the number of cases with this diagnosis will probably increase in the future. This could help in better understanding of the pathogenesis of this amazing condition.

Rhinitis/bronchopneumonia syndrome in Irish wolfhounds

Clercx C, Reichler I, Peeters D, et al. J Vet Intern Med 2003; **17**(6): 843–9

B ACKGROUND. Rhinitis/bronchopneumonia syndrome in the Irish wolfhound is characterized by respiratory signs that range in severity from slight transient rhinorrhoea present from birth, to continuous intractable purulent nasal discharge with recurrent bronchopneumonia. A primary immunodeficiency, such as IgA deficiency, is suspected to underlie this condition. Other possible causes of this syndrome include a viral aetiology (see Hotston Moore, 2003) or a primary congenital ciliary defect; however, these hypotheses have not been examined. This study describes the clinical, immunological, genetic and pathological features of Irish wolfhounds with rhinitis/bronchopneumonia syndrome. The dogs examined were from Belgium, the Netherlands, the United Kingdom, Canada, Germany and Switzerland.

I NTERPRETATION. Affected Irish wolfhounds included four from Belgium and the Netherlands, six from the United Kingdom, 10 from Canada, six from Germany and two from Switzerland. Radiographic, rhinoscopic and bronchoscopic findings were variable. Analysis of ciliary ultrastructure was performed in five affected dogs but no characteristic PCD was detected. Analysis of serum and BALF concentrations of IgA, IgG and IgM showed that the serum IgA concentration was below the reference range in five of eight affected dogs tested, while BALF IgA level was above the normal range in two affected adult dogs. The CD4 to CD8 lymphocyte subset ratio (CD4/CD8) in the peripheral blood was within the normal range

(n = 3) but higher than the normal range in the BALF (n = 1). Decreased neutrophil phagocytosis was observed in one of the four patients tested. Analysis of pedigrees of the Belgian, Canadian, German and Swiss dogs revealed common ancestry, suggesting a heritable syndrome.

Comment

The clinical features of the disease typically include respiratory signs that range in severity from slight transient rhinorrhoea from birth, although this sign can be delayed in onset, to continuous intractable purulent discharge with bouts of recurrent bronchopneumonia. The disease appears to be episodic in nature, but this likely reflects the repeated administration of antibiotic therapy to affected dogs. The clinical picture described in those dogs (rhinosinusitis, bronchitis, bronchopneumonia) is very similar to the one reported in dogs with PCD. However, in the present study, there was no ultrastructural evidence of primary ciliary abnormality, while secondary ciliary abnormalities were frequently observed.

Some dogs had low serum IgA concentration, but some also had BALF IgA level above the normal range, when compared with a population of healthy dogs, matched for age and breed. Measurement of serum immunoglobulin concentrations is the most widely available means of assessing immune competence in the dog. A likely candidate defect would be IgA deficiency, as affected individuals may have a weakened mucosal defence, thus predisposing to infection. It has recently been documented that serum IgA concentrations in the dog are not an adequate reflection of mucosal immunity as shown by analysis of various secretions [31] and the findings of the present study corroborate this fact; the elevated IgA concentration in BALF of affected dogs may in fact reflect a heightened immune response at the respiratory mucosal surface.

In conclusion, the aetiology of the rhinitis/bronchopneumonia syndrome in dogs such as the Irish wolfhound remains unclear. A simple ciliary defect or primary immunodeficiency has not been identified, and the finding of normal concentrations of respiratory IgA suggests that IgA deficiency *per se* is unlikely to play a part in the disease pathogenesis. This study provides support for the hypothesis that this syndrome has a hereditary component. The aetiology of this disease should be further investigated, the ultimate goal being to identify the genetic basis of the disease, in order to develop a means of detecting and eliminating carrier dogs from the Irish wolfhound population.

Conclusion

At the moment there are no perfect treatment strategies in canine aspergillosis. A better knowledge of immunopathogenesis of this disease is warranted to elucidate better the relationship between the host and the mycosis, and new treatment strategies are proposed in order to improve the success rate. Such investigations probably will be the subject of many more publications in future years.

In most chronic nasal diseases in both dogs and cats, a specific aetiology cannot be evidenced, despite a full diagnostic work-up. In most cases, a lymphoplasmacytic infiltration is seen; in dogs idiopathic LPR is now described as a well-defined condition, in which both nasal cavities are generally affected. Aetiology and pathogenesis still need to be elucidated, and could potentially help the clinician in the future in the choice of the best therapeutic strategy, which is at present empirical and a real challenge in many cases.

Whenever clinical signs are compatible with a laryngeal dysfunction, the choice of anaesthesia should be conditioned by the effects of the drugs on the laryngeal motion. Videolaryngoscopy together with the use of an image analysis software program can help in the assessment of laryngeal motion. The use of doxapram hydrochloride to stimulate vigorous respiratory motion during laryngoscopy can also be of some help in the diagnosis of suspected laryngeal disease.

For the management of tracheal collapse, which is a very common and progressively worsening condition, the endoscopic placement of intratracheal stents is an interesting alternative approach.

Despite complete diagnostic work-up, including radiography, CT scan, bronchoscopy and analysis of BAL, lower airways disorders in cats are poorly differentiated. They include infectious diseases (which remain rare in this species but difficult to confirm clinically), and non-infectious diseases, including so-called feline asthmatic bronchitis. However, not all bronchial disorders refer to asthmatic disease. Although immunological investigations are being carried out in cats with experimental asthma, immunological characterization of spontaneous cases of FBDs are needed to improve the accuracy of the diagnosis in these diseases. Moreover, the use of non-invasive tests of lung function and of hyperreactivity tests in spontaneous cases will be required in order to distinguish real asthmatic cases from cases with bronchial disease of other origin, and to choose the most appropriate therapeutic regimen.

In atypical and chronic and/or recurrent lower airways diseases in dogs, the use of *in vitro* functional testing, ultrastructural examination, and immunological investigation (at both blood, BAL and tissue levels) will have to be added to more conventional diagnostic tools, including the use of CT scans, in order to warrant approaching the most accurate diagnosis and therefore prognosis and therapy in those diseases.

References

1. Pavletic MM. Open frontal sinus treatment of chronic canine aspergillosis. *Vet Surg* 1991; 20: 43–8.
2. Sharp NJH, Sullivan M, Harvey CE. Treatment of canine nasal aspergillosis. *J Vet Intern Med* 1993; 7: 40–3.

3. Mathews KG, Koblik PD, Richardson EF, Komtebedde J, Pappagianis D, Hector RF, Kass PH. Computed tomographic assessment of non-invasive intranasal infusions in dogs with fungal rhinitis. *Vet Surg* 1996; **25**: 309–19.

4. McCullough SM, McKiernan BC, Grodsky BS. Endoscopically placed tubes for administration of enilconazole for treatment of nasal aspergillosis in dogs. *J Am Vet Med Assoc* 1998; **212**: 67–9.

5. Zonderland JL, Störk CK, Saunders J, Hamaide A, Balligand M, Clercx C. Intranasal infusion of enilconazole for treatment of sinonasal aspergillosis in dogs. *J Am Vet Med Assoc* 2002; **221**: 1421–5.

6. Tomsa K, Glaus TM, Zimmer C, Greene CE. Fungal rhinitis and sinusitis in three cats. *J Am Vet Med Assoc* 2003; **222**: 1380–4.

7. Forbes Lent SE, Hawkins EC. Evaluation of rhinoscopy-assisted mucosal biopsy in diagnosis of nasal disease in dogs: 119 cases (1985–1989). *J Am Vet Med Assoc* 1992; **201**(9): 1425–9.

8. Burgener DC, Slocombe RF, Zerbe CA. Lymphoplasmacytic rhinitis in 5 dogs. *J Am Anim Hosp Assoc* 1987; **23**: 565–8.

9. Tasker SC, Knottenbelt M, Munro EA, Stonehewer J, Simpson JW, Mackin AJ. Aetiology and diagnosis of persistent nasal disease in the dog: a retrospective study of 42 cases. *J Small Anim Pract* 1999; **40**: 473–8.

10. Codner EC, Lurus AG, Miller JB, Gavin PR, Gallina A, Barbee DD. Comparison of computed tomography with radiography as a non-invasive diagnostic technique for chronic nasal disease in dogs. *J Am Vet Med Assoc* 1993; **202**: 1106–110.

11. Saunders JH, van Bree H, Gielen I, de Rooster H. Diagnostic value of computed tomography in dogs with chronic nasal disease. *Vet Radiol Ultrasound* 2003; **44**(4): 409–13.

12. Peeters D, Day MJ, Clercx C. An immunohistochemical study of canine nasal aspergillosis. *J Comp Pathol*, in press.

13. Polizopoulou ZS, Koutinas AF, Papadopoulos GC, Saridomichelakis MN. Juvenile laryngeal paralysis in three Siberian husky x Alaskan malamute puppies. *Vet Rec* 2003; **153**: 624–7.

14. Miller CJ, McKiernan B, Pace J, Feldman MJ. The effects of doxapram hydrochloride (Doparm-V) on laryngeal function in healthy dogs. *J Vet Intern Med* 2002; **16**: 524–8.

15. Radlinsky MG, Mason DE, Hodgson D. Transnasal laryngoscopy for the diagnosis of laryngeal paralysis in dogs. *J Am Anim Hosp Assoc* 2004; **40**: 211–15.

16. Peeters D, McKiernan B, Weisiger R, Schaeffer D, Clercx C. Quantitative bacterial cultures and cytological examination of bronchoalveolar lavage specimens in the diagnosis of lower respiratory tract disease in dogs: a retrospective study of 48 cases. *J Vet Intern Med* 2000; **14**: 534–41.

17. Foster SF, Martin P, Braddock JA, Malik R. A retrospective analysis of feline bronchoalveolar lavage cytology and microbiology (1995–2000). *J Fel Med Surg* 2004; **6**: 189–98.

18. Corcoran BM, Foster DJ, Fuentes LV. Feline asthma syndrome: a retrospective study of the clinical presentation in 29 cats. *J Small Anim Pract* 1995; **36**: 481–8.

19. Dye JA, McKiernan BC, Rozanski EA, Hoffmann WE, Losonsly JM, Homco LD, Wesiger RM, Kakoma I. Bronchopulmonary disease in the cat: historical, physical, radiographic, clinicopathologic, and pulmonary functional evaluation of 24 affected and 15 healthy cats. *J Vet Intern Med* 1996; **10**: 385–400.

20. Padrid P. Feline asthma. Diagnosis and treatment. *Clin North Am Small Anim Pract* 2000; **30:** 1279–93.

21. Norris C, Gershwin L, Schelegle E, Hyde D. Experimental model of asthma in cats sensitized to house dust mite or Bermuda grass allergen. *Am J Respir Crit Care Med* 2001; **163:** A602.

22. Norris C, Leutenegger C, Gershwin L, Hyde D. Cytokine profiles in peripheral blood mononuclear cells and bronchoalveolar lavage cells in cats with experimental feline asthma. In: Proceedings of the 19th Annual ACVIM Forum, Denver, 2001.

23. Norris CR, Decile KC, Berghaus LJ, Berghaus RD, Walby WF, Schelegle ES, Hyde DM, Gershwin LJ. Concentrations of cysteinyl leukotrienes in urine and bronchoalveolar lavage fluid of cats with experimentally induced asthma. *Am J Vet Res* 2003; **64**(11): 1449–53.

24. Padrid P, Snook S, Finucane T, Shiue P, Cozzi P, Solway J, Leff AR. Persistent airway hyperresponsiveness and histologic alterations after chronic antigen challenge in cats. *Am J Respir Crit Care Med* 1995; **151:** 184–93.

25. Kirschvink N, Leemans J, Delvaux F, Clercx C, Snaps F, Gustin P. Preventive use of bronchodilators in bronchoscopy-induced airflow limitation in cats. *J Vet Intern Med*; accepted for publication.

26. Kirschvink N, Leemans J, Delvaux F, Snaps F, Clercx C, Gustin P. Bronchial reactivity assessed by whole body barometric plethysmography is correlated with lower airway inflammation in cats. Proceedings of the 14th ESVIM Meeting, Barcelona, September 2004.

27. Kirschvink N, Leemans J, Delvaux F, Billen F, Clercx C, Gustin P. Preventive use of bronchodilators reduces bronchoscopy-induced airflow limitation in cats. ACVIM meeting, June 2004.

28. Brissot HN, Dupré GP, Bouvy BM, Paquet L. Thoracoscopic treatment of bullous emphysema in 3 dogs. Proceedings of the 12th Annual Scientific meeting of the ECVS, 2003.

29. Lord PF. Neurogenic pulmonary edema in the dog. *J Am Anim Hosp Assoc* 1975; **11:** 778–83.

30. Bartsch RC, McConell EE, Imes GD, Schmidt JM. A review of exertional rhabdomyolysis in wild and domestic animals and man. *Vet Pathology* 1977; **14:** 314–24.

31. German AJ, Hall EJ, Day MJ. Measurement of IgG, IgM and IgA concentrations in canine serum, saliva, tears and bile. *Vet J Immunol Immunopathol* 1998; **64:** 107–21.

6

Endocrinology

JACQUIE RAND, LINDA FLEEMAN, ANNETTE LITSTER

Introduction

Hyperadrenocorticism and diabetes mellitus are commonly recognized endocrine disorders of dogs, while hyperthyroidism and diabetes are the most frequent feline endocrinopathies. Publications in the scientific veterinary literature during 2003 reported many major advances specifically relating to clinical management of these diseases. The most difficult task was to choose a short-list of those that have the potential to most influence clinical practice, and unfortunately many excellent papers could not be included within the scope of this review. The 10 publications finally chosen represent those most likely to change the currently accepted methods of diagnosing and treating the more common endocrine disorders of dogs and cats.

Canine hyperadrenocorticism can be diagnosed by measuring serum cortisol concentrations after stimulating the adrenal gland with exogenous adrenocorticotrophic hormone (ACTH). Adrenal-derived hormones other than cortisol may also be stimulated by ACTH, and measurement of these hormones has diagnostic potential. The first paper provides reference values in healthy dogs, dogs with confirmed hyperadrenocorticism, and dogs with non-adrenal illness.

Medical treatment of hyperadrenocorticism in dogs requires that clinicians monitor and manage the adverse effects and variable efficacy of currently available drugs. Trilostane has recently been suggested as an alternative for the treatment of this disease. Before clinicians begin to regularly offer this alternative, it is important that the safety and efficacy of trilostane be first compared with current therapies. In the second paper, a comparison is made between trilostane and mitotane for the long-term management of canine hyperadrenocorticism.

Diabetes in cats is analogous to human type 2 diabetes. Better understanding of the pathogenesis of feline diabetes has stimulated tremendous research interest in the potential of diet to improve glycaemic control of these patients. The third paper in this review reports the clinical outcomes of changing the diet of treated diabetic cats to a low-carbohydrate formulation.

The next three papers all deal with the important clinical problem of monitoring glycaemic control in diabetic dogs. While clinical hyperglycaemia can be reliably recognized in dogs using a number of methods, the only available test for the past 30 years to assess the risk of hypoglycaemia in diabetic dogs has been the serial blood glucose concentration curve. Several publications in 2003 have provided new information on this commonly performed diagnostic test. The first paper on monitoring glycaemia in dogs evaluates the clinical reliability of the traditional serial blood glucose curve, while the next two articles describe practical alternatives.

The number of dogs receiving treatment for diseases such as diabetes has increased as a result of improvements in the level of clinical care, which allow for longer survival after diagnosis. Consequently, more information is now required on the possible long-term sequelae of chronic endocrine diseases. The next article in the review reports the prevalence of atherosclerosis in dogs with diabetes, hypothyroidism and hyperadrenocorticism.

While hyperthyroidism continues to be the most common endocrine condition diagnosed in cats, there has been little recent advance in available treatment methods. The two papers reviewed in the section on hyperthyroidism provide information on alternative administration regimens for methimazole, and both aim for improved owner compliance while maintaining efficacy.

The final publication reviewed in this series evaluates a non-invasive, reversible method of controlling fertility in female cats. Alternative options to those currently available to control reproduction in cats have long held appeal and have the potential to influence feline clinical practice to a great extent.

Advances in the diagnosis and treatment of dogs with hyperadrenocorticism

Hyperadrenocorticism is one of the most commonly recognized endocrine disorders of dogs. Cortisol is the principal hormone implicated in the clinical signs of hyperadrenocorticism, although the adrenal cortex may also produce excessive amounts of other hormones. Hyperadrenocorticism can be diagnosed by stimulating the adrenal gland with exogenous ACTH. In 80–95% of dogs with pituitary-dependent disease and 60% of dogs with adrenocortical tumours, stimulation with ACTH results in high cortisol concentrations. Failure of the ACTH stimulation test to accurately identify some dogs with hyperadrenocorticism may be because of variations in the degree of adrenocortical hyperplasia, failure of expression of ACTH receptors on adrenal cortex cells, or because other adrenal-derived hormones may be contributing to the clinical signs of hyperadrenocorticism. To identify these conditions, it would be useful to know reference values for adrenal-derived hormones other than cortisol in healthy dogs and in dogs with non-adrenal illness.

Medical treatment with mitotane or ketoconazole can be unsatisfactory because of drug side effects or lack of efficacy, and trilostane has been recently suggested as an alternative. This is particularly relevant for clients unable to monitor dogs satisfactorily during the induction phase of mitotane treatment, and in countries where mitotane is no longer available. Trilostane is a competitive inhibitor of the enzyme hydroxysteroid dehydrogenase, inhibiting the conversion of pregnenolone to progesterone, thereby inhibiting steroid hormone production in adrenal glands. Before clinicians begin to regularly offer trilostane as an alternative for treating dogs with hyperadrenocorticism, it is important that its safety and efficacy be compared with current therapies.

Evaluation of the basal and post-adrenocorticotrophic hormone serum concentrations of 17-hydroxyprogesterone for the diagnosis of hyperadrenocorticism in dogs

Chapman PS, Mooney CT, Ede J, et al. Vet Rec 2003; **153**(25): 771–5

BACKGROUND. 17-hydroxyprogesterone is a progestin and a precursor of cortisol in the steroid synthesis pathway. Progestins have intrinsic glucocorticoid activity and may also increase the availability of cortisol by displacing it from its binding proteins. The concentration of 17-hydroxyprogesterone is increased in dogs with hyperadrenocorticism, suggesting that it may be a useful screening test for the diagnosis of the disease, although it has not been evaluated in dogs with non-adrenal illness. In addition, dogs with signs of hyperadrenocorticism that respond to surgical removal of an adrenal mass, but pre-operatively did not develop hypercortisolaemia following ACTH stimulation, may be identified by measuring hormones other than cortisol after ACTH stimulation. The aim of this study was to evaluate the sensitivity and specificity of measurements of basal and post-ACTH concentrations of 17-hydroxyprogesterone for the diagnosis of hyperadrenocorticism in dogs by studying groups of healthy dogs, dogs with non-adrenal disease, and dogs with confirmed hyperadrenocorticism. Serum concentrations of 17-hydroxyprogesterone and cortisol were measured before and after the administration of exogenous ACTH to three groups of dogs: (i) 27 healthy dogs; (ii) 19 dogs with non-adrenal illness in which there had been an initial clinical suspicion of hyperadrenocorticism, but this disease was ruled out by testing and another diagnosis was reached; and (iii) 46 dogs with confirmed hyperadrenocorticism.

INTERPRETATION. There were no significant differences in the basal or post-ACTH concentrations of cortisol or 17-hydroxyprogesterone between healthy dogs and dogs with non-adrenal illness. The post-ACTH concentrations of 17-hydroxyprogesterone in dogs with hyperadrenocorticism were significantly (P <0.001) greater than those in the other two groups combined (Fig. 6.1). The area under the receiver operating curve (ROC) for the post-ACTH concentration of cortisol (0.94) was significantly greater than that for the post-ACTH concentration of 17-hydroxyprogesterone (0.76). Using a two-graph ROC analysis, a cut-off of 8.5 nmol/l was found to maximize both the sensitivity and specificity of the post-ACTH concentration of 17-hydroxyprogesterone for the diagnosis of hyper-adrenocorticism at 71%. With a cut-off of 4.5 nmol/l the sensitivity increased to 90% but the specificity decreased to 40%; with a cut-off of 16.7 nmol/l the specificity increased to 90% but the sensitivity decreased to 47%.

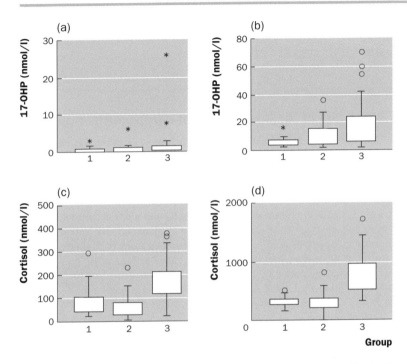

Fig. 6.1 (a) Basal 17-hydroxyprogestrone (17-OHP), (b) post-adrenocorticotrophic hormone (ACTH) 17-OPH, (c) basal cortisol, (d) post-ACTH cortisol concentrations (all in nmol/l) in the three groups of dogs. The 'box' represents the 25th to 75th percentile range and is bisected by a line representing the median. The 'whiskers' represent the main body of data which in most cases is equal to the range. Outlying data points are represented by open circles and extreme cases by asterisks. Group 1 = 27 clinically healthy dogs; Group 2 = 19 dogs with non-adrenal illness in which there was an initial clinical suspicion of hyperadrenocorticism, subsequently ruled out on testing and diagnosis of another disease; Group 3 = 46 dogs with hyperadrenocorticism. Source: Chapman et al. (2003).

Comment

The results of this study support earlier findings that in many dogs with hyperadrenocorticism, the post-ACTH concentration of 17-hydroxyprogesterone is increased. However, because of the overlap in the test results from dogs with hyperadrenocorticism with results from both healthy and sick dogs, the post-ACTH concentration of 17-hydroxyprogesterone cannot be recommended as a routine screening test for hyperadrenocorticism. Its measurement may be useful in some cases of atypical adrenocortical neoplasia, which is characterized by clinical signs of hyperadrenocorticism without hypercortisolaemia, because these dogs may have increases in steroid intermediates that are responsible for clinical signs.

Trilostane treatment in dogs with pituitary-dependent hyperadrenocortism

Braddock JA, Church DB, Robertson ID, Watson ADJ *Aust Vet J* 2003; **81**(10): 600–7

BACKGROUND. Trilostane is a potentially valuable alternative for dogs with hyperadrenocorticism that tolerate other medical therapies poorly and/or those that are not able to have surgical treatment. The objective of this study was to evaluate the efficacy of trilostane in treating dogs with pituitary-dependent hyperadrenocorticism. The trial was designed as a prospective clinical trial with 30 client-owned dogs with pituitary-dependent hyperadrenocorticsm. Dogs were monitored at 10, 30, 90 days, and then 3-monthly by clinical examination, ACTH stimulation testing, urinary cortisol/creatinine ratio measurement, and client questionnaire.

INTERPRETATION. Twenty-nine dogs were successfully treated with trilostane. The median dose used was 16.7 mg/kg with a range of 5.3–50 mg/kg administered once daily. Trilostane was safe, effective and free of side effects at the doses required. Most dogs were initially quite sensitive to the drug for 10–30 days, then required higher doses until a prolonged phase of stable dose requirements occurred. Some dogs treated for more than 2 years required reduction or temporary cessation of drug because of hypoadrenocorticsm.

Comment

This paper provides further valuable information on use of trilostane in dogs, and builds on the data published by Neiger's group |1|. It is important because it provides clearer guidelines for managing hyperadrenocorticism successfully with trilostane. It suggests that a higher success rate is achieved if the dose rate is increased based on lower post-ACTH stimulation cortisol concentrations, compared to dose rates used in some previous studies that had lower success rates. Because trilostane has a relatively short duration of effect, ACTH stimulation testing should be performed 3–8 h after drug administration. Assessment outside of this period may alter results.

Based on this study, dogs should be checked after beginning trilostane at 10, 30, 90 days and then 3-monthly using client information, clinical examination, and ACTH stimulation testing. The authors recommend a starting dose of 10 mg/kg and increasing the dose by 60 mg for dogs weighing more than 10 kg, and 30 or 60 mg for smaller dogs, depending on the degree of adrenal suppression. Most dogs were controlled on 16–19 mg/kg, but the range of dose rates was 5.3–50 mg/kg, with a trend for larger dogs to require a lower dose rate than smaller dogs. Table 6.1 shows cortisol concentrations used for the interpretation of ACTH stimulation testing. If a poor response to therapy occurs, duration of action of trilostane should be assessed with a urine cortisol/creatinine ratio measured in a sample collected at home just before the next dose of drug. The duration of action of trilostane in some dogs is too short for once-daily administration, and needs to be changed to a twice-daily

Table 6.1 Interpretation of cortisol concentrations at baseline and after stimulation with ACTH in treated patients

Treated hyperadrenocorticoid patient

Baseline cortisol	25–75 nmol/l	Normal baseline
Baseline and 1-h cortisol	≤15 nmol/l	Excessive control of hyperadrenocorticism
1-h cortisol	25–75 nmol/l	Tight control of hyperadrenocorticism
1-h cortisol	75–125 nmol/l	Acceptable control of hyperadrenocorticism

Source: Braddock et al. (2003).

regimen. The advantages of using trilostane are the less intensive monitoring compared with mitotane particularly in the induction period, and the theoretical reversibility of trilostane. However, cost is two to three times higher for trilostane than mitotane. Hypoadrenocorticism occurred in four of 29 dogs and developed 12–22 months after beginning therapy, with most dogs developing it at about 20 months. Only two dogs developed clinical signs of hypoadrenocorticism, one of which had signs and biochemical abnormalities supporting glucocorticoid and mineralocorticoid deficiency. Adrenal suppression persisted for up to 4 months, although dogs eventually required reinstitution of trilostane.

Advances in the management of dogs and cats with diabetes mellitus

The incidence of diabetes in the pet dog and cat populations is increasing. Successful management presents challenges in both species, and new treatment modalities are being explored, especially in cats because glycaemic control is usually less than ideal. The majority of cats have type 2 diabetes mellitus, characterized by a combination of inadequate insulin secretion and impaired insulin action (insulin resistance). The most successful outcome of therapy for cats is diabetic remission, and this requires that both insulin deficiency and insulin resistance be managed. Many factors contribute to insulin resistance and poor glycaemic control in cats including genotype, obesity, physical inactivity, drugs, illness, gender, diet, and hyperglycaemia [2]. Of these, diet effects are of particular interest because there is greatest potential for modulation. Dietary intervention that results in the reduction of glucose absorption from the gastrointestinal tract, thereby decreasing the postprandial glycaemic load, offers most promise for the management of feline diabetes.

Most diabetic dogs have a form of diabetes analogous to human type 1 diabetes and have absolute insulin deficiency. Consequently, nearly all diabetic dogs require lifelong treatment with exogenous insulin. Determination of an appropriate insulin dose for individual diabetic dogs, which will control hyperglycaemia without inducing iatrogenic hypoglycaemia, remains one of the greatest challenges when managing diabetic dogs. Poor glycaemic control can be readily identified in diabetic dogs by monitoring clinical signs, especially changes in water intake and body weight. Measurement of fructosamine or glycosylated haemoglobin provides an additional way of assessing glycaemic control. While clinical hyperglycaemia can be reliably recognized, identification of insulin-induced hypoglycaemia is much less straight-forward. Dogs with transient hypoglycaemia may show no clinical signs, or may have signs of hyperglycaemia. For several decades, the only available test for the assess-ment of risk of hypoglycaemia in diabetic dogs has been the serial blood glucose concentration curve, where multiple blood glucose measurements are obtained in hospital over 12–24 h following the dog's usual insulin dose and meal. Thus, the serial blood glucose curve is currently the only means of evaluating whether the insulin dose can be safely increased in a diabetic dog without risk of inducing hypo-glycaemia. However, several important problems are associated with this diagnostic test. These include stress-induced hyperglycaemia and hypoglycaemia related to inappetence induced by anxiety associated with hospitalization and repeated veni-puncture. In addition, clinical interpretation of the curves tends to be very subjective and vary considerably among practitioners.

Major improvements have been made over the past 30 years in the level of care and therapy available for diabetic dogs and cats, with the result that the survival rate is now much higher. There has been a decline in the initial case-fatality rate and an increase in the long-term survival after diagnosis. More information is now required on the possible long-term sequelae of diabetes mellitus in dogs and cats. In human patients, atherosclerosis and angiopathy are recognized as important sequelae of diabetes, and predispose to numerous vascular problems, including coronary artery disease, retinopathy, and nephropathy. Little is currently known about the incidence of atherosclerosis and angiopathy in managed diabetic dogs and cats.

Treatment of feline diabetes mellitus using an α-glucosidase inhibitor and a low carbohydrate diet
Mazzaferro EM, Greco DS, Turner AS, Fettman MJ. *J Feline Med Surg* 2003; **5**(3): 183–9

BACKGROUND. The most common form of diabetes in cats is analogous to human type 2 diabetes, previously called non-insulin-dependent or adult-onset diabetes. Although diets high in complex carbohydrates and fibre have been traditionally recommended for people and cats with diabetes, recent data suggest that diets with restricted carbohydrate content improve glycaemic control. The purpose of this study was to determine if treatment with an α-glucosidase inhibitor (acarbose), combined with a low carbohydrate diet was effective in improving glycaemic control, reducing insulin requirements, and changing body composition in cats with naturally-occurring diabetes mellitus. Client-owned cats (24) with diabetes mellitus were studied, of which 20 had been previously treated with insulin for 2 weeks to 3 years, but were not well controlled, and four were newly diagnosed cats. Cats were treated either with a low carbohydrate diet (Hill's Science Diet—canned Feline Growth with approximately 5% of calories from carbohydrate) and acarbose (18 cats), or the low carbohydrate diet alone (six cats). Additional twice-daily treatment provided for all cats was lente insulin (18 cats) or protamine zinc insulin (six cats).

INTERPRETATION. Patients were classified as responders (insulin was discontinued, $n = 15$) or non-responders (continued to require insulin or glipizide, $n = 9$). There was no difference in the proportion of responders between cats treated with diet and acarbose compared with cats treated by diet alone. Responders were initially obese (>28% body fat) and non-responders had significantly less body fat than responders (<28% body fat). Serum fructosamine and glucose concentrations decreased significantly in both responder and non-responder cats over the course of the 4 months of therapy, but the greatest improvement was in the responder cats. In cats continuing to require insulin, the dose was decreased from 5 to 2 U/cat administered twice daily. Percentage lean body mass was significantly increased in both responders and non-responders after 4 months of therapy. All responders tended to have a decrease in body fat, and non-responders tended to have an increase of body fat with therapy, although the results were not significant over the course of the study.

Comment

This paper is important because 60% of cats went into diabetic remission after switching to an ultra-low carbohydrate diet, even though the majority of these cats had previously been treated with lente insulin without attaining good glycaemic control. Although there was no control group to demonstrate the benefit of improved glycaemic control associated with closer monitoring in a clinical trial, this rate of remission is higher than that reported previously in a clinical trial of cats treated with lente insulin (approximately 30%). Importantly, the addition of acarbose, which decreases absorption of glucose from the gastrointestinal tract, appeared not to offer any benefit over diet alone, although the numbers were small. Notable for clinicians was that for cats continuing to require insulin, the dose was decreased by half. Therefore, for cats being switched from dry food diets to an ultra-low carbohydrate diet, it would be prudent to advise that that insulin dose should be initially reduced by half to avoid hypoglycaemia, and then increased as necessary.

Evaluation of day-to-day variability of serial blood glucose concentration curves in diabetic dogs
Fleeman LM, Rand JS. *J Am Vet Med Assoc* 2003; **222**(3): 317–21

BACKGROUND. Diabetes mellitus is a common endocrine disease of dogs and management requires lifelong, daily insulin administration. Regular reappraisal of this treatment is vital if optimal control of the disease is to be achieved. The current recommendation is that adjustment of the insulin dose should be based on history and physical examination findings in addition to results of serial blood glucose measurements after the dog's usual insulin injection and meal |3,4|.

When interpreting the curves, clinicians typically assume that the serial blood glucose curve for an individual dog will be similar on different days if insulin and meal factors are kept constant. The purposes of the study were to test the hypothesis that there is minimal day-to-day variability of serial blood glucose curves in diabetic dogs when insulin and meal factors are kept constant, and determine the clinical implications if significant day-to-day variability was found. Ten client-owned diabetic dogs were used. Paired 12-h serial blood glucose curves performed during two consecutive days were obtained on three occasions from each dog. Dogs received the same dose of insulin and meal every 12 h on both days. For each pair of curves, comparison was made between the results of days 1 and 2. The study also included comparison of theoretical recommendations for days 1 and 2 regarding insulin dosage adjustment, which were based on rigorously defined objective data from the curves.

INTERPRETATION. Large day-to-day variation in results of the serial blood glucose curves was found. Coefficient of variation of the absolute difference between days 1 and 2 for each parameter measured ranged from 68 to 103% (Table 6.2). Evaluation of the 30 paired curves led to an opposite recommendation for adjustment of the dog's insulin dose on day 2, compared with day 1, on 27% of occasions. For 17% of the curves, a different but not opposite recommendation resulted. The same recommendation for dosage adjustment on both days was made in only 57% of the paired curves. Disparity between the dosage recommendations was more pronounced when the glucose nadir was <180 mg/dl (10 mmol/l) on one or both days. In this subset of curves, an opposite recommendation for dosage adjustment was made on 40% of occasions, a different but not opposite

Table 6.2 Parameters of paired 12-h serial blood glucose concentration curves obtained on 3 occasions from 10 dogs with diabetes mellitus

Parameter	Overall mean	Mean absolute difference between days 1 and 2	SD of absolute difference	Coefficient of variation (%)	95% CI
Minimum blood glucose (mg/dl)	187	63	43	68	47–79
Mean blood glucose (mg/dl)	283	54	41	78	38–70
J-index	137	43	36	82	30–58
Difference between morning pre-insulin blood glucose and nadir (mg/dl)	148	115	99	86	79–151
Morning pre-insulin blood glucose (mg/dl)	335	115	101	88	77–153
Time from insulin injection to nadir (h)	7	3.3	2.9	90	2.2–4.4
SD blood glucose (mg/dl)	77	29	29	97	18–40
Evening pre-insulin blood glucose (mg/dl)	310	101	99	98	63–139
Maximum blood glucose (mg/dl)	398	68	68	101	43–94
Area under the curve (in h.mg/dl)	3287	776	803	103	476–1076

Source: Fleeman and Rand (2003).

recommendation resulted 25% of the time, and the same recommendation for both days occurred in only 35% of the sets of paired curves. This indicates that the day-to-day variability of serial blood glucose curves has important clinical implications, particularly in dogs with good glycaemic control.

Comment

This study demonstrates that the serial blood glucose curve appears to be an unreliable clinical tool for the evaluation of insulin dose in individual diabetic dogs. Thus, it would be expected that attempts to adjust a diabetic dog's insulin dose on the basis of serial blood glucose assessment alone might prove unreliable. It would seem advisable to always consider additional indicators of glycaemic control, such as changes in the dog's water intake, body weight, and the presence or absence of glucosuria, when appraising the insulin dose. The large day-to-day variability of the curves and the serious sequelae that may result from insulin overdose also justify the need for a conservative approach to dosage recommendations.

Evaluation of a continuous glucose monitoring system in diabetic dogs

Davison LJ, Slater LA, Herrtage ME, *et al*. *J Small Anim Pract* 2003; **44**(10): 435–42

BACKGROUND. Sensors that continuously measure subcutaneous or interstitial glucose concentration are now being used to monitor glycaemic control in human diabetic patients and offer great potential for monitoring diabetic dogs. Interstitial glucose concentration results are recorded every 5 min with these devices and monitoring can continue for periods up to 72 h. The monitor can be attached to a harness worn by the dog and so may be used while the dog is at home with its owner. This provides a potential alternative to the hospital-based serial blood glucose curve and offers a means of avoiding the problems of hospital-induced stress and subsequent inappetence, as well as patient discomfort due to repeated venipuncture. The aim of this study was to evaluate a continuous interstitial glucose monitoring system (Medtronic MiniMed, Northridge, California, USA) for use in diabetic dogs. Interstitial fluid glucose concentrations were recorded in 10 diabetic dogs with unstable glycaemic control every 5 min for up to 48 h, using a subcutaneous sensor attached to the monitoring device. Results from 183 time-points across 428 h of recording were statistically compared with blood glucose concentrations that were measured simultaneously with a portable glucose meter. Clinical comparison was also made between curves generated with the continuous glucose monitoring system and standard serial blood glucose curves.

INTERPRETATION. The correlation between interstitial fluid and blood glucose values was 0.81 ($P < 0.01$), which is higher than the minimum correlation recommended by the manufacturers for 'optimal accuracy' (>0.79). The device appeared to be more reliable in some dogs than others ($P < 0.05$). The largest discrepancies between the two sets of data occurred at higher glucose concentrations, particularly during the 1–3 h period following feeding, and the authors suggested that postprandial hyperglycaemia might not be reflected in the interstitial fluid. One limitation of the system is that it must be calibrated with blood glucose concentration several times every 24 h, so there is still a requirement for some blood sampling during monitoring. After initially receiving error messages in the 2 h following feeding, the researchers elected to calibrate the system just four times per 24 h, avoiding the postprandial period. Importantly, the system was shown to be able to detect episodes of hypoglycaemia. However, one disadvantage is that results from the continuous monitoring system are not available in real time. Although clinical interpretation of the serial glucose measurements in this study tended to be very subjective, it was found that similar clinical recommendations regarding insulin dosing adjustment would be made in the majority of cases if the continuous glucose monitoring system were used instead of a standard serial blood glucose curve.

Comment

The Medtronic MiniMed system is a potentially valuable tool for the management of canine diabetic patients. Further testing in diabetic dogs is needed before reliance on this method as the sole monitoring tool. Caution is required because this device does not reliably detect hypoglycaemia in insulin-treated human diabetics and performs well only for normal or increased glucose concentrations |5|. It is also yet to be determined whether the interstitial glucose concentration parallels blood glucose concentration during very rapid changes in dogs, such as occur during the Somogyi phenomenon. The main advantage is that this system collects and automatically analyses a large amount of glycaemic data. This allows for clinical assessment of glycaemic control in diabetic dogs to be based on a far greater number of measurements than is usual for a standard serial blood glucose curve.

Home monitoring of blood glucose concentration by owners of diabetic dogs

Casella M, Wess G, Hassig M, Reusch CE. *J Small Anim Pract* 2003; **44**(7): 298–305

BACKGROUND. Repeated evaluation of serial blood glucose curves performed in a hospital environment contributes a significant proportion of the cost of stabilizing a diabetic dog and has inherent problems. Many diabetic dogs will become anxious when separated from their owners and admitted into the hospital environment. This anxiety may be associated with inappetence or stress-induced elevation of their blood glucose values. Recent development of techniques for sampling capillary blood glucose from the pinna |6| potentially allow owners of diabetic dogs to obtain data at home regarding their pet's level of glycaemic control. This may provide an economical alternative to the hospital-based serial blood glucose curve and offer another means of avoiding the problems of inappetence and stress-induced hyperglycaemia. The objective of this study was to investigate whether home monitoring of blood glucose concentration of diabetic dogs by owners would be possible on a long-term basis. The owners of 12 recently diagnosed diabetic dogs were each asked to generate four serial glucose curves by taking capillary blood samples from their dog's pinna, at 3–4-week intervals. Within 1 week of each curve being produced by the owner, an additional curve was produced by a veterinarian in the hospital. The owners were also required to respond to a questionnaire regarding problems that they may have encountered while performing the curves at home.

INTERPRETATION. Ten of the 12 owners were able to generate blood glucose curves; three of them needed a second demonstration, and two telephoned for further guidance. The blood glucose concentrations obtained from the first two 'hospital' curves were significantly lower than those measured at home; however there was no difference between the nadir glucose concentrations. Overall, in 42% of cases, the clinical recommendation based on the 'hospital' curves would have been different from that based on 'home' curves. In the majority of cases, the clinical decision was based on the home-generated curves, with the result that clinical signs improved in all dogs and serum fructosamine concentration decreased in nine of the dogs during the study period. Technical problems experienced by the owners decreased over the study period. Additionally, owners reported that most of the dogs that did not tolerate the procedure well at the outset became accustomed to it during the first day of testing at home. It was also noted that any hospital-induced inappetence of the dogs resolved by the third or fourth 'hospital' curve, as the dogs became accustomed to the hospital and staff.

Comment

This is the first study to demonstrate that long-term monitoring of blood glucose concentrations of diabetic dogs can be successfully performed by their owners at home. It was emphasized that this monitoring option should be introduced gradually to owners and that thorough explanation and demonstration of the technique, as well as ongoing telephone support, is required to minimize technical problems and improve compliance. In 42% of the 'hospital' curves, the clinical recommendation would have been different from the recommendation based on 'home' curves. This is a similar result to that obtained in the previous study that compared hospital-generated serial blood glucose curves performed on two consecutive days, and so may be due to the inherent day-to-day variability of serial blood glucose curves in diabetic dogs, rather than a difference between 'home' and 'hospital' curves.

Association between diabetes mellitus, hypothyroidism or hyperadrenocorticism, and atherosclerosis in dogs
Hess RS, Kass PH, van Winkle TJ. *J Vet Intern Med* 2003; **17**(4): 489–94

BACKGROUND. Atherosclerosis is a leading cause of mortality and is responsible for much of the morbidity in human beings. Spontaneous atherosclerosis in dogs has been reported mainly in association with hypothyroidism, and is thought to develop because of hypercholesterolaemia. Anecdotally atherosclerosis has also been reported in association with canine diabetes mellitus. However, controlled studies of the association between atherosclerosis and these endocrinopathies have not been reported in dogs. The objective of this study was to determine whether dogs with atherosclerosis were more likely to have concurrent diabetes mellitus, hypothyroidism, or hyperadrenocorticism than dogs that do not have atherosclerosis. A retrospective mortality prevalence case–control study was performed. The study group included 30 dogs with histological evidence of atherosclerosis. The control group included 142 dogs with results of a complete post mortem examination, a final post mortem examination diagnosis of neoplasia, and no histological evidence of atherosclerosis. Control dogs were frequency matched for age and year in which the post mortem examination was performed. Proportionate changes in the prevalence of diabetes mellitus, hypothyroidism, and hyperadrenocorticism were calculated by exact prevalence odds ratios, 95% confidence intervals (95% CI), and P values. Multiple logistic regression analysis was used to examine the combined effects of prevalence determinants while controlling for age and year of post mortem examination.

INTERPRETATION. Dogs with atherosclerosis were over 53 times more likely to have concurrent diabetes mellitus ($P = 0.002$) and over 51 times more likely to have concurrent hypothyroidism than dogs without atherosclerosis ($P < 0.001$). Dogs with atherosclerosis were not found to be more likely to have concurrent hyperadrenocorticism than dogs that did not have atherosclerosis ($P = 0.59$). In summary, diabetes mellitus and hypothyroidism, but not hyperadrenocorticism, were more prevalent in dogs with atherosclerosis compared with dogs without atherosclerosis on post mortem examination.

Comment

The significance of this study for practitioners is that atherosclerosis is more frequent than previously thought, and it is associated with diabetes mellitus and hypothyroidism, but not hyperadrenocorticism. Thirty of 6300 dogs (0.5%) met the inclusion criteria for the study, although the true prevalence may be higher because 50 dogs with histological evidence of atherosclerosis were initially identified (0.8%), and some of these were eliminated from the study because of missing records or slides. This makes atherosclerosis as prevalent as diabetes mellitus (0.6%) in this population. Most dogs with atherosclerosis had hypothyroidism (60%) or diabetes mellitus (20%), and some had multiple endocrinopathies all including diabetes. Hypercholesterolaemia was also a risk factor for atherosclerosis with 63% of atherosclerotic dogs having hypercholesterolaemia, and 40% being hyperlipidaemic. Four of the 30 dogs with atherosclerosis did not have an endocrinopathy or hypercholesterolaemia, indicating that some dogs develop spontaneous atherosclerosis for reasons other than the identified risk factors. Although the mean age of dogs with atherosclerosis was 9 years, the range was very wide (0.5–18 years). Of the dogs with atherosclerosis, 20 of 30 dogs had coronary artery lesions. The relevance of this finding to clinical cardiovascular disease in dogs is unknown. Further studies are needed to determine whether spontaneous atherosclerosis is associated with impaired cardiovascular function in hypothyroid dogs.

Advances in the management of feline hyperthyroidism

While hyperthyroidism continues to be the most common endocrine condition diag-
nosed in cats |7|, the treatment methods available have remained virtually unchanged
during the last decade. As medical management using daily oral anti-thyroid drugs is
relatively affordable and safe, this treatment is commonly used in feline practice.
However, once diagnosed, feline hyperthyroidism requires lifelong treatment, which
challenges owner compliance. If drug administration is irregular, clinical remission
will almost certainly not occur, leading to an exacerbation of the presenting clinical
signs and perhaps secondary cardiovascular and renal degenerative disease. New
methods of administration of anti-thyroid drugs and dosage regimens are being
investigated, in the hope of improving owner compliance and clinical outcome for
the hyperthyroid cat.

Transdermal methimazole treatment in cats with hyperthyroidism
Hoffmann G, Marks SL, Taboada J, Hosgood GL, Wolfsheimer KJ. *J Feline Med Surg* 2003; **5**(2): 77–82

BACKGROUND. Hyperthyroidism is the most common endocrinopathy in cats over
8 years old. Medical management options include lifelong daily oral administration of
drugs that inhibit hormone synthesis. The objectives of this study were to assess
serum thyroxine concentrations and clinical response in hyperthyroid cats to
treatment with transdermal methimazole, and to determine if further investigation is
indicated. Clinical and laboratory data from 13 cats with hyperthyroidism were
retrospectively evaluated. Methimazole (Tapazole, Eli Lilly) was formulated in a
pleuronic lecithin organogel-based vehicle and was applied to the inner pinna of the
ear at a dosage ranging from 2.5 mg per cat every 24 h to 10.0 mg per cat every
12 h. The dose rates reflected the clinical choice of the veterinarians who managed
the cases. During the treatment period, cats were re-evaluated at a mean of
4.3 weeks (recheck-1), and again at a mean of 5.4 months (recheck-2).

INTERPRETATION. Owners reported that clinical improvement was observed in all cats.
Attending veterinarians reported resolution of the following clinical signs: weight loss (five of
eight), inappetence (four of five), mental changes (three of four), vomiting (three of four), dry
hair-coat (two of two). Significant decreases in total thyroxine concentrations were measured
at recheck-1 (mean 39.57 nmol/l; SEM 14.40; SD 41.2) and recheck-2 (mean
36.71 nmol/l; SEM 13.90; SD 45.56) compared with pre-treatment concentrations (mean
97.5 nmol/l; SEM 11.42; SD 39.5). No adverse effects were reported. Three cats did not
show improvements in serum total thyroxine concentrations at the rechecks, and in two of
the three this was probably because of poor owner compliance, as drug application was
irregular and/or not performed daily.

Comment

This paper is important because hyperthyroidism is the most common endo-crinopathy of cats and the advantages and disadvantages of treatment options are juggled every day in small animal practice. Permanent therapeutic modalities include surgical thyroidectomy, but this is regularly associated with either life-threatening post-operative complications such as hypoparathyroidism, or failure to permanently resolve the hyperthyroidism. Radioactive iodine treatment may also result in treatment failure and requires access to an approved facility. Both of these permanent treatments need careful consideration before recommendation in elderly cats, which often have intercurrent renal and/or cardiac disease. Also, the cost of these treatments is prohibitive for some owners. For these reasons, many owners choose to control their cat's hyperthyroidism with long-term, daily, oral administration of an anti-thyroid drug, usually methimazole |8|. However, it is often difficult to reliably administer oral medication to cats, especially long-term, resulting in poor owner compliance and a suboptimal therapeutic response. A transdermally absorbed formulation of methimazole that could be applied topically may dramatically improve owner compliance and overall management of this widespread feline condition. In this report, cat numbers were quite low ($n = 13$) and the study was conducted over a relatively short period (approximately 6 months). However, all cats showed clinical improvement; there were significant decreases in serum total thyroxine at rechecks, and there were no adverse effects reported. This seems an ideal basis for future prospective long-term studies in a larger population, paired with pharmacokinetic evaluation.

Efficacy and safety of once versus twice daily administration of methimazole in cats with hyperthyroidism

Trepanier LA, Hoffman SB, Kroll M, Rodan I, Challoner L. *J Am Vet Med Assoc* 2003; **222**(7): 954–8

BACKGROUND. Hyperthyroidism is the most common feline endocrinopathy and is commonly treated with long-term daily oral administration of the anti-thyroid drug methimazole. While the plasma half-life of methimazole is relatively short (approximately 2-6 h) |9|, it is actively concentrated in its target site, the thyroid gland, producing a prolonged effect. Studies with human hyperthyroid patients have shown similar rates of remission to euthyroidism between once daily and more frequent administration of methimazole. The objective of this randomized clinical trial was to determine whether once-daily administration of methimazole was as effective and safe as twice-daily administration in cats with hyperthyroidism. Forty cats with newly diagnosed hyperthyroidism were randomly assigned to receive 5 mg of methimazole, per os, once daily ($n = 25$) or 2.5 mg of methimazole, per os, twice daily ($n = 15$). A complete physical examination was carried out, including measurement of body weight, and blood was drawn for haematology and serum biochemical analyses, including measurement of serum total thyroxine concentration. Urinalysis was also performed, and systolic blood pressure was measured before and 2 and 4 weeks after initiation of treatment.

INTERPRETATION. Serum thyroxine concentration was significantly higher in cats given methimazole once daily, compared with cats given methimazole twice daily, 2 weeks (3.7 vs 2.0 µg/dl; $P = 0.005$) and 4 weeks (3.2 vs 1.7 µg/dl; $P = 0.01$) after initiation of treatment. In addition, the proportion of cats that were euthyroid after 2 weeks of treatment was lower for cats receiving methimazole once daily (54%) than for cats receiving methimazole twice daily (87%). However, after 4 weeks of treatment, the percentage of cats treated once daily that were euthyroid (12 of 17; 71%) was no longer significantly different from the percentage of cats treated twice daily that were euthyroid (11 of 12; 92%; $P = 0.17$). There were no significant differences between the groups at any time in regard to heart rate, systolic blood pressure, or body weight. Ten of the 24 cats evaluated in the once-daily group (42%) and six of 15 cats in the twice-daily group (40%) developed adverse effects attributed to methimazole administration during the 4 weeks of the study. Percentages of cats with adverse effects (primarily gastrointestinal signs and facial pruritus) were not significantly different between groups.

Comment

Long-term management of feline hyperthyroidism is a common problem in small animal practice. Once diagnosed, affected cats require treatment for the rest of their lives, and as daily oral methimazole is a relatively cheap and convenient treatment, it is commonly used. However, many owners find oral dosing regimens difficult to achieve and this problem is exacerbated if treatment is required twice rather than once daily. If not controlled satisfactorily, feline hyperthyroidism may lead to progressive renal, cardiac, and even ocular complications, so an effective treatment regimen that results in remission to euthyroidism is important for the cat's health and quality of life. Human studies have shown that once-daily methimazole is just as effective as more frequent dosing, because methimazole is concentrated in the thyroid gland, producing an extended anti-thyroid effect. It was for these many reasons that once-daily methimazole dosing was investigated for cats, in the hope that a less frequent dosing scheme may be just as efficacious and encourage higher owner compliance. While there was no difference in the rate of adverse effects when once-daily and twice-daily dosing were compared, the percentage of cats that became euthyroid on the twice-daily schedule was higher than on the once-daily schedule. This difference was statistically significant after 2 weeks of oral methimazole, but not after 4 weeks. Relatively low group numbers may have been the reason for the lack of statistical difference between the groups after 4 weeks, but there may have been a time effect and it would be interesting to conduct a more long-term study, especially as feline hyperthyroidism requires lifelong treatment once diagnosed. While all cats in this study were newly diagnosed, there was no attempt made to vary the dosage of methimazole according to the level of serum total thyroxine at diagnosis, as is usually done in practice, as all cats received 5 mg methimazole daily. However, there were clear differences in the rate of remission to euthyroidism and serum total thyroxine concentrations between the once-daily and twice-daily groups, and the results of this study do not support the routine administration of methimazole on a once-daily rather than twice-daily basis in newly-diagnosed hyperthyroid cats.

Advances in reproductive control in cats

Cat overpopulation is widespread and leads to the euthanasia of huge numbers of cats every year. The key to management of this problem is reproductive control that is affordable and easy to administer. Such control measures would facilitate the successful implementation of more extensive cat population management schemes by municipal animal control bodies. However, in breeding establishments, such control should also be reversible, to enable later use of valuable breeding stock.

Effect of immunization with bovine luteinizing hormone receptor on ovarian function in cats

Saxena BB, Clavio A, Singh M, *et al. Am J Vet Res* 2003; **64**(3): 292–8

BACKGROUND. The methods currently available to control reproduction in cats are invasive, expensive and irreversible. A non-invasive and reversible contraceptive vaccine has long held great appeal as it has the potential to reduce the problem of cat overpopulation. The purpose of this study was to test inhibition of the binding of luteinizing hormone (LH) and chorionic gonadotrophin (CG) to their common receptor site, in cats that had been immunized to produce LH receptor (LH-R) antibody. A total of nine adult female domestic cats were housed separately and provided with a lighting schedule of 12 h light/12 h dark. Seven of the cats (treatment group) were immunized with 0.5 mg of adjuvanted LH-R encapsulated in a silastic subdermal implant (3 × 10 mm). The remaining two cats (control group) were implanted with an implant containing only adjuvant and saline. During the post-implantation period, adjuvanted LH-R was injected intramuscularly into treatment group cats on days 98, 139, 160 and 193 to sustain immunogenic stimulation and maintain antibody titres. Control group cats were injected at the same times with adjuvant and saline solution. To assess their state of fertility, all cats were induced to ovulate with LH releasing hormone on day 345. Samples of venous blood were collected for determination of serum concentrations of oestradiol, progesterone, thyroid gland hormones, LH and LH-R antibody prior to implantation on day 0 and at intervals of 14–21 days thereafter to day 395. Vaginal cells were obtained for cytological examination on the same days as the collection of blood samples. Observation of oestrus behaviour continued from before day 0 until day 516.

INTERPRETATION. LH-R antibody was detected in the sera of immunized cats within 21 days after implantation. Detection of LH-R antibody was associated with suppression of serum progesterone to ≤0.5 ng/ml during the study period, compared with concentrations of 5–10 ng/ml in control cats. Immunized cats did not display signs of oestrus. Release of LH after administration of LH-releasing hormone in all cats indicated an intact hypothalamic–pituitary axis. Eight days after injection of LH-releasing hormone, the mean serum progesterone concentrations rose to 2.74 ng/ml in control cats, but little progesterone was detected in the sera of the immunized cats, possibly indicating poor corpus luteum function. Serum oestradiol concentrations remained between 30 and 40 pg/ml in both immunized and control cats during the entire experimental period. With the decrease in LH-R antibody titres in treatment group cats towards the end of the experimental period, hormone concentrations returned to a pattern consistent with that during fertility.

Comment

The contraceptive effect of the vaccine reported here is reversible, in contrast to currently available permanent surgical contraceptive methods. Progesterone-based contraceptive agents have been associated with a relatively high rate of complications in cats, such as cystic endometrial hyperplasia, pyometron, and mammary hyperplasia. Prolonged use has also been linked with insulin resistance and diabetes mellitus, which is sometimes permanent. Because of these side effects, progestogens have not been recommended for use in valuable future breeding queens. The androgen mibolerone is contraindicated in cats because of reports of hepatotoxicity and thyrotoxicosis. The study reported here was conducted over a relatively long period (516 days) and no reproductive or other side effects of immunization were reported. There was a return to hormone concentration patterns consistent with fertility when LH-R antibody titres declined, although experimental cats were not tested by breeding after the conclusion of the trial. Immunocontraception shows promise as a temporary method of contraception in queens that are intended for future breeding. Because of extensive structural homology of LH-R among species and cross-species non-specificity of antibodies against LH-R, the vaccine described in this report may have application in other species.

Conclusion

A wealth of new information on the clinical management of endocrine disorders in dogs and cats has resulted from publications in 2003. The major findings and their likely impact upon clinical practice are summarized below.

• Although many dogs with hyperadrenocorticism have elevation of the post-ACTH concentration of 17-hydroxyprogesterone, there is overlap with results from both healthy dogs and dogs with non-adrenal illness. Therefore, the post-ACTH concentration of 17-hydroxyprogesterone cannot be recommended as a routine screening test for canine hyperadrenocorticism, although its measurement may be useful in some cases of atypical adrenocortical neoplasia characterized by clinical signs of hyperadrenocorticism without hypercortisolaemia.

• The advantages of using trilostane for the medical management of canine hyperadrenocorticism, compared with mitotane, are the less intensive monitoring during the induction period, and the theoretical reversibility of trilostane. One major disadvantage is that cost is two to three times higher for this drug than for mitotane. The paper by Braddock *et al.* (2003) provides clear guidelines for managing hyperadrenocorticism successfully with trilostane. Although it has a relatively short duration of effect, which can be expected to end before the next dose is due, iatrogenic hypoadrenocorticism can be induced with trilostane therapy.

- Diabetic remission occurred in 60% of diabetic cats when their diet was changed to one with an ultra-low carbohydrate content, even though the majority of these cats had previously been treated with insulin without attaining good glycaemic control. Although there was no control group to demonstrate the benefit of improved glycaemic control associated with closer monitoring in a clinical trial, this rate of remission is twice as high as that reported previously for diabetic cats treated with insulin alone. Notable for clinicians was that for cats continuing to require insulin, the dose was decreased by half.

- Large day-to-day variability occurs in serial blood glucose curves in diabetic dogs, making this an unreliable clinical tool on which to base decisions regarding insulin dose. Therefore, it is advisable to always consider additional indicators of glycaemic control, such as changes in the dog's water intake and body weight, and to adopt a conservative approach to dosage recommendations.

- The subcutaneous continuous glucose monitoring system described in the paper by Davison *et al.* (2003) is a potentially valuable tool for the management of canine diabetic patients. Further testing in diabetic dogs is needed before reliance on this method as the sole monitoring tool. The main advantage is that this system collects and automatically analyses a large amount of glycaemic data, and provides a far greater number of measurements than is usual for a standard serial blood glucose curve.

- Casella *et al.* (2003) are the first to demonstrate that long-term monitoring of capillary blood glucose concentrations of diabetic dogs can be successfully performed by the majority of owners at home, thus providing a means for reducing the cost of stabilizing diabetes. It was emphasized that this monitoring option should be introduced gradually to owners and that thorough explanation and demonstration of the technique, as well as ongoing telephone support, is required to minimize technical problems and improve compliance.

- Atherosclerosis is more frequent than previously realized in dogs with diabetes mellitus and hypothyroidism, but not hyperadrenocorticism. Two-thirds of the dogs with atherosclerosis had coronary artery lesions, although the relevance of this finding to clinical cardiovascular disease in dogs is unknown.

- A transdermally absorbed formulation of methimazole applied topically to the inner pinna was found to be efficacious and safe for the treatment of hyperthyroidism in cats. This has the potential to dramatically improve owner compliance and overall clinical management of cats with hyperthyroidism, compared with long-term, daily, oral administration of methimazole.

- While it is an appealing option for management of feline hyperthyroidism, the routine administration of methimazole on a once-daily rather than twice-daily basis to newly diagnosed cats is not supported by the study by Trepanier *et al.* (2003). The percentage of cats that achieved remission to euthyroidism on the twice-daily schedule was higher than on the once-daily schedule, and there were clear differences in the serum total thyroxine concentrations between the two treatment groups.

- Immunocontraception using adjuvanted bovine LH-R encapsulated in a silastic subdermal implant shows promise as a temporary method of contraception in queens that are intended for future breeding. Immunized cats did not display signs of oestrus, and no reproductive or other side effects were reported. There was a return to hormone concentration patterns consistent with fertility when LH-R antibody titres declined.

References

1. Neiger R, Ramsey I, O'Connor J, Hurley KJ, Mooney CT. Trilostane treatment of 78 dogs with pituitary-dependent hyperadrenocorticism. *Vet Rec* 2002; **150**: 799–804.
2. Rand JS, Fleeman LM, Farrow HA, Appleton DJ, Lederer R. Canine and feline diabetes mellitus: nature or nurture? *J Nutr* 2004; **134**(8 Suppl): 2072S–80S.
3. Fleeman LM, Rand JS. Management of canine diabetes. *Vet Clin North Am Small Anim Pract* 2001; **31**: 855–80.
4. Feldman EC, Nelson RW. Canine diabetes mellitus. In: *Canine and Feline Endocrinology and Reproduction*, 3rd edn. St Louis, MO: Saunders, 2004; 486–538.
5. The Diabetes Research in Children Network (DirecNet) Study Group. Accuracy of the GlucoWatch G2 Biographer and the Continuous Glucose Monitoring System during hypoglycemia. *Diabetes Care* 2004; **27**: 722–6.
6. Wess G, Reusch C. Capillary blood sampling from the ear of dogs and cats and use of portable meters to measure glucose concentration. *J Small Anim Pract* 2000; **41**: 60–6.
7. Feldman EC, Nelson RW. Feline hyperthyroidism (thyrotoxicosis) In: *Canine and Feline Endocrinology and Reproduction*, 3rd edn. St Louis, MO: Saunders, 2004; 152–218.
8. Retsios E. Methimazole. *Compen Contin Educ Pract Vet* 2001; **23**: 36–41.
9. Trepanier LA, Peterson ME, Aucoin DP. Pharmacokinetics of methimazole in normal cats and cats with hyperthyroidism. *Res Vet Sci* 1999; **50**: 69–74.

7

Neurology

SIMON PLATT

Introduction

Neurology and neurosurgery knowledge in small animal veterinary medicine has exponentially increased over the last three decades. This is a subject that has evolved from teachings based upon exquisite pathological reports, to the present day, where we are now able to accumulate information pre-mortem with the aid of the profound advancements of the various diagnostic modalities. Evidence-based studies have correlated electrophysiological testing with a plethora of neuromuscular and some central neurological conditions. Advancements in the capabilities of laboratory testing, particularly in the field of neuromuscular disease have opened the door to the diagnosis of multiple diseases, which have only previously been suspected and or reported in human medicine. The recent establishment of the canine genome has enabled new life to be injected into the area of inheritable diseases, which make up a respectable proportion of neurological cases presenting at a young age. There may be certain diseases that we can address in the future via the manipulation of breeding programmes and so such genetic investigation is essential. The advent of more routine access to advanced imaging modalities such as magnetic resonance imaging (MRI) has greatly expanded neurological knowledge and enabled a more definitive work-up of the neurological case to be performed. However, such advancements have complicated the decision-making processes that we undertake on a daily basis for neurology cases, as it has become imperative to understand which diagnostic modality is indicated for each case. The improved sensitivity of MRI increases the need to perform a thorough and accurate clinical evaluation of the patient in order to avoid misinterpretation of clinically insignificant lesions visible on MR images. Despite the recent advancements in knowledge and diagnostic techniques, it remains essential to approach the neurological patient in a consistent manner; performing the neurological examination, localizing the lesion and developing a differentials list of possible diseases that may be responsible; from this point, a diagnostic, treatment and prognostic plan can be formulated. An index of suspicion for the various diseases can be based upon signalment and the manner in which the disease presents; however, such indices can only be utilized with the benefit of evidence-based medicine, which stems from the likes of the studies included in this chapter. The selection of the following 10 papers has not been an easy task. Their selection by no means implies that papers not included here have a lower worth; there has been a wealth of new science, both clinical and experimental, which valuably contributes to this field. The papers reviewed in this chapter attempt to be broad in their range of subjects addressed as well as practical based on their present day relevance. Disk disease, epilepsy and congenital/heritable disease are three areas that have a major prominence in clinical neurology and these topics have been enhanced by the papers addressed below. The chapter starts though with a topic that has not received much attention until recently, being that of feline intracranial disease.

Feline intracranial disease

The advent of advanced imaging has tremendously benefited the diagnosis and treatment of feline brain diseases. The aetiology of brain dysfunction in cats is generally similar to those causes documented in dogs; there are degenerative, anomalous, metabolic, neoplastic, nutritional, idiopathic, inflammatory, toxic, traumatic and vascular causes. Specifically, however, there are some notably different diseases such as neurological feline infectious peritonitis, feline immunodeficiency virus and feline ischaemic encephalopathy |1|. There has been a lack of information on the pathogenesis, natural history, diagnosis and treatment of many of these diseases until recently. One of the most devastating of intracranial diseases is neoplasia, which appears to be less common in cats than in dogs; an incidence in cats of approximately 3.5 per 100 000 population has been reported |2|. While there have been a few case series documenting the diagnosis and treatment of feline intracranial meningiomas |3,4|, and a couple of large pathological studies |5,6|, there have not been any large clinicopathological studies in this area. Meningioma is reportedly the most common primary brain tumour of the cat |3|, which may occur as multiple tumours |7| and may be incidental findings at autopsy in approximately 30% of cases |3|. An unusually high incidence of meningiomas has been reported in cats with mucopolysaccharidosis Type I |8|. Information about other types of feline intracranial tumours is currently very poor. Two of the papers presented in this section, both written by Troxel *et al.*, go hand-in-hand to advance the clinical knowledge on feline intracranial neoplasia, assisting with the problematic issue of accurately diagnosing the tumour type, which will ultimately help with an appropriate treatment regimen and an accurate prognosis.

In addition, a case series by Shamir *et al.* is discussed documenting 11 cases of post-anaesthetic cerebellar dysfunction in cats. Intracranial disease subsequent to routine anaesthesia has been poorly documented in cats, even though this is potentially a catastrophic occurrence.

Feline intracranial neoplasia: retrospective review of 160 cases (1985–2001)

Troxel MT, Vite CH, Van Winkle TJ, *et al. J Vet Int Med* 2003; **17**: 850–9

BACKGROUND. The ability to diagnose feline intracranial neoplasia and provide specific treatment is increasing in private practice and referral practices alike. Therefore, additional information regarding the clinicopathological characteristics of these diseases is necessary and would assist in the evidence-based decision making processes. The primary aims of this study were to (i) determine the frequency of different tumour types within a large cohort of cats with intracranial neoplasia, and (ii) attempt to associate signalment, tumour size and location with survival for each tumour type. Post mortem or surgical biopsy samples of feline intracranial neoplasia (1985–2001) were evaluated along with case signalment, infectious disease status, clinical signs and their duration, treatment, survival time, number of tumours, tumour location and tumour size.

INTERPRETATION. During the study period, 244 intracranial neoplasms were diagnosed in 228 cats; however, medical records were only available for 160 cats with 185 tumours. Ninety-six (60%) cases were obtained at autopsy. Comparison of the clinical signs and lesion location with the tumour type was made with χ^2 test. Analysis of variance was used to compare age with tumour type. Kruskal–Wallis testing was used to compare duration of clinical signs at diagnosis and until death due to the tumour. Overall, 70.6% of tumours were classified as primary and 29.4% secondary. However, pituitary tumours and lymphomas were classed as secondary tumours, with <6% ($n = 9$) of the total tumour numbers being metastases and approximately 4% being due to direct extension of osseous or soft tissue neoplasia. The most common tumour documented was meningioma (58%), with lymphoma (14.4%) and pituitary tumours (8.8%) accounting for the second and third most common lesions. Seventeen per cent of the meningiomas were incidental and 14% were present with another type of tumour type. The nine metastases were of variable origin and included three pulmonary adenocarcinomas. Table 7.1 documents a summary of the clinicopathological characteristics of each tumour confirmed by histopathology. Treatment data for cats with meningioma revealed that those treated with surgery had a significantly longer median survival time after diagnosis (685 days) than those that did not (18 days). Median survival time of the cats with lymphoma treated with steroids was 21 days (range 9–270 days); for cats with pituitary tumours treated with steroids was 52.5 days; survival time for cats with ependymoma varied from 272 to 685 days.

Comment

This paper provides useful information on the relative frequencies of feline intra-cranial neoplasia from a large group of cats, the most common clinicopathological characteristics and survival data of each tumour type. However, there are low numbers of some of the tumours and so the information may not be as helpful in these cases. Overall, meningiomas were the most common tumours (58.1%). Lymphoma was the next most common neoplasm of the brain in cats (14.4%); this is occasionally seen as a primary neoplasm (33% in this study), but diffuse cerebral or brainstem disease was significantly more likely to indicate lymphoma than other tumour types. Primary tumours made up 70% of the sample population. However, the tumour classification system over-emphasizes the quantity of secondary, potentially metastatic, tumours seen in cats, because both pituitary neoplasia and lymph-

Table 7.1 Feline intracranial neoplasia. A summary of the data presented on the most frequent individual tumours investigated

Parameters	All tumours	Meningioma	Neuro-epithelial	Glioma*	Glioma†	Lymphoma	Pituitary mass
Numbers		93	7	6	6	23	14
Age median (years)	11.3 ± 38	12.1 ± 3.2	8.2 ± 3.3	12.9 ± 31	9.3	10.5	10.1
Gender							
Intact female	2.5%	34/93	3/7	1/6	3/6	2/23	3/14
Spayed	38%	57/93	4/7	5/6	3/6	11/23	11/14
Castrated	60%					10/23	
Signs							
Obtunded	26%	26%	57%	2/6	2/6	4/23	28%
Circling	22.5%	22%	–	6/6	2/6	–	–
Seizures	22.5%	24.7%	42.9%	4/6	3/6	–	–
Ataxia	17%	–	–	–	2/6	7/23	–
Behaviour	16%	–	–	–	–	3/23	–
Non-specific	21%	21.5%	–	–	–	–	–
Lethargy	20%	16%	1/7	–	–	7/23	28%
Inappetance	18.1%	13%	1/7	–	–	8/23	21%
Incidental	20%	22.6%	–	–	–	–	35%
Duration of signs (days)							
Median	21	24.5	21	5.5	–	14	37.5
Range	1–1095	1–1095				1–270	1–253
CSF							
No.	28	15	2	2	3	6	
Median TP	38.0	59.5	63.5	25	21	54.5	
TP range	16–427	16–403	–	–	20–427	35–404	
Median NCC	5	5	49.9	55	3	14.5	
NCC range	0–162	–	4–95	–	2–45	0–162	
Location‡							
Extra-axial	82.7%	100%	0%	0%	0%	7/23	100%
Intra-axial	11.8%	–	100%	100%	100%	16/23	–
Both	5.4%	–	–	–	–	–	–
Supratentorial	87%	92.4%	28.6%	100%	5/6	7/23	100%
Infratentorial	3%	5.4%	71.4%	–	1/6	8/23	–
Both	9.4%	2.1%	–	–	–	–	–

* Astrocytomas.
† Oligodendrogliomas.
‡ Location of mass based on MR images.
CSF, cerebrospinal fluid analysis; TP, total protein; NCC, nucleated cell count.
Source: Troxel et al. (2003).

oma are classed as secondary tumours in this study. The true prevalence of metastases in this study was only 6%.

The most useful information retrieved from the signalment, was the significant difference noted between the median age of cats with meningiomas (12.2 years) and those with neuroepithelial tumours such as ependymomas (8.2 years). Concomitant infection with feline leukaemia virus and feline immunodeficiency virus was <4%. When lymphoma was specifically evaluated, 17.6% (three of 17) cats were feline leukaemia virus positive.

Clinically, there were some similarities noted to dogs with intracranial neoplasia |9|, but there were differences in the prevalence of specific clinical signs associated with the tumours. In this study, the most common clinical signs were altered consciousness (26.2%), circling (22.5%), seizure (22.5%), lethargy (20.0%) and inappetence (18.1%); according to a recent study, the most common clinical signs documented in dogs with brain tumours are seizures (46%), circling (23%) and ataxia (21%) |10|. However, clinical signs alone are not very helpful in discerning the underlying aetiology of brain disease and with the same type of neoplasia, the signs can be very dependent on the location of the lesion, the size of the lesion and the presence of peritumoral changes such as oedema. It was interesting to note that 50% of all the feline pituitary tumours ($n = 14$) had clinical endocrine disease due to their tumour, which is higher than that seen in dogs with these tumours. Additionally, while it is documented to be an infrequent occurrence in dogs, pituitary tumours were associated with visual dysfunction in 35.7% of cats.

Cerebrospinal fluid (CSF) was supportive of the diagnosis of intracranial neoplasia in most cases, but CSF analysis did not provide a definitive diagnosis; albuminocytological dissociation was noted in eight cats (28.6%); this is compared with 39.6% of 77 dogs with primary brain tumours |11|. The remaining 20 cats (71.4%) had varied increases in nucleated cell counts. The median CSF total protein and nucleated cell counts were 38.0 mg/dl (range 16–427) and five cells/μl (0–162) respectively, which can be helpful in developing an index of suspicion for neoplasia as a differential; the wide ranges though mean that their contribution to the diagnosis can never be absolute. The sensitivity of MRI in the detection of an intracranial neoplasia was documented as 98% (45 of 46 cats) but the authors acknowledge that this may not be accurate as it comes from a retrospective study that positively selected for intracranial neoplasia from post mortem or biopsy results.

Survival data are always difficult to interpret in veterinary medicine, especially from a retrospective uncontrolled case series. This is because the outcome is variably influenced by the wishes of the owners and their financial constraints as well as welfare issues that arise in debilitated animals. In addition, the type of treatment offered can be determined by the neurological status and age of the patient, which means that treatment data are never randomized and there is limited control data. Most previous reports have documented an improved outcome for cats with intracranial meningiomas, which are treated surgically |12,13|. This study provided similar results, with the median survival time post-surgery being 685 days (23 months). The median survival time for nine cats with lymphoma treated with systemic corticosteroids was 21 days. The median survival time of five cats with pituitary tumours treated with palliative corticosteroids was 52.5 days in this study. More preferable results have been documented following radiation therapy of these lesions |14|. Gliomas were uncommon tumours in this study and so limited valuable information can be gained about survival data.

Magnetic resonance imaging features of feline intracranial neoplasia: retrospective analysis of 46 cats
Troxel MT, Vite CH, Massicotte C, *et al. J Vet Int Med* 2004; **18**: 176–89

BACKGROUND. Routine diagnostic tests are not specific for the diagnosis of brain tumours. Even though the clinicopathological characteristics of feline intracranial tumours can help with their diagnosis, advanced imaging is necessary to confirm the presence of a structural brain lesion. At present, very little information regarding the MRI features of feline intracranial tumours is available. The purpose of this study was to review the MRI features of histologically confirmed brain tumours in cats and to determine whether or not these characteristics could be used to accurately predict tumour type. MRI scans of cats with histologically confirmed intracranial neoplasia (1985–2001) were reviewed. For inclusion, the MR series had to consist of at least: (i) sagittal and transverse pre-contrast (gadolinium dimeglumine) T1-weighted images (T1–WI); (ii) sagittal and transverse post-contrast T1-weighted images; (iii) transverse pre-contrast T2-weighted images (T2–WI). Several of the cats also had proton density weighted images performed and were therefore included in the evaluation. The following characteristics were recorded: axial origin; neuroanatomic location; tumour shape and margins; signal intensity and regularity; degree of contrast enhancement; presence of peritumoral oedema; mineralization and haemorrhage; cyst formation; herniation; presence of mass effect and involvement of the calvarium. All the images were independently and blindly re-evaluated to determine the accuracy of correct identification of each histological tumour type on the basis of MR characteristics alone.

INTERPRETATION. MRI scans of 46 cats with histologically characterized brain tumours were evaluated; the tumours included four gliomas, six lymphomas, 33 meningiomas, two olfactory neuroblastomas, and one pituitary tumour. Thirty-four MRI scans were independently re-evaluated to determine accuracy of tumour identification. Differences in MRI characteristics among tumour types are summarized in Table 7.2. The following patterns of MRI characteristics among tumour types assisted with the prediction of histological tumour type. Approximately 92% of all extra-axial masses that had moderate-to-marked contrast enhancement and a dural tail were meningiomas (Fig. 7.1). Extra-axial masses that caused mild oedema and showed evidence of chronic haemorrhage or mineralization were always meningioma. Extra-axial masses with hyperintense signal on T2–WI, isointense or hypointense signal on T1–WI, and moderate-to-marked contrast enhancement were meningiomas 90% of the time. All intra-axial masses with ring enhancement and cystic regions were gliomas.

Comment

The rapid evolution of advanced imaging techniques such as computed tomography and MRI, has enabled the veterinary profession to detect more accurately structural abnormalities of the brain. MRI is the imaging modality of choice for most central nervous system (CNS) diseases, due to its superior soft-tissue contrast resolution, its multiplanar capability, high sensitivity to oedema, and the absence of 'beam-hardening' artefacts in the caudal fossa. The sensitivity for detecting tumours in dogs is close to 100% |15|. In this study, the accuracy for detection of feline intracranial

Table 7.2 A summary of the MRI characteristics of the feline intracranial tumours most commonly identified

MRI characteristics	Meningioma	Lymphoma	Glioma
Case numbers	33	5	4*
Extra-axial location	33/33 (100%)	3/5 (60%)	0/4 (0%)
Tumour margin			
Regular	70%	Varied	
Distinct	100%		
T2–WI signal			
Hyperintense	29/33	4/5	4/4
Heterogeneous	27/33	3/5	
T1–WI signal			
Isointense	14/33	3/5	0/4
Hypointense	19/33	2/5	4/4
Homogeneous	33/33	5/5	
PD–WI signal			
Hyperintense	15/33	2/3	
Post-contrast T1–WI			
Marked enhancement	97%	5/5	4/4 Variable
Homogeneous	50%	0/5	4/4
Ring enhancement	4/33		
Peritumoral oedema			
None	21%	–	
Mild	58%	–	
Moderate	6%	2/5	
Marked	15%	3/5	
Mass effect	97%	3/5	2/4
Dural tail	64%	1/5	0/4
Calvarium involved	73%	2/3	0/4
Cystic component	6%	–	3/4
Ventriculomegaly	64%	1/5	2/4
Transtentorial herniation	42%	0/5	0/4
Cerebellar herniation	21%	0/5	0/4

* Of the four gliomas, three were oligodendrogliomas and one was an astrocytoma.
Source: Troxel et al. (2004).

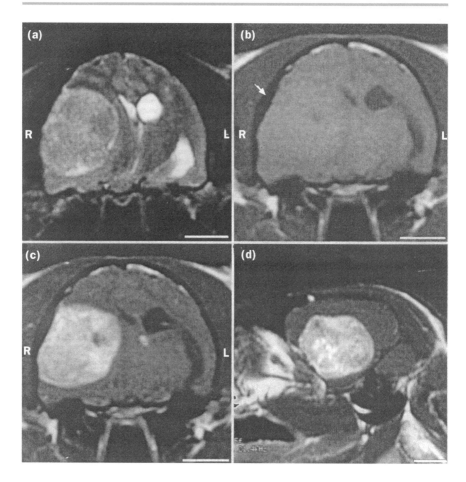

Fig. 7.1 Meningioma involving the right temporoparietal region of a cat. There is a marked mass effect with a compression of the right lateral ventricle and thalamus as well as a deviation of midline structures from right to left. The mass is ovoid with a regular, distinct margin. The tumour has a hyperintense, heterogeneous signal on transverse T2-weighted images (T2–WI) (a) and an isointense, homogeneous signal on transverse T1-weighted images (T1–WI) (b) and shows a marked, heterogeneous contrast enhancement on the transverse (c) and sagittal (d) post-contrast T1–WI. A small region with a hypointense signal on both the T2–WI and T1–WI is suggestive of mineralization or chronic haemorrhage. Mineralization was confirmed on histologic examination. There was no peritumoral oedema associated with this meningioma. Hyperostosis of the calvarium (*arrow*) overlying the neoplasm is visible (b).

Bar = 1 cm. (GE Signa 1.5-T, extremity coil, 3 mm slice thickness with 0.3 mm interslice distance, T2–WI: FSE 3083/96, transverse T1–WI: FSE 600/21, sagittal T1–WI: FSE 400/16). Source: Troxel *et al.* (2004).

neoplasia was 98%. However, as the authors acknowledge, caution must be used in interpreting this kind of data as both canine and feline studies were retrospective. Tissue was obtained from patients based on their MR images or from those which were euthanized which may affect the accuracy of the data. MRI features of intracranial tumours in dogs can provide a specific tumour diagnosis with approximately 90% accuracy |15|. In the present feline study, there was an overall success rate of 82%. Specifically, there was a 96% success rate for the accurate diagnosis of meningiomas, based on imaging characteristics that included identification of an extra-axial mass (differentials include lymphoma, pituitary tumour and olfactory neuroblastoma), lack of destruction of the cribriform plate, mild peritumoral oedema, mass effect, broad-based appearance, marked contrast enhancement, or dural tail sign. Tumour shape, margin and size were not characteristic of any particular tumour type; however, plaque-like lesions were always meningiomas in this study. As in dogs, most of the tumours in this study were hyperintense on T2–WI and hypointense or isointense on T1–WI |15|. The signal pattern was generally heterogeneous on T2–WI and was either homogeneous or heterogeneous on T1–WI. All of the brain tumours in this study exhibited some degree of contrast enhancement, except for one diagnosed as meningeal lymphoma. Marked contrast enhancement was noted in five of six lymphomas, in the majority (91%) of the meningiomas, in both olfactory neuro-blastomas and one pituitary tumour; all of these tumours are derived from tissues lacking a blood–brain barrier and, therefore, should be expected to contrast-enhance. Contrast enhancement was variable in the gliomas. Involvement of the calvaria (hyperostosis) was noted in the majority (73%) of meningiomas in this study. Peritumoral oedema was more notably associated with intra-axial lesions, with mild to moderate oedema associated with the extra-axial lesions. Hydrocephalus and herniation was not associated with any particular tumour type. Owing to the small numbers of the tumours in all groups apart from the meningiomas, statistical significance could not be attached to any of the above characteristics. Without 100% association of any specific MR characteristics to a specific tumour type, they can only increase the index of suspicion for a definitive diagnosis and must be combined with the clinicopatholgical characteristics to narrow down the differential diagnosis list.

Post-anesthetic cerebellar dysfunction in cats

Shamir M, Goelman G, Chai O. *J Vet Int Med* 2004; **18**: 368–9

BACKGROUND. Several cerebellar disorders have been described that affect cats in different age groups with congenital, infectious, neoplastic, anomalous, traumatic and toxic aetiologies |1|. The age of the cat, sometimes the breed of cat, the onset and progression of the clinical signs and the presence of other neurological abnormalities can help determine the underlying disease mechanism. A unique acute onset of cerebellar dysfunction subsequent to uncomplicated anaesthesia is described in this report. The cats had not had any evidence of neurological disease

prior to the anaesthesia. The clinical course of the disease was described in addition to the signalments of the cases involved and the anaesthetic regimens in order that specific risk factors could be identified.

INTERPRETATION. A retrospective study with follow-up observations of 11 cats is described. The cats all experienced an acute onset of cerebellar dysfunction following uncomplicated anaesthesia. Clinical signs were compatible with diffuse cerebellar disease including mild to severe ataxia of all four limbs, intentional tremor, lack of menace response and delayed hopping. The medical records were reviewed for the following details: CBC and serum blood chemistry at the onset of clinical signs (6 of 11); current follow-up; serology for *Toxoplasma*, feline immunodeficiency virus and feline leukaemia virus infections; and MRI examination ($n = 1$). All cats were long-haired Persian cross-breeds; eight were females and three were males. The age range was wide (8 months–10 years). All cats were born in Israel where they were examined. None of the cats had previously had any neurological disease and eight were considered healthy at the time of the anaesthesia; three of the cats had an illness that led to the need for anaesthesia; all blood tests were normal. All procedures were classed as routine such as ovariohysterectomy ($n = 6$). Ketamine was the only anaesthetic agent common to the procedures in all cats. Follow-up revealed that six of the animals were alive 6 months–8 years after the onset of the clinical signs; the signs had not reversed. Three cats were euthanized, and two cats died of unknown causes.

Comment

An acute onset of cerebellar disease in cats can be due to ischaemia, parasitic migrations (Cuterebra), toxicity, and metabolic aberrations such as hypoglycaemia. In young animals, when it is difficult to evaluate the time of onset of cerebellar disease with accuracy (due to the naturally expected poor co-ordination), other causes such as congenital cerebellar dysfunction due to panleucopenia virus infection, hereditary cerebellar degeneration, neuraxonal dystrophy and storage disease should be considered. However, most of these diseases in young cats are slow progressive disorders. This study describes a unique situation of sudden onset cerebellar disease following routine anaesthesia; the regulation of the anaesthesia was not discussed and so whether there were any problems such as hyoptension or hypoxic periods cannot be discerned. Such a report is useful in documenting the outcome of patients; however, this report is fascinating on account of (i) the fact that all 11 cats were long-haired Persian cross cats, and (ii) there is a potential link between the use of ketamine and cerebellar disease. These risk factors may only be of interest in Israel, where the study was performed, if the predisposition to post-anaesthetic cerebellar disease following ketamine is indeed genetic; however, this cannot be stated and so concern about the use of ketamine in Persians and their crosses should remain. The authors briefly discuss the potential mechanism of the non-reversible cerebellar dysfunction; ketamine is a non-competitive antagonist at the excitatory neurotransmitter (*N*-methyl-D-aspartate) receptor |16|, and has been purported to be a neuroprotectant. These receptors exist throughout the nervous system; potentially a mutation of this receptor in the cerebellum in these cats may have predisposed the cerebellum to a cytotoxic process. However, there is no explanation as to why three of the cats had been anaesthetized with ketamine before and not had any problems. It is obvious that further work in this area needs to be done to elucidate the pathophysiology and confirm the risk factors. Histopathology may have helped but then again it can often just represent a uniform reaction to a multitude of insults.

Epilepsy

An epileptic seizure results from abnormal electrical activity in the cerebral cortex |1|. The majority of epileptic seizures described and witnessed in veterinary medicine are those that affect the whole body in a generalized uncontrolled and erratic manifestation of skeletal muscle activity. We as veterinarians and owners may miss the more subtle, focal seizures and so have been slower to gain an understanding of this disorder when compared with the human field. Most concern relating to epilepsy revolves around the treatment and management of patients with seizure activity. We must not ignore the issue that effective treatment is only possible when we have identified an aetiology, but even then there are a plethora of cases that are difficult for us to treat and help improve their quality of life. This failure may stem from both limited veterinary drug availability as well as a poor understanding of the pathophysiology of this disorder. A better understanding may enable better drug selection and as more human anticonvulsant drugs are used in veterinary medicine, such an understanding is likely to become invaluable. The two papers reviewed here cover the use of a new human anticonvulsant drug for canine refractory epilepsy and an investigation into the neurotransmitter status in dogs with epilepsy.

Zonisamide therapy for refractory idiopathic epilepsy in dogs
Dewey CW, Guiliano R, Boothe DM, et al. J Am Anim Hosp Assoc 2004; **40**: 285–91

BACKGROUND. Up to 30% of idiopathic canine epileptics are refractory to appropriate doses of phenobarbital (PB) and potassium bromide (KBr) used in combination |17|. There are few additional anticonvulsants that can be used in this situation in dogs, as most human drugs have a short half-life in dogs or are potentially toxic. Therefore, there is a recognized need for safe and effective alternative anticonvulsant drugs that can be used in addition to PB and KBr, in dogs with refractory seizures. Zonisamide is a sulphonamide-based anticonvulsant drug recently approved for human use in the USA, with multiple potential mechanisms of action. It is effective for both focal and generalized seizures in humans, and side effects are minimal, including sedation and ataxia. It is metabolized by hepatic microsomal enzymes and is reported to be well tolerated in dogs, even when used at very high doses for extended periods of time. Its clinical use has not been reported in dogs and there is no pharmacokinetic information available for the use of this drug. The purpose of this study was to evaluate the efficacy, tolerance and pharmacokinetic properties of zonisamide when it is used as an additional anticonvulsant in dogs with refractory idiopathic epilepsy. Inclusion criteria for the study were: (i) dogs with idiopathic epilepsy based upon characteristic signalment and features of the disease; advanced imaging was not performed unless the dogs were outside of a 1–5-year age range, in which case they also needed to have normal CSF analysis; (ii) dogs with seizure activity that was considered 'uncontrolled' (uncontrolled implied a minimum average of two seizures per month and a total of >6); (iii) all dogs must have been on at least one of PB or KBr and have 'adequate' serum levels; subtherapeutic serum levels were only considered eligible if unacceptable side effects attributable to these drugs were reported by the owner. The dose of zonisamide used initially in each dog was 5–10 mg/kg every 12h, which was estimated to be that necessary to achieve a therapeutic serum range (10–40 μg/ml). Dosages were adjusted until the therapeutic reference range was reached in each dog based on the serum levels, which were taken at least 1 week after any dose changes at time 0 h (trough) and 3 h (peak) post-pill. Each dog's seizure frequency was recorded for equivalent times of at least 8 weeks pre- and post-medication. A positive responder was defined as a dog that experienced at least a 50% reduction in seizures after the initiation of zonisamide. Trough and estimated peak serum zonisamide concentrations were compared for all animals using a paired Student's t test and compared between responders and non-responders using an unpaired Student's t test. Owners were questioned about the side effects noted since the introduction of the anticonvulsant.

INTERPRETATION. Twelve dogs, all with generalized tonic-clonic seizures (median duration = 20.5 months; range 2–82 months), were included and were treated with a mean dose of 8.9 mg/kg every 12 h. Ten of the dogs were already on PB and KBr at the start of the study (median duration 5.8 months; range 1–31 months) and all serum bromide levels were within the designated therapeutic range. Three of these dogs had serum PB levels below the therapeutic laboratory range. Median follow-up time was 37 weeks (8–71 weeks) at which time 11 of the dogs achieved peak and trough serum levels which were within the therapeutic range. (Median trough 18.4 μg/ml; median peak 21.2 μg/ml). There was no evident difference between the serum concentrations of responders and non-responders for peak or trough values. Seven of the 12 dogs (58%) experienced at least a 50% decrease in seizures while on zonisamide; within these dogs the median seizure reduction was 84.5% and two dogs were considered seizure free. The five dogs that were non-responders all experienced an increase in seizure frequency. A reduction or elimination of concurrent antiseizure drugs was possible in seven of the responders. Fifty per cent of all the dogs had side effects, which included generalized ataxia, transient lethargy, transient vomiting and keratoconjunctivitis sicca. One dog experienced lameness due to polyarthropathy during the treatment period, but this could not be confirmed to be due to the use of zonisamide. No abnormalities were detected in any of the haematology samples, although there were mild elevations of alanine aminotransferase and alkaline phosphatase, noted in the serum biochemistry samples.

Comment

Overall, this study demonstrated that zonisamide is a useful adjunctive anticonvulsant drug in dogs with idiopathic refractory generalized tonic-clonic epilepsy. It was well tolerated and effective at twice daily dosing in reducing seizure frequency by 50–100% in 58% of dogs, when used at doses that are well within those described to be safe |**17**|. Several of the dogs had the concurrent anticonvulsant drug doses reduced, which has the potential of further improving the dogs' and the owners' quality of life. The side effects were mild and not severe enough to warrant termination of the drug. However, it is suggested that this drug be used with caution based on the limited number of dogs that have been treated and its poorly tested use as an adjunctive medication. As it is a sulphonamide-based drug, the dogs should be monitored for keratoconjunctivitis sicca, dermatitis, arthropathies and blood dyscrasias. The authors acknowledge that this is a small study but that additionally it is part retrospective and part prospective; such studies, although common and necessary in veterinary medicine, are notoriously difficult to interpret without urging caution. The trial is not placebo controlled and all the dogs have variations in their onset and duration of clinical signs, seizure frequency, current medical regimen and even signalment. These are important differences, which may effect the response to this drug. Crucial to these studies is the definition of *idiopathic* and *refractory* when referring to epilepsy. There is always the potential in this study that the dogs were true idiopathic (inferred heritable epilepsy) epileptics, but there may be some, which were actually cryptogenic epileptics, i.e. a case with an underlying structural abnormality responsible for the seizures but which cannot be identified by way of the current diagnostic methods. This latter type is more likely in dogs older than 5 years. Advanced imaging and CSF analysis would ideally be necessary to rule out other causes of seizure activity in dogs. The effect on response of different underlying aetiologies is undetermined. Refractory epilepsy in dogs is that which cannot be controlled adequately with acceptable serum levels of both PB and KBr. Exactly what is adequately controlled and what serum levels are adequate is also poorly documented. Those dogs with cluster seizure activity or frequent weekly seizures may be more difficult to control than those with four seizures a month, but both could be considered refractory. The therapeutic ranges of the anticonvulsant drugs should serve as markers for decision making in dose alterations but should not be over-utilized; the side effects of the drugs and the success of the therapy are more important factors. Monitoring seizure frequency is a good measure of outcome for the evaluation of drug effect. However, the seizure frequency after the initiation of medication is likely to be more accurate than that estimated before this time as the owners are more likely to keep a written record. Given these limitations accepted by the authors, this study is a valuable advance to the treatment of epilepsy in dogs. Whether this drug is effective as sole therapy and whether it is effective against focal seizure activity will remain to be seen.

Inhibitory and excitatory neurotransmitters in the cerebrospinal fluid of epileptic dogs

Ellenberger C, Mevissen M, Doherr M, Scholtysik G, Jaggy A. *Am J Vet Res* 2004; **65**(8): 1108–13

BACKGROUND. The precise underlying aetiology of epilepsy is poorly understood; a greater understanding would lead to therapy, which may be more appropriately targeted and ultimately more effective. The proposed pathophysiology in human epilepsy focuses on an imbalance between excitatory and inhibitory neurotransmitter mechanisms and specifically includes changes in neurotransmitter function and or concentrations, and alteration in the expression of neurotransmitter receptors |18|. A decrease in the CSF concentration of γ-aminobutyric acid (GABA), the predominant inhibitory neurotransmitter in the brain, may lead to seizures, and an increase may have anticonvulsant effects |18|. In the veterinary literature, low concentrations of CSF GABA have been documented in dogs with generalized tonic-clonic seizures and those with confirmed idiopathic epilepsy |19,20|. The purpose of this study was to compare the CSF concentrations of both excitatory and inhibitory amino acids in Labrador retrievers (LR) with genetic epilepsy and non-Labrador retrievers (non-LR) with idiopathic epilepsy. As mentioned, in the comment on the zonisamide therapy section, there may be differences between such groups with respect to their pathophysiologies and their response to therapy. Criteria for inclusion in this study were a history of >1 episode of seizure activity; no physical or neurological abnormalities; normal haematology, serum chemistry, bile acids, urinalysis and CSF analysis. A group of 129 dogs were evaluated retrospectively and divided into a non-LR group ($n = 94$) and a LR group ($n = 35$), which originated from a defined population of epileptics with a polygenic recessive mode of inheritance. In each group, the numbers of dogs treated with anticonvulsant drugs were recorded for statistical evaluation. A control group of 20 healthy 1-year-old beagles were also evaluated in this study and proven to be normal on subsequent histopathology. All CSF analysed was procured at least 72 h after the last recorded seizure activity from the cerebellomedullary cistern and stored in −70°C until thawed and evaluated by high-powered liquid chromatography (HPLC). Intergroup differences for measured CSF concentrations of glutamate (the predominant excitatory neurotransmitter in the CNS), GABA, and aspartate (an excitatory neurotransmitter) were evaluated using ANOVA (analysis of variance); this was also used to test the effect of gender and drug treatment on the CSF levels.

INTERPRETATION. CSF GABA concentrations were significantly lower in the LR group compared with the control group and the non-LR group; however, there were no significant differences between the control group and all dogs combined (Fig. 7.2). CSF glutamate in the LR group and all dogs combined was significantly lower when compared with control, but there was no difference between the control group and non-LR (Fig. 7.2). CSF aspartate levels were lower in the LR group and non-LR group when compared with control dogs, but not significantly. When all dogs were combined, the CSF aspartate levels were significantly lower than the controls. The glutamate to GABA ratio was significantly higher in the LR group than in the non-LR group but was not significantly different from the control dogs. Besides

there being a lower CSF glutamate concentration in female LR dogs, there were no gender
influences on the results. There was also no significant effect of PB treatment on the
neurotransmitter levels when the LR group was compared with the controls; however, there
was a significant reduction in the glutamate, aspartate and GABA concentrations in the
treated subset of the non-LR group.

Comment

This relatively large study demonstrates that there may be a role of altered excitatory
and inhibitory neurotransmitters in the pathogenesis of epilepsy and that this role
may be different in genetic epileptic LRs and other idiopathic epileptics. For too long,

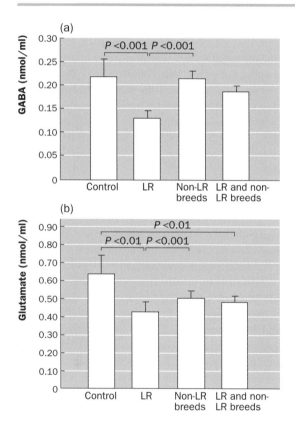

Fig. 7.2 Mean (± SEM) CSF concentrations (nmol/ml) of γ-aminobutyric acid (GABA; (a))
and glutamate (b) in control dogs ($n = 20$), Labrador retrievers with genetic epilepsy (35),
non-Labrador retrievers with idiopathic epilepsy (94), and all dogs with epilepsy (either
idiopathic or genetic epilepsy; 129). LR, Labrador retrievers with genetic epilepsy; non-LR,
non-Labrador retrievers with idiopathic epilepsy. Values of $P < 0.05$ represent significant
differences between groups. Source: Ellenberger *et al.* (2004).

veterinary medicine has dealt with all idiopathic epileptic dogs as being similar in terms of their underlying pathophysiology and treatment requirements. As time moves on, we are understanding that idiopathic epileptic dogs can be separated based upon their clinical manifestations of the seizure focus and the underlying cerebral abnormality. Not until this time, will we be able to more specifically tailor a therapy to an individual and know what to expect. This study goes some way to investigating subsets of epileptic dogs as well as normal controls and in doing so produces an excellent insight into the pathophysiology of this disease. The finding of decreased CSF GABA levels in the LR group, compared with control dogs, is in agreement with results of previous veterinary studies |19,20| confirming the important part that GABA plays in epilepsy. Decreased activity of glutamic acid decarboxylase, which synthesizes GABA via decarboxylation of L-glutamate, may result in low levels of CSF GABA. The finding of decreased CSF GABA in the LR group when compared with the non-LR group though is new and exciting information as this suggests that LRs may have different pathophysiological mechanisms as the cause of epilepsy when compared with other idiopathic epileptics as a whole. Confirmation that not all epileptics should be dealt with in the same manner! Concentrations of CSF glutamate in LR dogs were decreased when compared with normal dogs, but no significant difference in CSF concentrations of glutamate was found in non-LR group dogs when compared with control group dogs. Although similar results have been reported in humans with epilepsy |21|, this result is in contradiction to the results in another veterinary study |20|. The justifiable explanation for this given by the authors relates to the vastly different control levels of glutamate in each study. HPLC analysis of glutamate is notoriously difficult and the veterinary reports in the literature have given rise to normal values that vary by factors of 10 or more! The authors offer an explanation for the low level of CSF glutamate, which relates to transient alterations in glutamate transporter expression; however, it is unclear whether the alterations are the cause of seizure activity or the result of it and so further investigations will be necessary. The low glutamate to GABA ratio in the non-LR group of dogs supports the hypothesis that an imbalance between GABAergic inhibition and excitation by glutamate is involved in epilepsy pathogenesis. It has been proposed that an imbalance between excitatory and inhibitory synaptic transmission that favours excitation leads to the initiation of epileptic discharges. Because the glutamate to GABA ratio was found to be significantly higher in LR-group dogs, compared with non-LR group dogs, this ratio is proposed by the authors to be a marker of genetic epilepsy in Labrador retrievers.

Inherited/congenital central nervous system disease

Both the CNS and peripheral nervous systems are affected by disorders that are either congenital or heritable in their origin. The establishment of the canine genome has now enabled fervent investigation into these diseases, both as an aid to understanding the disease in animals and humans as well as potentiating treatment via breeding programmes. Congenital or heritable disorders of the CNS can be structural in nature such as the Chiari-like malformations and hydrocephalic dogs described below or they can be degenerative, such as is the situation with deafness, also discussed below. A degenerative condition implies a process whereby CNS tissue matures normally but then degenerates prematurely due to an error of metabolism. Most of the affected animals are normal at birth and then have an onset of progressive neurological signs later in life. Part of the problem with congenital and/or heritable diseases in veterinary medicine has been in establishing what is acceptable or 'normal' between the plethora of breeds that we deal with. Both the Chiari-like and hydrocephalic papers below, attempt to address this by investigating imaging associations with clinical disease. In a disorder such as deafness where clinical diagnosis can be more objective, investigations have previously attempted to associate phenotypic parameters of individual breeds with the presence of deafness so that future breeding programmes can be developed. This is furthered by the investigation below.

Neurologic signs and results of magnetic resonance imaging in 40 cavalier King Charles spaniels with Chiari Type 1-like malformations

Lu D, Lamb CR, Pfeiffer DU, Targett MP. *Vet Rec* 2003; **153**; 260–3

BACKGROUND. In humans, a Chiari Type 1 malformation is a developmental condition characterized by cerebellar herniation through the foramen magnum and syringohydromyelia. Associated abnormalities include a small posterior fossa, inferior displacement of the medulla and/or the fourth ventricle, angulation of the cervicomedullary junction, hydrocephalus, syringohydromyelia and various osseous abnormalities |22|. A similar syndrome has been reported in cavalier King Charles spaniels (CKCS) |23|. The purported pathophysiology involves an underdevelopment of the occipital bone leading to 'overcrowding' of the posterior fossa; in addition to herniation of the cerebellum through the foramen magnum, this has the effect of altering the circulation of CSF at the foramen magnum and preventing the equilibration of the pressure between the intracranial and spinal subarachnoid spaces |22|. Ultimately this leads to the development of syringohydromyelia as the transiently increased intracranial pressure (ICP) during each systole forces the cerebellum against and through the foramen, inducing a pressure wave that acts on the surface of the spinal cord and promotes the leakage of CSF into the cord |23|. The most common clinical sign in CKCS is a persistent scratching of the shoulder and neck |23|. Other neurological signs may include lower motor neurone deficits, proprioceptive abnormalities and facial nerve paresis |23|. The diagnosis is on the basis of MRI results; however, with such modalities, evidence-based decisions can only be made after the relationships between structural changes and neurological dysfunction have been established. The aim of this study was to describe the range of neurological signs observed in 40 CKCS with a Chiari Type-1-like malformation and to examine the relationship between these signs and results of MRI. The medical

records of 40 CKCS, which had brains and cervical spines examined with MR, were
reviewed. The MR series included T1- and T2-weighted transverse and sagittal
images. The following parameters were evaluated: degree of deformity of the
cerebellum; the presence of hydrocephalus; the presence of syringohydromyelia;
degree of cerebellar herniation; degree of compression in the spinal cord by the
cerebellar vermis; relative size of the cerebellum; and the degree of hydrocephalus.
The clinical signs were split up into cranial and spinal lesions. The association
between cranial or spinal signs and the variables was assessed with χ^2 analysis and
Mann–Whitney U-test.

INTERPRETATION. Thirty-nine clinical dogs were evaluated; 22 dogs were in the cranial
group (median age 6 years) and 17 dogs were in the spinal group (median age 4 years). One
neurologically normal dog was evaluated. Within the cranial group, nine had facial paresis,
seven suffered seizures, and seven had vestibular syndrome. Within the spinal group, 16 of
17 had spinal hyperaesthesia, eight had proprioceptive deficits, and three persistently
scratched their shoulder and neck regions. The median duration of clinical signs was
1.5 months for the dogs in the cranial group and 4.5 months for the dogs in the spinal group.
All the dogs had herniation of the cerebellum compatible with a Chiari Type 1 malformation.
Twenty-six of the 40 dogs had hydrocephalus, and 26 had syringohydromyelia. There were no
significant differences between the two groups in terms of signalment; severity of cerebellar
indentation and herniation; severity of hydrocephalus; severity of syringohydromelia; the
proportion of the foramen magnum occupied by the spinal cord; and the size of the
cerebellum. Each of the three dogs with neck scratching had marked syringohydromyelia;
however, four other dogs in the spinal group and five other dogs in the cranial group had a
similar degree of syringohydromyelia. A log-linear analysis for associations between multiple
factors revealed no statistically significant interactions. Follow-up information over a median
period of 20 months revealed that the neurological signs decreased in severity or resolved in
20 of the dogs, of which 13 received no treatment, two had surgery, and five had various
medical therapies. The neurological signs were considered to have remained unchanged in
severity in 10 of the dogs, and in six they were considered to have increased in severity or
become more frequent than when the condition was diagnosed.

Comment

All 40 CKCS had an abnormal shaped cerebellum; a consistent concave caudal aspect
and a pointed vermis, with the tip directed caudally towards or through the foramen
magnum, similar to Chiari Type 1 in humans. In humans, computed tomography
is the best method of evaluating the misshapen occipital bones, especially with the
3-dimensional reconstruction capability. MR imaging is the best manner in which to
evaluate CNS parenchymal changes secondary to the osseous abnormalities. However, the significance of these parenchymal changes has not been certain and without
such information, therapeutic decisions cannot be appropriately made. The importance of this study is in its evaluation of the MRI abnormalities with the aim of trying
to associate them with the neurological signs in 39 affected CKCS, with the need
being to define criteria that make it possible to recognize clinically significant abnormalities. On the basis of the results, the authors state that 'it is uncertain whether
the observed malformations contribute to the observed neurological signs or have no

clinical effect'. Unfortunately, there was only one clinically normal dog in this study, which makes it difficult to compare the extent of parenchymal abnormality that may be present in the absence of clinical signs. The prevalence of this condition in CKCS has not been documented, and as clinically affected dogs are the only ones that are diagnostically evaluated, we may be over-interpreting the abnormalities that we identify on MR images. One of the difficulties with this syndrome is the variability of the clinical signs. Scratching has been documented as one of the most common clinical signs |23|; however, this was not the case in this study and it did not represent a consistent sign of syringohydromyelia. The most common sign in this study was spinal hyperaesthesia on vertebral palpation—this may be similar to people with the condition who present with suboccipital headaches or neck pain. Although this sign did not correlate with any of the structural variables evaluated in the study, ruling out the other differentials of neck pain such as meningitis, disc disease and neoplasia may help to establish the disease as a clinical problem. It is likely that future investigations into the disease will attempt to find a diagnostic variable that correlates well with the clinical signs; this study has established there to be no such association with static structural abnormalities, and so with this in mind and based upon the pathophysiology of this syndrome, a dynamic assessment such as CSF flow studies and Doppler ultrasound may be helpful.

Deafness prevalence and pigmentation and gender associations in dog breeds at risk

Strain GM. *Vet J* 2004; **167**: 23–32

BACKGROUND. Canine deafness can be hereditary or acquired. Deafness has been associated with skin pigmentation patterns in dogs and has been observed in over 80 breeds; hereditary components are assumed but not proven for most breeds and are associated with skin pigmentation genes conferring either white pigment or light versus dark patterns. There is little doubt that white pigmentation is a risk factor for deafness in dogs but the mechanisms are not understood. The canine locus or gene designated by S is most associated with deafness. This locus affects the distribution patterns of pigmented and non-pigmented areas of the body; other genes determine the actual colour of the pigmented areas |24|. The S locus has at least four alleles, three of which are recessive and are responsible for white colouring by acting on differentiation and/or migration of melanocyte precursor cells from the neural crest during embryogenesis |24|. Data from many studies demonstrate that pigment-associated deafness is the result of absent melanocytes in the stria vascularis of the cochlea, which leads to early post-natal degeneration of the stria and secondary degeneration of the cochlear hair cells and neurons. Most studies of congenital deafness in dogs have focused on the dalmation, which have demonstrated the prevalence in the USA to be approximately 8% bilateral deafness and 22% unilateral deafness, or 30% affected |25|. This study documents deafness prevalence in eight dog breeds in which pigment-associated congenital sensorineural deafness occurs—dalmation, English setter (ES), English cocker spaniel (ECS), bull terrier (BT),

Australian cattle dog (ACD), whippet, Catahoula leopard dog and Jack Russell terrier
(JRT). It also evaluates the potential influence of gender and pigmentation
phenotypes on hearing status. Hearing results and phenotype data were recorded
from dogs ($n = 11\,300$) of eight breeds, during the period 1986–2002. The data were
collected in clinics or at dog shows, performed on litters to rule out deafness or
because of the suspicion of hearing deficits. Brainstem auditory evoked responses
(BAER) were performed and deafness was classified as unilateral or bilateral.
Hearing status of both parents were additionally recorded. Gender and iris colour
measurements (pigmented or blue) were recorded from animals in all breeds. Other
pigmentation phenotype measures were recorded that varied by breed. These
included: (i) the presence of a patch in dalmations; (ii) colour varieties in those
breeds where some white is always present, such as spot colour in dalmations; and
(iii) white versus non-white pigmentation in those breeds where those varieties exist.
Deafness prevalence data and association analyses were performed using the
c^2 test with SAS statistics software. As pedigree relationships were not known for
most subjects, pedigree-based analyses could not be performed.

INTERPRETATION. The presence of congenital deafness is reported in 80 dog breeds at
the time of this report. Prevalence data for the dogs from the eight breeds examined in this
study ranged from a high of 29.9% affected in the dalmation breed to a low of 6.9% affected
in the ECS (Table 7.3). Prevalence data for the whippet, Catahoula, and JRT are reported, but
the rates are not necessarily representative for those breeds due to the low numbers of dogs
tested and the fact that these breeds were more likely to be presented for evaluation on
suspicion of deafness rather than as a routine evaluation by a breeder such as occurs in
dalmations. The ratio of unilaterally deaf to total affected ranged from a high of 0.904 in BT
to a low of 0.733 in dalmations (Table 7.3). This ratio reflects the proportion of deaf dogs
within a breed with unilateral deafness, which may go undetected in the absence of BAER
testing (i.e. 73.3% in the dalmation). For the five breeds analysed, no gender difference in
deafness prevalence was seen; however, the percentage of total affected females exceeded
the percentage of total affected males in the dalmation, ECS, BT and ACD. The coat
pigmentation varieties that are unrelated to the genes that produce white were not
significantly associated with deafness. There were no statistical differences in deafness
prevalence between black and liver-spotted dalmations, or among blue, orange or tricolour
roan ES, or the four-colour varieties of the ACD. Significant differences were seen for coat
pigmentation varieties linked to white genes. Dalmations without a patch were statistically
more likely to be deaf than dalmations with a patch. White BT were statistically more likely to
be deaf than coloured BT. The prevalence of blue eyes (one or both) in the dalmation was
comparatively high at 10.6%, while in ES it was 0.5%, in ECS it was 0.4% and in BT it was
0.2%. Deafness prevalence was statistically related to iris colour with blue-eyed dogs more
likely to be deaf. Of the 554 dalmations with one or two blue eyes, 32.3% were unilaterally
deaf and 18.4% were bilaterally deaf, or 50.7% were affected. English setters with blue eyes
were more likely to be deaf than those with brown eyes. BT iris colour did not exhibit a
consistent significant association with deafness prevalence and none of the ACD had a blue
eye. A significant association between hearing status and parent hearing status was seen for
the dalmation, ES and ECS breeds, where dogs had a higher likelihood of deafness if one or
both parents were also affected.

Table 7.3 Deafness prevalence in 11 300 dogs from selected breeds

Breed	n	Bilaterally hearing*	Unilaterally deaf (U)	Bilaterally deaf (D)	Total deaf [U + D]	Ratio (U/[U + D])
Dalmatian	5333	70.1% (3740)	21.9% (1167)	8.0% (426)	29.9% (1593)	0.733
English setter†	3656	92.1% (3368)	6.5% (236)	1.4% (52)	7.9% (288)	0.819
GMS	662	87.6% (580)	10.3% (68)	2.1% (14)	12.4% (82)	
ESAA	2994	93.1% (2788)	5.6% (168)	1.3% (38)	6.9% (206)	
English cocker spaniel	1136‡	93.1% (1057)	5.9% (67)	1.1% (12)	6.9% (79)	0.848
Parti-coloured	1067	93.0% (992)	5.9% (63)	1.1% (12)	7.0% (75)	
Solid	60	98.3% (59)	1.7% (1)	0.0% (0)	1.7% (1)	
Bull terrier	665‡	89.0% (592)	9.9% (66)	1.1% (7)	11.0% (73)	0.904
White	346	80.1% (277)	18.0 (62)	2.0% (7)	19.9% (69)	
Coloured	311	98.7% (307)	1.3% (4)	0.0% (0)	1.3% (4)	
Australian cattle dog	296	85.5% (253)	12.2% (36)	2.4% (7)	14.5% (43)	0.837
Whippet§	80	98.8% (79)	0.0% (0)	1.3% (1)	1.3% (1)	–
Catahoula leopard dog§	78	37.2% (29)	23.1% (18)	39.7% (31)	62.8% (49)	–
Jack Russell terrier§	56	83.9% (47)	7.1% (4)	8.9% (5)	16.1% (9)	–

* Percentage and (n).
† Values collected by GMS and from the English Setter Association of America hearing registry.
‡ n values for colour varieties do not sum to the n values for all dogs in a breed due to missing data.
§ Insufficient numbers of animals tested for percentage to be reliable.
Source: Strain (2004).

Comment

The size of this study makes this the largest deafness investigation so far carried out in veterinary medicine, examining eight breeds of the at least 80 documented, for phenotypic factors associated with hearing loss; the importance of the study is ultimately that we can improve on our index of suspicion for those unilateral cases that may be difficult to detect subjectively as well as have a better understanding of the gravity of the situation in certain breeds, which is necessary if we are going to advise on breeding programmes attempting to reduce the prevalence in certain breeds. The vast majority of the breeds documented carry white pigmentation or merle genes, strengthening our preconceptions of the link between coat colour and deafness. It has been clear for a long time now that deafness is hereditary in the dalmation, and that coat pigmentation is an important component as in other species carrying white, but the exact mechanism of inheritance is still not determined. Studies such as this advance our knowledge closer to the point where this mechanism will become clear, which is essential for breeding programmes in these dogs. As this study confirms again, there is an extremely high rate of deafness in dalmations (29.9%), which would be a concern for any other health problem. In the absence of a genetic marker for the gene or genes responsible for pigment-associated deafness, the remaining strategy to reduce deafness prevalence has been to not breed affected dogs and to breed away from pedigrees with high prevalence rates. Unfortunately, unilaterally deaf dogs exhibit little if any behavioural evidence of their defect, so affected dogs and bitches that are not BAER tested as puppies or prior to being bred will, when bred, continue to increase the prevalence of the disorder. The percentage of unilateral deafness was 73% for dalmations, 82% for ES, 84% for ACD, 85% for ECS, and 90% for BT (Table 7.3); in the absence of BAER testing these are percentages of affected animals potentially available for breeding, and hence for worsening the prevalence of deafness. In this large study there were no evident gender influences on hearing status. Although several investigators have identified a significant excess of deafness in dalmation females, this is potentially suggested to be due to the voluntary nature of hearing testing in this breed, with females being of primary interest for breeding purposes. Colour variations resulting from genes producing white demonstrated significant associations with deafness; patched dalmations were less likely to be deaf than unpatched and white BT were more likely to be deaf than coloured BT. Statistical inferences could not be made between roan and solid ECS because only one of the solid dogs was affected. Suppression of iris pigmentation by white genes was significantly associated with deafness in the dalmation, ES and ECS. Although blue eyes in the non-dalmation breeds were rare, their presence carried a high association with deafness. The findings of this study suggest a significant association between deafness and parental hearing status, supporting that deafness has a high heritability. Further work can now progress in the identification of genes responsible for deafness in dogs, which will help in reducing the prevalence of this disease by utilization of DNA testing.

Relationship among basilar artery resistance index, degree of ventriculomegaly, and clinical signs in hydrocephalic dogs

Saito M, Olby N, Spaulding K, Munana K, Sharp NJH. *Vet Rad Ultrasound* 2003; **44**(6): 687–94

BACKGROUND. Hydrocephalus accounts for 3% of the congenital anomalies diagnosed in dogs. Congenital hydrocephalus is characterized by increased CSF volume and associated dilation of the ventricular system of the brain |1|; it is usually the lateral ventricles which are dilated and this results from failure of CSF drainage. Canine congenital hydrocephalus is often asymptomatic and dilated lateral ventricles are a common incidental finding in small, toy and brachycephalic breeds. However, the dilemma that exists is that some of these dogs will have neurological signs related to the ventriculomegaly, and that this abnormality can progress causing an increase in ICP, decreased brain perfusion and subsequent tissue destruction. Currently, there is a poor correlation between the severity of clinical signs and the presence of hydrocephalus and so a need has arisen for a non-invasive test that can be used both to determine the clinical significance of hydrocephalus and for ongoing patient monitoring |26,27|. Doppler ultrasonography is a non-invasive means of assessing hydrocephalus in humans that measures systolic and diastolic blood flow velocity in specific intracranial arteries. Cerebrovascular (CV) resistance index (RI) is a measure of vascular resistance (RI = systolic velocity – diastolic velocity/systolic velocity). In humans, there is a positive relationship between RI and increasing severity of hydrocephalus, and thus provides a useful monitoring tool for this condition. In experimental dogs, RI is directly related to ICP values. The aims of this project were to: (i) assess whether degree of ventriculomegaly and/or CV RI correlate with the clinical severity of congenital hydrocephalus and/or other intracranial diseases; (ii) determine whether measurement of the degree of ventriculomegaly and/or CV RI enables identification of clinically significant congenital canine hydrocephalus; and (iii) determine whether measurement of ventriculomegaly and/or CV RI in asymptomatic dogs is predictive of future neurological deterioration. Thirty-six dogs that had clinical signs consistent with hydrocephalus or that were small breeds known to be predisposed to hydrocephalus (e.g. chihuahua) with or without signs of intracranial disease were evaluated (1999–2002). The severity of the neurological signs were scored and ultrasound was performed via a temporal window, the foramen magnum and the bregma in awake dogs or following mild sedation with diazepam if necessary. Dorsoventral measurements of the lateral ventricles and brain were made on transverse images. The ratio of the height of the ventricles to the height of the brain (VB ratio) was categorized as a percentage (<15% normal; 15–25% moderate; >25% severe). Peak systolic and end diastolic blood flow velocity in the basilar artery were measured in each dog via the foramen magnum while the heart rate was calculated from the Doppler ultrasound trace. Four groups were evaluated: (I) dogs with a normal neurological examination and no ventriculomegaly on ultrasound images; (II) dogs with ventriculomegaly with a normal neurological examination; (III) dogs with ventriculomegaly and neurological examination abnormalities; (IV) dogs with intracranial disease other than hydrocephalus and with neurological examination abnormalities. Dogs with seizures and cardiovascular disease were excluded. The mean VB ratio and RI were calculated for each group and compared using the Tukey-Kramer pairwise comparison. Sensitivity and specificity were calculated for the VB ratio and RI and a combination of both.

INTERPRETATION. Forty-four studies were performed in 36 dogs, with five dogs having more than one study. The mean age of the 15 males and 21 female dogs was 18 months (7 months–10 years). The mean body weight was 3.0 kg (0.5–21.8 kg). Of the breeds investigated there were 10 CKCS and 13 Chihuahuas. The mean RI of all the dogs was 0.68 (0.50–0.81). The VB ratio ranged from 5.5 to 80.3%. Diastolic velocity through the same Doppler waveform sequences seen in many dogs was related to heart rate; as heart rate increased, end diastolic velocity increased. A significant positive correlation was identified between the RI and the systemic blood pressure but there was no statistical difference in the mean systemic blood pressure recordings among the groups. This was the only extracranial variable found to correlate with the RI. RI was significantly increased in both Groups III and IV compared with I and II. The VB ratio was significantly increased in Group III when compared with the others and Group II when compared with Groups I and IV. There was substantial overlap in the VB ratio when Groups II and III were compared but minimal overlap in the RI of these groups. In Groups II and III, the neurological score significantly positively correlated with both the RI and the VB ratio. The majority of controls and the asymptomatic hydrocephalic dogs had RI values less than the mean, therefore values in excess of the mean could be considered abnormal, which implied a 92% sensitivity and a 63% specificity for detection of symptomatic hydrocephalus. When VB ratios of more than 28% were considered abnormal, the sensitivity and specificity for detection of symptomatic hydrocephalus was 85% and 88%, respectively; when the VB and RI factors were combined, there was a resulting 77% and 94% sensitivity and specificity for the detection of symptomatic hydrocephalus. Follow-up took place at 2–28 months later (mean = 15 months). Eight dogs with asymptomatic hydrocephalus were rechecked (five by phone consult) and two were recorded as symptomatic. The mean VB ratio of these two dogs was 65% compared with 22% in the rest; the mean RI of these two groups of dogs was the same (0.6). In all 36 dogs, those with a VB ratio >60% developed neurological signs.

Comment

Based on the results of this study, a clear relationship exists between RI and the severity of the hydrocephalus in dogs, as has been seen in humans. The calculation of this ratio is independent of the angle of insonation (which should be parallel with the direction of blood flow); it has been shown to correlate closely to the ICP in humans and dogs and has been evaluated in normal dogs prior to this study. The basilar artery is readily accessible in dogs and so this represents a diagnostic technique, which may become a practical non-invasive application. As there are no regional variations in intracranial RI, the basilar artery is the easiest vessel to evaluate in order to obtain this value. Previous reports of RI values prove that this gives tremendous interevaluator consistency |28|. In this study, basilar artery RI was significantly higher in dogs with symptomatic hydrocephalus (Group III) and with the other intracranial diseases studied (Group IV), than in the dogs without neurological signs (Group I and II).

There was overlap between Groups I and II, and Groups III and IV, but in both Groups I and II, this was the result of high RI values in a single dog. Basilar artery RI was significantly correlated to neurological status in hydrocephalic dogs, which infers that there is an increase in CV resistance in dogs with clinically significant hydrocephalus, either as a result of ICP elevations or of structural changes in the brain parenchyma. In individual dogs in which repeated measurements of RI were made over time, changes in neurological status were reflected in the RI values, whereas changes in VB ratio did not consistently occur. The authors acknowledge that the measurement of basilar artery RI was not useful for predicting whether an asymptomatic hydrocephalic dog would develop clinical signs or for differentiation of hydrocephalus from other intracranial diseases. In fact, increased RI values have been reported in many intracranial disorders, such as inflammatory disease, and so it is not a very specific test. Additionally, there are some technical problems with RI measurement, which are mainly due to the fact that RI is influenced by factors such as systolic blood pressure, heart rate, drugs that affect the cardiovascular system and/or ventilation, and underlying cardiovascular disease. In this study, there was a significant positive correlation between the VB ratio and the severity of neurological signs in the symptomatic and asymptomatic hydrocephalic dogs, which is in contrast to a previous study that reported a poor correlation between degree of ventriculomegaly and severity of neurological signs in hydrocephalic dogs [27]. This may be due to the different neurological scoring systems used in each study, and so one should use caution in interpreting whether the VB ratio correlates with the presence of neurological deficits, or the actual degree of the deficits. However, the VB ratio is a useful tool to help differentiate symptomatic hydrocephalus from other intracranial diseases in dogs with elevated RI.

Intervertebral disc disease (IVDD)

The diagnosis and treatment of IVDD are very controversial topics in veterinary medicine. Direct comparisons of study results for diagnostic and treatment modalities are difficult because of the variability of neurological dysfunction, duration of clinical signs and lack of long-term follow-up studies. The outcome for an individual patient can be dependent on a multitude of different factors, not all of which we can control for, and hence the prognostication for an individual can be difficult. An owner's decision to pursue therapy may be solely based upon such prognostic advice and so we desperately need continued investigation into this area and more in the way of long-term studies. The two studies reviewed below are important on account of the high number of dogs included as well as the long-term follow-up. Both studies address extremely important issues relating to IVDD; the first paper assists in the decision-making process for large breed dogs with acute onset and often debilitating disc disease; the second paper investigates the prognosis for patients with paraplegia and loss of deep pain perception (DPP).

A retrospective comparison of cervical intervertebral disk disease in nonchondrodystrophic large dogs versus small dogs

Cherrone KL, Dewey CW, Coates JR, Bergman RL. *J Am Anim Hosp* Assoc 2004; **40**: 316–20

BACKGROUND. Cervical disc disease accounts for approximately 15% of all intervertebral disc extrusions, with dachshunds, beagles and poodles accounting for approximately 80% of the cases |29|. Hansen Type I and II disc disease occurs in the neck but Type I is more common. The amount of disc that extrudes, the force of the extrusion or protrusion and the duration of the compression all contribute to the severity of neurological deficits |30|. Older non-chondrodystrophoid breeds are classically described as having slowly progressive, Hansen Type II disc disease but they do get Type I disease as well, although this has not been previously evaluated in the literature. The purpose of this study was to compare the historical and clinical features of two sizes of dogs (<15 and >15 kg) with Hansen Type I cervical disc extrusion. Generally, the authors wanted to assess any differences in presentation and outcome in the two sizes of dogs after acute disc extrusion; the <15 kg group broadly represented chondrodystrophoid dogs and the >15 kg group broadly represented non-chondrodystrophoid dogs. The medical records of 190 dogs with surgically confirmed Hansen Type I cervical intervertebral disc extrusion (1998–2002) were reviewed. The information recorded included: signalment; body weight; pre-surgical clinical signs; onset and duration of clinical signs; type of diagnostic imaging performed; type of surgery performed; and post-operative neurological status. The specific location of the disc extrusion was identified at surgery or autopsy. The distinguishing criterion between Hansen Type I or II lesions was the presence or absence of apparent extruded disc material in the vertebral canal at surgery or necropsy. Dogs with dynamic compressive lesions were excluded from the study. Acute onset was defined as less than 24 h; chronic onset was defined as more than 24 h. Recovery time was classed as the time from surgery until unassisted ambulation or resolution of pain. Follow-up was performed by direct physical examination, telephone conversation, written questionnaire or all three. Outcome was classed as successful if the dog regained or retained its ability to ambulate unassisted post-surgery and was free of cervical spinal hyperaesthesia. Recurrence of any clinical signs was recorded.

INTERPRETATION. Complete information was available for 190 dogs; 24% (46 of 190) of the cases were larger, non-chondrodystrophic dogs, with 16 different breeds represented in this category (Labrador retrievers accounted for 20% of all large breed dogs, with rottweilers and German shepherd dogs each accounting for 13%). Seventy-six per cent (144 of 190) of the dogs were small, chondrodystrophic dogs (dachshunds accounted for 36% of all small dogs). The characteristics of all dogs, specifically the small and large breed dogs, are represented in Table 7.4.

Table 7.4 Summary of the data where available of dogs with Hansen Type I cervical intervertebral disc disease

Clinical parameters	All dogs	Large dogs (>15 kg)	Small dogs (<15 kg)
Speed of onset			
Acute	45%	43%	46%
Chronic	55%	57%	54%
Spinal hyperaesthesia	87%	80%	90%
Pain as only sign	33%	24%	36%
Nerve root signature	8%	13%	7%
Tetraparetic/ambulatory	42%	30%	46%
Tetraparetic/non-ambulatory	22%	39%	16%
Tetraplegic	3%	7%	2%
Disc space affected			
Most common	C2–C3	C6–C7	C2–C3
2nd most common	C3–C4	C3–C4	C3–C4
Mean time to ambulation (days)			
Non-ambulatory pre-surgery	6	7	4.5
Acute onset	5		
Chronic onset	4		
Recurrence of pain	10%	13%	8%
Mean time to recurrence (days)	91	49	112
Second surgery necessary	4%	8.7%	2.1%

Source: Cherrone *et al*. (2004).

Comment

In the study reported here, Type I cervical IVDD is reported in 46 medium to large non-chondrodystrophic dogs; this is a group of dogs not previously described with Type I disease and this study additionally compares them with the more 'classic' syndrome of Type I disease seen in small chondrodystrophic breeds. Previously it has been suggested that cervical disc disease in large breed dogs usually occurs from a Hansen Type II protrusion in the caudal cervical spine |**31**|. Additionally, the doberman pinscher is the main non-chondrodystrophic breed described to be affected by cervical disc disease, and this is associated with cervical spondylomyelopathy. Although no general comparison with the incidence of hospital admissions for this breed was made, only three of the 46 large dogs were dobermans. This low number may also be because dogs with dynamic compressive lesions were excluded from the study. No dog of either group was less than 2 years of age, which implies that other differentials should be investigated in young dogs with neck pain and/or tetraparesis. The most common clinical sign in this study was cervical spinal hyperaesthesia; the reason for this is likely to be related to the greater diameter of the cervical vertebral canal; however, the location of extruded disc fragments within the vertebral canal is the most important factor in determining whether affected dogs have pain or tetraparesis |**30**|. The data in this study suggest, perhaps surprisingly, that the majority of clinical parameters assessed were similar in both groups of dogs. The notable differences included the finding that nearly 40% of large dogs presented non-ambulatory compared with 16% of small dogs and additionally the fact that the most common disc affected in large dogs was C6–C7 whereas it was C2–C3 in small dogs. Previous studies have suggested that dogs with caudal cervical disc extrusions respond less favourably and are more severely affected than dogs with cranial cervical disc extrusions |31|. However, this was not the case in this study, which demonstrated that outcomes were no different. As long as DPP was present, the outcomes were good and no different between ambulatory and non-ambulatory dogs. Success of surgical therapies in dogs with disc disease is a difficult factor to evaluate as ability to walk is not always sufficient for owners and normality may be their objective. To truly evaluate the success of therapy, a more structured and stratified neurological examination scale would be needed. Although, the onset and duration of disease were included in the parameters measured, there was no notable effect on outcome, which is slightly different from other studies |31|. It would be difficult to truly evaluate the effect of duration of disease in this study as the dogs were divided into <24-h duration and >24 h. The latter group evidently could compare dogs with a 24-h duration and a 10-day duration, but the pathophysiology of the disease would have changed by this time. Also, the onset of disease can be complicated in large dogs as acute signs could follow chronic intermittent signs implying that onset of signs is a different parameter to onset of disease. Ten per cent of dogs in this study had recurrence of spinal pain, lower than that reported in previous studies (33%) |29|, and it was more often at a different site from the initial lesion. The prophylactic use of fenestration was not discussed or evaluated. More large dogs than small dogs required a second surgery, but with small numbers no inferences can be made about this fact.

Long-term functional outcome of dogs with severe injuries of the thoracolumbar spinal cord: 87 cases (1996–2001)

Olby N, Levine J, Harris T, Munana K, Skeen T, Sharp N. *J Am Vet Med Assoc* 2003; **222**(6): 762–9

BACKGROUND. Dogs with spinal cord injuries resulting from intervertebral disc herniation or vertebral fracture that result in complete functional transection of the cord are considered to have an extremely grave prognosis for return of hind-limb function. This is in contrast to the prognosis for those dogs without a functional transection of the spinal cord. At present this degree of injury is judged based on the subjective assessment of the dog's DPP in the pelvic limbs. However, the absence of DPP does not help us assess whether the injury is permanent or not. The lack of DPP is accepted to be a poor prognostic indicator; approximately 25–76% of dogs with IVDD and less than 10% of dogs with a spinal fracture, all with loss of DPP, are expected to recover |31,32|. Therefore, the outcome for individual patients is difficult to predict and the advice that can be given to owners is limited. Two studies addressing this issue have separately demonstrated (i) that the speed of onset of clinical signs was related to outcome, with a peracute onset of clinical signs being associated with a worse outcome, and that (ii) the amount of spinal cord swelling evident on a myelogram correlated with outcome |31|. Both studies were limited in numbers and the question about which factors are associated with speed of recovery in dogs which regain motor function still remains. The present study evaluated the long-term outcome and secondary health problems of paraplegic dogs that had lost hind-limb DPP as a result of traumatic injury or intervertebral disc herniation and evaluated factors potentially associated with recovery of function. The specific aims were to: (i) determine the long-term (>6 months) outcome of dogs with paraplegia and loss of DPP due to IVDD or spinal cord trauma; (ii) identify factors associated with recovery of pelvic limb function and speed of recovery of pelvic limb function; and (iii) determine the incidence of long-term health problems (i.e. urinary and faecal incontinence, urinary tract infection, and recurrence of signs of pain and pelvic limb paresis). Dogs with acute onset of paraplegia and no DPP, due to IVDD or trauma were retrospectively evaluated (1996–2001). Dogs were only included in the study if a complete work-up, including a serum biochemical panel, a CBC, CSF analysis, and computed tomography of the spine or thoracolumbar myelography had been performed and if there was a documented follow-up (>6 months). Dogs with spinal trauma had at least a minimum work-up that included a serum biochemical panel, a CBC, and plain spinal radiographs. Dogs with IVDD had their onset of signs classed as peracute (<1 h), acute (1–24 h) or gradual (>24 h). Duration of disease prior to surgery was classed as <12 h, 12–24 h, 24–48 h or >48 h. All dogs with IVDD underwent hemilaminectomy while dogs with spinal trauma underwent a conservative or surgical treatment regimen. Dogs in both groups were classed as: (i) euthanized at the time of the initial examination; (ii) euthanized within 1 month after the initial examination; (iii) having recovered DPP; or (iv) as having never recovered DPP despite being maintained by the owners for at least 2 months after initial examination. The reason for and timing of euthanasia was reported where applicable. Time (1 week; 1–2 weeks; 2–4 weeks, or >4 weeks) after injury for recovery of DPP and for return of the ability to walk without support and without falling was also recorded. Outcome was classified as successful if the dog regained DPP and the ability to walk without support or falling, or unsuccessful if the dog did not regain DPP or the ability to walk unaided. Additionally, any dogs that regained the ability to walk without support or falling but with persistent DPP absence, were documented, and classed for statistical purposes as unsuccessful if due to IVDD and successful if due to trauma. The two aetiological groups were separately evaluated. The association between the various individual variables and recovery of the ability to walk was evaluated by use of logistic regression. Odds ratios significantly >1 were considered indicative of an association with recovery of the ability to walk.

INTERPRETATION. Eighty-seven dogs were evaluated (70 with IVDD and 17 with traumatic injury). Nine of the 17 dogs with trauma were treated medically ($n = 6$) or surgically ($n = 3$); none recovered DPP but two were able to walk after 2 and 6 months, with intermittent faecal and urinary incontinence. Sixty-four of the 70 dogs with IVDD were treated surgically (the others were euthanized at presentation); seven (11%) were euthanized within a week of the surgery because of the clinical signs of myelomalacia. Thirty-seven (58%) regained DPP and the ability to walk; 41% regained DPP within 1 week after surgery,

14 (38%) regained DPP during the second week after surgery, seven (19%) regained DPP during the third or fourth week after surgery and one dog (3%) regained DPP 36 weeks after surgery. The mean time to regain the ability to walk was 7.5 weeks; however, 62% (23 of 37) were walking within 4 weeks after surgery. Fifteen of the 37 (41%) dogs that regained DPP and the ability to walk had intermittent faecal incontinence but this was infrequent in 11 of these dogs. Twelve of the 37 (32%) dogs that regained DPP and the ability to walk had mild urinary incontinence; nine of the 37 (24%) had a urinary tract infection during the 3 months after surgery, and two (5%) had recurrent urinary tract infections. Eighteen dogs (28%) did not regain DPP. Four of these dogs were euthanized (2–36 months) after the injury; seven of the remaining dogs regained the ability to walk despite a lack of DPP (mean time was 37.6 weeks; 16–72 weeks). Overall, a successful outcome was obtained in 44 of 64 (69%) dogs with IVDD that underwent surgery, although only 37 of the 64 (58%) dogs regained DPP. None of the factors evaluated were associated with whether dogs would regain the ability to walk again, but in dogs that regained DPP and the ability to walk, both age and weight were significantly associated with time required to walk again; dogs less than 3 years of age and 5 kg in body weight were able to walk within a shorter time period than older dogs and dogs over 10 kg in body weight respectively. Finally, it was clear from the results that dogs with IVDD had a significantly better outcome than dogs with traumatic spinal cord injuries.

Comment

This is an extremely important study that indicates that dogs with paraplegia and loss of DPP due to traumatic spinal cord injury have a grave prognosis for recovery of motor function when compared with similarly affected dogs with IVDD. This may imply that these dogs are more likely to have a structural transection associated with accompanying fractures and luxations. For those dogs that recovered motor function without recovery of DPP, possible explanations include (i) the development of spinal reflex walking due to local spinal circuit function, or (ii) survival of axons crossing the injury site especially following severe damage to the central cord and its grey matter, which may spare peripheral subpial descending axons. Therefore, although the loss of DPP is a sign of severe spinal cord injury, it should not be taken as evidence of complete structural cord transection. This would imply a future role for electrophysiological studies in determining whether descending impulses can traverse an injury site. Based on this study and a previous investigation, it seems that approximately 10% of dogs with paraplegia and loss of DPP may experience progressive neurological deterioration due to myelomalacia. The authors state (based on the variable published results on recovery of function following loss of DPP) that this group of dogs is probably incorrectly assigned to the same group and that a critical revision of the neurological grading scale may assist in more accurate prognoses. Based on this study, it may not be possible to utilize the speed of onset and duration of disease to make a prognostic assessment in paraplegic dogs with no DPP, as has been demonstrated in a previous study. Therefore, an immediate surgical decompression of the cord cannot be justified but intuitively one would still suggest the sooner the cord is decompressed, the more ideal will be the recovery. Certainly dogs with this severe neurological compromise should be given enough time to demonstrate a chance of recovery, but the loss of DPP for greater than a month after surgery implies that recovery of function is unlikely. Long-term follow-up of the 18 dogs with IVDD that had persistent paraplegia with no DPP, revealed that, although none of them regained DPP, seven regained the ability to walk over a mean time of 37.6 weeks; all of these dogs, however, had long-term problems with urinary and faecal incontinence. This finding highlights the fact that persistent absence of DPP does not necessarily indicate that a dog will be persistently paraplegic; the development of a voluntary tail wag was a useful early prognostic sign for recovery of voluntary function in these dogs. The problems of incontinence will be unacceptable to many owners; even with successful recovery after the loss of DPP, 40% of dogs will experience faecal incontinence and 32% will experience mild urinary incontinence. A quarter of the successfully recovered dogs will also experience a urinary tract infection within the first 3 months after surgery; this is evidently better than the group of dogs that failed to regain DPP, with all of the group having recurrent urinary tract infections.

Conclusion

It is impossible in one chapter to address all of the subject areas that have been investigated over the last year in veterinary neurology; however, the papers reviewed above attempt to cover several important ones and some emerging ones, which include IVDD, epilepsy, congenital or inheritable disease, and feline intracranial disease. Despite recent and profound advancements in the use of advanced diagnostic modalities, the decision-making process when faced with a veterinary neurology case should still be based upon a thorough neurological examination and an incisive history. All recent studies aim to provide a piece of an evidence-based 'jigsaw', which should be utilized to assist with diagnostic interpretation, treatment choices and prognostication. The above papers were chosen because they each result in an advancement of the clinical understanding of their respective subject areas, but also serve as another step in the direction to more proficient neurological case handling.

References

1. Braund KG. *Clinical Neurology in Small Animals: Localization, Diagnosis and Treatment*, 2003; http://www.ivis.org/special_books/Braund/toc.asp
2. Vandevelde M. Brain tumors in domestic animals: an overview. In: *Proceedings: Brain Tumors in Man and Animals*. Research Triangle Park, North Carolina USA: National Institute of Environmental Sciences, 1984.

3. Nafe LA. Meningiomas in cats: a retrospective clinical study of 36 cases. *J Am Vet Med Assoc* 1979; **174**: 1224–7.

4. Engle GC, Brodey RS. A retrospective study of 395 feline neoplasms. *J Am Anim Hosp Assoc* 1969; **5**: 21–5.

5. Zaki FA, Hurvitz AI. Spontaneous neoplasms of the central nervous system of the cat. *J Small Anim Pract* 1976; **17**: 773–82.

6. Braund KG. *Clinical Syndromes in Veterinary Neurology*, 2nd edn. St Louis, MO: Mosby, 1994.

7. McGrath JT. Meningiomas in animals. *J Neuropathol Exp Neurol* 1962; **21**: 327–32.

8. Haskins ME, McGrath JT. Meningiomas in young cats with mucopolysaccharidosis. *J Neuropathol Exp Neurol* 1983; **42**: 664–70.

9. Heidner GL, Kornegay JN, Page RL, Dodge RK, Thrall DE. Analysis of survival in a retrospective study of 86 dogs with brain tumors. *J Vet Int Med* 1991; **5**: 219–26.

10. Bagley RS, Gavin PR, Moore MP, Silver GM, Harrington ML, Connors RL. Clinical signs associated with brain tumors in dogs: 97 cases (1992–1997). *J Am Vet Med Assoc* 1999; **215**: 818–19.

11. Bailey CS, Higgins RJ. Characteristics of cisternal cerebrospinal fluid associated with primary brain tumors in the dog: A retrospective study. *J Am Vet Med Assoc* 1986; **188**: 414–17.

12. Gordon LE, Thacher C, Matthiesen DT, Joseph RJ. Results of craniotomy for the treatment of cerebral meningioma in 42 cats. *Vet Surg* 1994; **23**: 94–100.

13. Gallagher JG, Berg J, Knowles KE, Williams LL, Bronson RT . Prognosis after surgical excision of cerebral meningiomas in cats: 17 cases (1986–1992). *J Am Vet Med Assoc* 1993; **203**: 1437–40.

14. Kaser-Hotz B, Rohrer CR, Stankeova S, Wergin M, Fidel J, Reusch C. Radiotherapy of pituitary tumors in five cats. *J Small Anim Pract* 2002; **43**: 303–7.

15. Thomas WB, Wheeler SJ, Kramer R. Magnetic resonance imaging features of primary brain tumors in dogs. *Vet Radiol Ultrasound* 1996; **37**: 20–7.

16. Reader JC, Stenseth LB. Ketamine: A new look at an old drug. *Curr Opin Anaesth* 2000; **13**: 463–8.

17. Walker RM, DiFonzo CJ Barsoum NJ, Smith GS, Macallum GE. Chronic toxicity of the anticonvulsant zonisamide in beagle dogs. *Fund Appl Toxicology* 1998; **11**: 333–42.

18. Sherwin AL. Neuroactive amino acids in focally epileptic human brain: a review. *Neurochem Res* 1999; **24**: 1387–95.

19. Loscher W, Schwartx-Porsche D. Low levels of gamma-aminobutyric acid in cerebrospinal fluid of dogs with epilepsy. *J Neurochem* 1986; **46**: 1322–5.

20. Podell M, Hadjiconstantinou M. Cerebrospinal fluid gamma-aminobutyric acid and glutamate values in dogs with epilepsy. *Am J Vet Res* 1997; **58**: 451–6.

21. Araki K, Harada M, Ueda Y, Takino T, Kuriyama K. Alteration of amino acid content of cerebrospinal fluid from patients with epilepsy. *Acta Neurol Scand* 1988; **78**: 473–9.

22. Milhorat TH, Chou MW, Trinidad EM, Kula RW, Mandell M, Wolpert C, Speer MC. Chiari I malformation redefined: clinical and radiographic findings for 364 symptomatic patients. *Neurosurgery* 1999; **44**: 1005–17.

23. Rusbridge C, MacSweeny JE, Davies JV, Chandler K, Fitzmaurice SN, Dennis R, Cappello R, Wheeler SJ. Syringohydromyelia in Cavalier King Charles spaniels. *J Am Anim Hosp Assoc* 2000; **36**: 34–41.

24. Sponenberg DP, Rothschild MF. Genetics of coat colour and hair texture. In: Ruvinsky A, Sampson J (eds). *The Genetics of the Dog*. Wallingford: CABI Publishing, 2001; pp 61–85.

25. Strain GM, Kearney MT, Gignac IJ, Levesque DC, Nelson HJ, Tedford BL, Remsen LG. Brainstem auditory evoked potential assessment of congenital deafness in Dalmations: associations with phenotypic markers. *J Vet Int Med* 1992; **6**: 175–82.

26. Spaulding KA, Sharp NJH. Ultrasonographic imaging of the lateral cerebral ventricles in the dog. *Vet Radiol* 1990; **31**: 59–64.

27. Hudson JA, Simpson ST, Buxton DF, Cartee RE, Steiss JE. Ultrasonographic diagnosis of canine hydrocephalus. *Vet Radiol* 1990; **31**: 50–8.

28. Hudson JA, Buxton DF, Cox NR, Finn-Bodner ST, Simpson ST, Wright JC, Takino T, Kuriyama K. Color flow Doppler imaging and Doppler spectral analysis of the brain of neonatal dogs. *Vet Radiol Ultrasound* 1997; **38**: 313–22.

29. Toombs JP. Cervical intervertebral disc disease in dogs. *Compend Contin Educ Pract Vet* 1992; **14**: 1477–86.

30. Seim HB. Surgery of the cervical spine. In: Fossum T (ed). *Small Animal Surgery*. Philadelphia, PA: Mosby, 2002; pp 1228–37.

31. Coates JR. Intervertebral disc disease. *Vet Clin North Am Small Anim Pract* 2000; **30**(1): 77–110.

32. Bagley RS. Spinal fracture or luxation. *Vet Clin North Am Small Anim Pract* 2000; **30**: 133–53.

8

Soft tissue surgery

JONATHAN BRAY

Introduction

The discipline of soft tissue surgery typically covers a diverse range of disease processes and organ systems. The literature this year has been peppered with a variety of interesting case reports and novel approaches to existing problems. It has proved difficult to select a representation for this chapter, but the author has chosen to present eleven papers which have resulted in a modification to his existing clinical practice or approach.

For this chapter, we will first examine recent papers on two neoplastic diseases where existing theories about treatment or conventional management have been challenged. Next, we will outline the latest advances in the treatments for two diseases for which consistently successful management has proven elusive. Then, the progress in minimally invasive therapy for two conditions where conventional surgery is challenging or technically demanding will be reviewed. Finally, we will review three isolated papers that examine some additional problems that may confront the soft tissue surgeon.

Apocrine gland adenocarcinoma

Canine anal sac adenocarcinoma is a relatively uncommon tumour. Textbook descriptions suggest the tumour is more common in old, ovariohysterectomized dogs |1|. It is also suggested that paraneoplastic hypercalcaemia is a common occurrence, and that the overall prognosis is poor. However, this knowledge is based on the results of a few small case series, and is often at odds with actual clinical experience. These two papers, one from the USA, the other from the UK, represent the largest case series reported for anal sac adenocarcinoma, and significantly alter our current understanding about the behaviour and prognosis of this tumour.

Carcinoma of the apocrine glands of the anal sac in dogs: 113 cases (1985–1995)
Williams LE, Gliatto JM, Dodge RK, et al. J Am Vet Med Assoc 2003; **223**: 825–31

B A C K G R O U N D . Apocrine gland adenocarcinoma is recognized as an aggressive and highly malignant neoplasm affecting the anal sac of both male and female dogs. This retrospective study reviewed the signalment, clinical signs, biological behaviour and clinical response to various treatments in 113 cases. Treatments included surgery alone, radiation therapy alone, chemotherapy alone, local therapy only (surgery, radiotherapy or a combination) and combination therapy.

INTERPRETATION. A roughly equal sex distribution was identified. Perianal swelling, faecal tenesmus or signs of perineal irritation were common presenting signs for dogs with tumour. Polyuria/polydipsia was inconsistently reported in animals with paraneoplastic hypercalcaemia, which itself occurred in only 27% of dogs. However, hypercalcaemia was a negative prognostic indicator with significantly reduced survival times evident in patients where it occurred (256 days median survival time [MST]). Iliac lymphadenopathy due to metastasis was a common finding (47%) yet did not appear to influence survival times. Pulmonary metastases were less common (8%) and their presence was reflected in reduced survival times (219 days MST). One hundred and four dogs underwent treatment consisting of surgery, radiation therapy, chemotherapy or multimodal therapy. The MST for all treated dogs was 544 days (range 0–1873 days) (Table 8.1). Surgical management was an important factor in improving patient survival (548 days MST compared with 402 days MST without surgery). Multimodality therapy (surgery, radiation, chemotherapy) appeared to provide optimal patient outcomes (742 days MST), although this finding was not significant. The study suggests that with aggressive management, this tumour may carry a more favourable prognosis than previously considered.

Table 8.1 Survival probabilities for 104 dogs treated for carcinoma of the anal sac

Treatment (No. of dogs)	Survival probability (95% confidence interval)				Median (d)	P value
	6 months	1 year	2 years	3 years		
Surgery alone (31)	0.90 (0.77, 1.00)	0.65 (0.43, 0.88)	0.29 (0.06, 0.53)	—	500	0.936
Radiation therapy alone (10)	0.85 (0.61, 1.00)	0.79 (0.52, 1.00)	0.38 (0.04, 0.74)	—	657	0.822
Local therapy alone (43)	0.91 (0.81, 1.00)	0.76 (0.60, 0.92)	0.37 (0.17, 0.57)	0.23 (0.06, 0.41)	544	0.999
Chemotherapy alone (11)	0.67 (0.35, 0.00)	—	—	—	212	<0.001
Surgery and chemotherapy (35)	0.86 (0.73, 0.99)	0.69 (0.50, 0.87)	0.36 (0.12, 0.59)	0.14 (0.00, 0.32)	540	0.964
Surgery, radiation, and chemotherapy (15)	0.86 (0.68, 1.00)	0.80 (0.59, 1.00)	0.56 (0.27, 0.85)	0.35 (0.05, 0.66)	742	0.098
Any surgery (81)	0.87 (0.79, 0.96)	0.72 (0.60, 0.84)	0.39 (0.25, 0.54)	0.28 (0.14, 0.42)	548	0.0495
Any radiation therapy (27)	0.88 (0.76, 1.00)	0.84 (0.69, 0.98)	0.48 (0.26, 0.70)	0.24 (0.04, 0.44)	719	0.164
Any chemotherapy (61)	0.85 (0.75, 0.95)	0.65 (0.51, 0.79)	0.38 (0.22, 0.55)	0.19 (0.05, 0.34)	539	0.999

—, no survivors
Source: Williams et al. (2003).

Anal sac adenocarcinoma in the dog—a series of 80 clinical cases

Polton GA, Brearley MJ. Scientific Abstracts, 47th Annual BSAVA Congress Proceedings, 2004; 563

BACKGROUND. This retrospective study described the signalment, clinical signs, treatment and clinical outcome of 80 cases with apocrine gland adenocarcinoma. Clinical records at Davies White Veterinary Specialists and the Animal Health Trust between 1996 and 2003 were reviewed. Survival analyses were performed using the Kaplan–Meier Product Limit estimation method, log-rank testing and Cox's Proportional Hazards estimations.

INTERPRETATION. An equal male/female incidence of tumour was identified, with a median age of presentation of 11.5 years. An increased risk of developing anal sac adenocarcinoma in cocker spaniels and in neutered animals was recognized. Common clinical signs included the presence of a perianal mass, perianal irritation, faecal tenesmus and polyuria/polydipsia. Paraneoplastic hypercalcaemia remained an inconsistent feature of the tumour, being reported in only 20% of patients in this study. Importantly, the tumour was an incidental finding in 40% of cases. A range of therapeutic interventions was used including surgery for the primary and/or secondary tumours, radiotherapy of the primary tumour site and chemotherapy using carboplatin or epirubicin. The MST for all patients was 537 days. Patients without metastases fared significantly better (MST 1229 days). The presence of regional nodal metastases reduced survival times by 75% (MST 334 days); the presence of distant metastases to the lung was a poor indicator of long-term survival (MST 107 days). Aggressive multimodality management (comprising surgery to remove primary and nodal metastases, radiotherapy to the primary tumour bed and chemotherapy) resulted in favourable outcomes, particularly where the tumour was confined to the primary site.

Comment

The results of these two large case series share similar themes and outcomes, and thus will be reviewed together. Together, they have provided a considerable shift in our previous understanding of anal sac tumours. Previously considered to be a tumour that occurred almost exclusively in the female dog, it now appears that the tumour will affect male and female dogs in equal numbers. The tumours may also develop to a significant size in some animals (>10 cm^2), causing perianal swelling that is evident to the owners. However, in 50% of cases, the tumours may not be detected without a rectal examination. Signs of perianal irritation (scooting the anus along the ground, or licking about the perineum) may be evident in some dogs. Occult anal sac tumour may occur in some animals, with clinical signs relating to a paraneoplastic hypercalcaemia, or due to the effect of iliac lymphadenopathy on faecal passage (tenesmus). Importantly, hypercalcaemia may occur in only about a quarter of neoplasms, and specific clinical signs (polyuria/polydipsia) may only be present in a proportion of these. Nevertheless, because hypercalcaemia was shown to be a significant predictor of reduced survival time, specific biochemical analysis should be an essential component of clinical investigation.

Apocrine gland adenocarcinoma remains a highly metastatic tumour. Lymphadenopathy of the iliac lymph nodes (likely due to metastasis) is common (47%) while more distant metastases (to lung, liver, etc.) are less common (8%). Interestingly, the presence of iliac lymphadenopathy did not appear to negatively influence patient survival in one paper, although the presence of more distant metastases (e.g. lung) was a consistently poor prognostic finding. Radiographs of the thorax and abdomen, in conjunction with abdominal ultrasonography, should therefore be performed in all animals to detect the presence of distant metastases. Despite their proximity to the aortic bifurcation, removal of enlarged iliac lymph nodes can usually be accomplished without difficulty in most patients, and may be an important element of management in patients where faecal tenesmus is a feature of their disease. Repeated metastatectomy for recurrent enlargements of iliac lymph nodes may be useful to prolong survival in some individuals (Pers. Comm., Polton G, 2004).

Apocrine gland adenocarcinoma was previously considered to carry a poor prognosis, with MSTs of only 6–8.3 months. Although apocrine gland adenocarcinoma is certainly an aggressive disease, the results of both studies would suggest that good survival is possible when aggressive multimodality treatment is applied. However, because this was a retrospective study, the use of specific treatments was not standardized across patients. The use (or disuse) of specific treatments in an individual would therefore have been influenced by a variety of factors, including the perceived impact of overall disease burden on outcome, the personal bias of the clinician, owner and financial issues. Nevertheless, optimal survival appears to be seen in animals treated with a combination of surgery (local tumour excision ± metastatectomy), radiotherapy (treatment of the local tumour wound bed), and chemotherapy, although these data were not statistically significant in this study. The role of surgery is important, as dogs treated with chemotherapy alone had a significantly poorer outcome than those where surgery or radiotherapy was utilized concurrently.

Margins for mast cell tumour resection

Mast cell tumours are the most common cutaneous neoplasm of the dog, accounting for between 7 and 21% of all tumours [2]. Mast cell tumours are more common in the older dog (mean age: 9 years). Some dog breeds have an increased incidence of tumour occurrence, including the English bull terrier, boxers, Boston terriers, Labradors, beagles and schnauzers. No sex predilection is reported.

In the dog, mast cell tumours typically have a cutaneous distribution, with visceral disease occurring secondarily. Systemic mastocytosis is rare. Cutaneous mast cell tumours most frequently occur on the trunk (50%), with the remainder on the extremities (40%) and head (10%).

For discrete mast cell tumours, the treatment of choice is wide surgical excision. It is recommended that a 3 cm margin of surrounding normal tissue should be removed, together with an extensive deep margin |2|. However, this clinical dictum has been questioned by a recent paper that observed no difference in survival times in dogs with 'tumour-free' and 'non-tumour-free' margins |3|. Although this finding was considered to be due to a small sample size, the results of the two papers presented here remain consistent with this observation.

Relationships between the histological grade of cutaneous mast cell tumours in dogs, their survival and the efficacy of surgical resection

Murphy S, Sparkes AH, Smith KC, Blunden AS, Brearley MJ. *Vet Rec* 2004; **154**: 743–6

BACKGROUND. The records of mast cell tumours diagnosed in tissue submitted by veterinary practices to a central diagnostic laboratory were evaluated. The tumours were graded according to the system of Patnaik, and margins evaluated. Margins were classified as incomplete, narrow (tumour-free margins less than 5 mm) or complete (tumour-free margin more than 5 mm). The original submitting practice was then contacted by telephone for additional information, in particular for evidence of tumour recurrence and survival times of the dogs.

INTERPRETATION. The histological grade of 340 cutaneous mast cell tumours derived from 280 dogs was determined; 87 of the tumours (26%) were well differentiated, 199 (59%) were intermediately differentiated and 54 (16%) were poorly differentiated. The histological grade of the tumour influenced the likelihood of recurrence more than the histological assessment of whether a resection was 'complete' or 'incomplete'. Dogs with high-grade tumours (poorly differentiated) had poor outcomes, with a high rate of recurrence (19%) and significantly shorter MST (278 days vs over 1300 days for other tumour types) (Fig. 8.1). Tumour regrowth was reported in only 8% of cases, despite more than 58% of resections being classified as narrow or incomplete. The results suggested that wide surgical margins are not a prerequisite for a successful long-term outcome in dogs with well-differentiated cutaneous mast cell tumours.

Comment

This paper is the largest retrospective study of canine cutaneous mast cell tumours to be published in the UK, and provides 3-year follow-up data on 340 cutaneous mast cell tumours resected from 280 dogs. No control was placed on the extent of the initial surgery or subsequent management of the patient following diagnosis, thus this paper attempted to represent the efficacy of tumour management within a first-opinion practice setting. Excisional biopsy was the treatment of choice in the majority (96%) of patients, with pre-operative fine needle aspiration performed in only a minority (14%) of these patients. As the diagnosis of the mass would have been unknown to the surgeon in the majority of cases, it is presumed that 'textbook' 3 cm margins may not have been obtained about the mass in all cases. Indeed, 'complete'

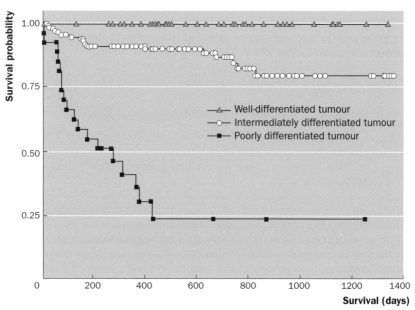

Fig. 8.1 Kaplan–Meier survival plot for the dogs with the three grades of mast cell tumour. Source: Murphy *et al.* (2004).

margins were obtained in only 42% of surgeries; 'narrow' or 'incomplete' margins were obtained in the remainder (19% and 39%, respectively).

In this paper, tumour regrowth was reported in only 8% of cases, despite more than 58% of resections being classified as narrow or incomplete. Adjunctive therapy following detection of an incomplete resection was only rarely applied in this study, suggesting that margin assessment does not necessarily correlate with potential recurrence. The status of the apparent tumour margin is therefore of some interest. The potential role of the immune system in clearing residual disease following surgery is discussed in the paper, as is the possibility that 'normal' mast cells are simply being recruited about the periphery of a tumour as a result of cytokine activity, thus increasing its apparent bulk. Because it is impossible to differentiate 'normal' mast cells from well-differentiated neoplastic cells, this may serve to explain the discrepancy in margin assessment and ultimate tumour regrowth in these tumour grades.

This was a retrospective paper, with poor control of a several crucial elements (e.g. precise treatment details, post-operative management, adjunctive treatment, detailed clinical examination) and a heavy reliance on telephone follow-up and owner interpretation of outcome. Significantly, follow-up data were not available for 30% of the original tumour submissions. This lack of follow-up data may have occurred because the owner chose to take their animal to a different practice, the animal was euthanized, or as a result of poor record keeping or archiving. Regardless of the cause, this 'lost' information may potentially affect the survival data and conclusions of this study.

Based on the available results, however, tumour grade appears more closely correlated with recurrence, with poorly differentiated tumours more likely to recur. Incisional biopsy prior to surgical resection of tumours, particularly those located in 'difficult to excise' regions, should allow the clinician to determine an optimal resection margin.

Evaluation of surgical margins required for complete excision of cutaneous mast cell tumors in dogs
Simpson AM, Ludwig LL, Newman SJ, Bergman PJ, Hottinger HA, Patnaik AK.
J Am Vet Med Assoc 2004; **224**: 236–40

BACKGROUND. This paper examined whether the accepted convention of including a 3 cm margin of normal tissue around a mast cell tumour is valid. Tumours were obtained from 21 client-owned dogs. After preparation for surgery, the skin around the tumour was marked at 1, 2 and 3 cm intervals from the tumour edge at 0°, 90°, 180° and 270°. After resection, which included a deep fascial plane, the tumour was graded and sections of tissue at each mark were examined histologically for neoplastic mast cells.

INTERPRETATION. There were three (13%) Grade I and 20 (87%) Grade II tumours. This paper suggests that all Grade I tumours can potentially be completely excised with 1 cm lateral margins. Seventy-five per cent of Grade II tumours can be completely excised with 1 cm margins, and 100% completely excised with 2 cm margins. A deep fascial plane must be included in all cases.

Comment

This paper challenged the conventional dictum that all mast cell tumours must be excised with a minimum 3 cm lateral margin of normal skin. This management can result in a significantly large defect, often requiring extensive reconstruction and associated patient morbidity. Quite how this '3 cm rule' became established within surgical oncology tenets is not clear, as the original literature citation cannot be identified.

By closely examining the tissues at 1 cm intervals about the circumference of the tumour, it was demonstrated that tumour does not extend beyond a 2 cm radius, even in spite of the original tumour size. Complete resection of these tumours could therefore have been obtained with 2 cm margins, which would have reduced the surgical morbidity considerably.

The results of this paper suggest that accurate histological grading by incisional biopsy prior to definitive treatment of a mast cell tumour is essential to permit accurate appraisal of surgical options. For Grade I tumours, excellent surgical outcome should be expected for a resection with 1–2 cm margins, including a deep fascial plane. For Grade II tumours, a wider 2 cm lateral margin would be more appropriate to achieve similar rates of success. However, because of the limited numbers of patients examined in these studies, continued clinical judgement and caution is essential, particular where a tumour demonstrates other known negative prognostic factors that may suggest a more invasive or aggressive biological behaviour.

Treatment of chylothorax

Idiopathic chylothorax is a frustrating disease, with consistently poor results reported for successful management by a variety of treatment strategies. Thoracic duct ligation is the most widely accepted surgical method for treating animals with chylothorax |4|.

Identification of the duct may be difficult in some animals, and a variable configuration of the duct is recognized, with some animals having multiple separate ducts |5|. These issues can lead to uncertainty as to whether complete thoracic duct ligation was successfully accomplished. The use of intra-operative mesenteric lymphangiography is recommended to improve recognition of the duct and its various anatomical configurations, and to document successful closure of the duct. Injection of methylene blue has also been advocated to improve recognition of the duct during surgery.

Thoracic duct ligation is associated with only a limited success (50–60% in dogs, <40% in cats) and is a technically demanding procedure |4|. In some animals, the chylous effusion changes to a serosanguineous effusion following surgery, which is equally intractable to treatment. Limited non-surgical treatment options are available and euthanasia is frequently performed in animals that do not respond to surgical therapy or medical palliation of clinical signs.

Thoracic duct ligation and pericardectomy for treatment of idiopathic chylothorax
Fossum TW, Mertens MM, Miller MW, et al. J Vet Intern Med 2004; **18**: 307–10

BACKGROUND. Chylothorax is a devastating disease, and the success rates from either medical or surgical management are less than satisfactory. This study reports on the results of a new surgical treatment for idiopathic chylothorax. Treatment included a combination of thoracic duct ligation and subtotal pericardectomy. Thoracic duct ligation was performed through a caudal intercostal thoracotomy (8th, 9th or 10th intercostal space). Subtotal pericardectomy was then performed through a separate intercostal incision (4th intercostal space) or by reaching cranially in the thorax from the original incision. Ten dogs and 10 cats were included in this study. Thoracic duct ligation and subtotal pericardectomy was performed concurrently in 13 animals. In a further four animals, pericardectomy was performed

several months after unsuccessful thoracic duct ligation, to enable complete resolution. Pericardectomy alone was performed in a three further animals in this study.

INTERPRETATION. Excellent success rates were achieved in this study with effusion resolving in 90% of patients (100% in dogs, 80% in cats). This represents a considerable improvement on current treatment methods. Pericardectomy alone was not consistently successful with one dog requiring subsequent thoracic duct ligation to resolve a continued chylous effusion. Success was also attributed to the role of an experienced surgeon. Previous surgery (attempted thoracic duct ligation) had been performed in nine animals by other surgeons. Resolution occurred in 100% of these animals, suggesting that clinical experience may have a positive influence on treatment outcome. The duration of 'reported' clinical signs was found to be a poor predictor of surgical success, as many owners may not be aware of low-grade clinical signs until the disease is quite advanced. Based on the results of this study the authors recommend the concurrent use of thoracic duct ligation and subtotal pericardectomy in any animal with idiopathic chylothorax, or when a serosanguineous effusion has occurred after thoracic duct ligation.

Comment

Chylothorax is thought to arise in association with conditions that increase right-sided venous pressure or from obstructions to the flow of thoracic duct lymph into the venous circulation (e.g. cardiomyopathy, right heart failure, cranial vena cava obstruction). In animals with chylothorax, it is frequently observed that the pericardium and pleural tissues can be considerably thickened, probably as a result of chronic irritation by the chyle. This study tested the hypothesis that this thickened pericardium would lead to continued elevations in systemic venous pressures and thus impede the drainage of chyle into existing lymphaticovenous communications following conventional thoracic duct ligation.

The surgical treatment of chylothorax in this study was more successful than previously reported. The impact of pericardectomy on disease resolution appears to be favourable, with chylous effusion resolving in two dogs where this was the only procedure performed. Pericardectomy also enabled resolution of a serosanguineous pleural effusion (a recognized complication following thoracic duct ligation) in one dog. A remarkably high rate of success was noted (100% in dogs, 80% in cats), which is a considerable improvement on current expectations.

This was a retrospective study, with considerable variation in treatment application. Only 13 animals received the combined treatments concurrently. The remaining study population received pericardectomy only when thoracic duct ligation had apparently failed, whereas three animals only had pericardectomy performed. Five animals were dead at the time of follow-up, but no information was provided on the cause of death in these cases. Data on post-operative management (time to resolution of effusion, complications, intercurrent medical treatment, etc.) were lacking.

Nevertheless, the results of this study suggest that thoracic duct ligation in combination with pericardectomy should be the recommended management strategy for animals with idiopathic chylothorax.

Management of advanced tracheal collapse in dogs using intraluminal self-expanding biliary wallstents

Moritz A, Schneider M, Bauer N. *J Vet Intern Med* 2004; **18**: 31–42

BACKGROUND. This study reported on the long-term results of 24 dogs with tracheal collapse refractory to conventional medical treatment that underwent management with an intraluminal self-expanding stainless steel endoprosthesis (Wallstent™) (Fig. 8.2) A diagnosis of tracheal collapse was established by physical examination, radiography and endoscopy. All animals were considered severely affected, and had failed attempts at conventional medical management. In the majority of patients, the trachea was collapsed throughout its entire length, especially in the region of the thoracic inlet. Grade 4 tracheal collapse was present in about half the patients (54.2%); Grade 3 collapse was present in a further third of the group. Concurrent bronchial collapse was present in 45.8% of dogs.

INTERPRETATION. Compared with conventional surgical management (placement of extraluminal polypropylene prosthesis), the implantation of biliary Wallstents was found to be atraumatic, comparatively quick and technically easy to perform. The initial post-operative survival rate (91.7%) was comparable with that reported for surgical (94–96%) and non-surgical management (93%). Significant clinical improvement occurred in more than 90% of patients; 30.4% were considered asymptomatic by their owners. Complications directly relating to placement of the endoprosthesis included death (8.3%), mild pneumomediastinum (8.3%), tracheal haemorrhage (4.2%) and steroid-responsive granuloma formation (28%). This minimally invasive method for the management of severe tracheal collapse appears to provide an attractive alternative to surgery. However, resolution of several technical elements of the endoprosthesis is necessary to reduce the incidence of life-threatening complications.

Comment

Collapsing trachea is a common disorder in middle-aged toy and miniature dogs |6|. Although medical management can be successful in some dogs, surgical stabilization of the trachea with extraluminal prosthesis is necessary in many animals |7|. The success of conventional surgery is reasonable, with clinical improvement noted in 75–85% of patients |7|. However, surgery is invasive and technically difficult, and is limited to the management of tracheal collapse affecting the cervical segment only. As many dogs with tracheal collapse may also have intrathoracic and bronchial airway collapse, conventional surgery offers limited prospects for these patients. Complications after surgery can be considerable, and include laryngeal paralysis, tracheal necrosis, loosening or failure of the implant, and persistent coughing. Intensive post-operative management is frequently necessary.

Previous reports on the placement of either Palmaz–Schatz stents or thermal shape-memory nickel titanium alloys in the trachea of both experimental and clinically affected dogs identified a high rate of significant complications, including

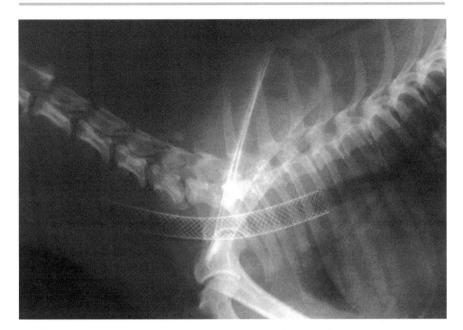

Fig. 8.2 Radiograph showing placement of stent across thoracic inlet.

pneumothorax, infection and tracheal obstruction due to mucus or granuloma formation about the stent |8|. Repeated endoscopy (every 2–3 months) was necessary in some animals to remove exuberant granulation tissue from the tracheal lumen with a laser.

By contrast, the results of this study are encouraging. Immediate improvements in clinical signs were observed in the majority of patients (95.8%) almost from the moment of deployment of the stent. Most patients continued to have marked improvement in their clinical signs, with follow-up periods averaging over 2.5 years following stent placement. A third of dogs were asymptomatic. Where signs persisted, these were often limited to a cough, which was subjectively assessed to be mild and occurred occasionally after a period of excitement. This persistent cough may have been due to incomplete tracheal contact by the stent, which occurred in 55.6% of patients. In contrast to conventional surgical techniques, patients with intra-thoracic and bronchial collapse were significantly improved by stent placement.

Despite this success, considerable complications remain associated with the physical deployment of the endoprosthesis within the tracheal lumen. Once released, the Wallstents cannot be removed or repositioned. Two dogs died in the immediate post-operative period; one due to intractable laryngeal spasm, which occurred as the endoprosthesis was placed too close to the larynx, and another due to severe emphysema likely due to perforation of the tracheal mucosa. Other complications directly relating to placement of the endoprosthesis included mild pneumo-mediastinum (8.3%), tracheal haemorrhage (4.2%) and steroid-responsive granul-oma formation (28%). This latter complication was severe in more than half of this group, resulting in annular narrowing of the trachea by 50–75%. Although these lesions regressed completely following treatment with corticosteroids, this complica-tion may remain a significant limitation of intraluminal stent placement.

Management of patent ductus arteriosus

Patent ductus arteriosus (PDA) is the most commonly performed corrective surgical procedure in dogs with congenital heart disease. Reported operative and overall mortality rates for surgical PDA repair of between 2–8% and 7–11%, respectively, have been reported |**9,10**|.

Traditional and usual methods for PDA management is open ligation via left intercostal thoracotomy. The most commonly reported problems associated with this method include death due to rupture of the ductus during dissection and resid-ual ductal flow post-operatively due to incomplete ligation or recanalization |**11**|. In addition, the relatively high morbidity and cost associated with thoracotomy can result in owners declining such intervention in their pet.

Alternatives to surgical ligation of PDA have been investigated for many years. The introduction of thrombogenic coils and other similar devices in the 1990s have provided a viable alternative to surgical intervention, and is now the preferred method of PDA repair in humans. The results of two papers on PDA are presented here. The first examines the success of two different surgical methods of PDA closure. Next, the development of thoracoscopic-assisted PDA closure is examined. Finally, the experience with a catheter-delivered self-expanding occluding stent for non-surgical closure of a PDA is described.

Minimally invasive patent ductus arteriosus occlusion in 5 dogs
Borenstein N, Behr L, Chetboul V, et al. Vet Surg 2004; **33**(4): 309–13

BACKGROUND. This study described and reported the results of a technique for minimally invasive occlusion of PDA and outcome in five dogs. Three dogs had video-enhanced mini-thoracotomy PDA occlusion. Two other dogs had thoracoscopic PDA occlusion using a custom-designed thoracoscopy clip applicator. Soft tissues were dissected cranial and caudal to the ductus in the usual fashion, but no attempt was made to dissect about the medial aspect. Titanium ligating clips were used for PDA closure in all dogs.

INTERPRETATION. Thoracoscopic PDA occlusion was successful in both dogs in which it was attempted. Complete PDA closure was achieved in four dogs. Three months after surgery, the largest dog had residual ductal flow that haemodynamically was insignificant. Although technically demanding, minimally invasive PDA occlusion appears to be a safe and reliable technique in dogs. The authors note that pre-operative measurement of the diameter of the PDA is crucial to determine if complete closure with metal clips can be achieved. Dogs with a PDA >11–12 mm are not suitable candidates for this technique as the haemostatic clips are not large enough to completely occlude the ductus.

Comment

Progressive development of skills in thoracoscopy will lead to attempts to utilize this process on procedures for which there is an accepted surgical alternative. Reported advantages of minimally-invasive surgery include reduced tissue trauma, minimal post-operative pain, shortened recovery period and improved cosmesis. The procedure is technically demanding, however. Compromises to established surgical principles are frequently necessary due to limitations of the procedure. It remains to be established whether these compromises in technique impact on clinical outcome. Although the use of thoracoscopy is considered innovative in veterinary surgery, thoracoscopic occlusion has been performed in human infants since 1991 and is associated with a success rate similar to open ligation but with a lower complication rate.

In this study, closure of the PDA was successfully achieved in four dogs, with minimal residual shunting occurring in another dog. Dissection of the shunt was limited to the cranial and caudal portions of the PDA, prior to placement of a haemostatic clip. Observation of the dissection was enhanced by intrathoracic illumination and by the magnified image on the television monitor. This is a notable advantage compared with the view often obtained during open ligation procedures in very small neonatal patients.

Minimally invasive PDA occlusion should be considered as an alternative to occlusion via conventional thoracotomy. However, the procedure requires considerable experience with thoracoscopic techniques.

Use of a self-expanding occluding stent for nonsurgical closure of patent ductus arteriosus in dogs
Sisson D. *J Am Vet Med Assoc* 2003; **223**(7): 999–1005

BACKGROUND. This study evaluated the clinical application of a catheter-delivered, self-expanding mushroom-shaped device specifically designed for closure of PDA. The device is manufactured in six sizes, and is filled with polyester patches designed to act as a thrombogenic sieve to obstruct blood flow. The diagnosis was confirmed by physical examination, electrocardiography, thoracic radiography, and two-dimensional, M-mode, spectral and colour-flow Doppler echocardiography. Vascular access was achieved via the femoral vein and artery. Ductal size and anatomy were established by means of angiography. The occluding stent, attached to a delivery cable, was manoeuvred with fluoroscopic guidance though the right side of the heart into the ductus via a prepositioned introducer sheath. The stent was released once its correct position was confirmed with angiography. Closure of the PDA was evaluated by means of angiography 15 min after stent deployment and by echocardiography 1 and 3 months after the procedure.

INTERPRETATION. There were 23 dogs in this study. Two morphological types of PDA were identified on the basis of angiography. In the majority of animals (20 of 23), the ductus resembled a funnel or cone. In the remaining dogs, the PDA resembled an elongated narrow tube. Angiography performed after stent deployment indicated PDA closure in 13 of 20 (65%) dogs. There were no operative deaths. There were two deployment failures, but both were attributable to operator error and inexperience. The misplaced stents could not be retrieved and further ductus closure was not attempted. There were two post-operative deaths in dogs with heart failure; both deaths were thought to be unrelated to use of the occluding stent. Complete PDA closure, determined by Doppler colour-flow echocardiography, was evident in 17 of 19 dogs within 3 months and in one additional dog within 1 year of stent deployment, resulting in closure in 18 of 19 dogs completing the study protocol.

Comment

Catheter-delivered techniques are attractive in the management of PDA because they are minimally invasive, and associated with a reduced risk of ductus rupture during dissection. A variety of transcatheter techniques have been reported using a number of thrombosis-inducing coils. Technical problems with the coils include uncontrolled release, misplacement, embolization and incomplete occlusion of the PDA. These problems occur particularly when the PDA is too large, or there is no focal narrowing of the ductus to allow lodgement of the coils |12|.

The mushroom-shaped device utilized in this study appears perfectly suited to conform to the ductal anatomy with minimal potential for dislodgement and embolization. A variety of sizes is available, thus ensuring that a perfect 'fit' can be accomplished for different morphological shapes of ductus and patient size. Significant operator-related errors occurred in this study, which compromised successful management of the patient. However, these errors occurred early in this clinical study, and none occurred in the last 16 of 23 dogs treated. The main complications were due to haematoma formation at the venous access site, and surgical ligation of these vessels after completion of ductal ligation is suggested.

Results suggest that a catheter-delivered occluding stent can be used successfully to close PDAs in dogs. The specific design of the stent used in this study appears to offer considerable advantages over other transcatheter techniques.

Suture placement in laryngeal paralysis

Biomechanical evaluation of suture pullout from canine arytenoid cartilages: effects of hole diameter, suture configuration, suture size, and distraction rate

Mathews KG, Roe S, Stebbins M, Barnes R, Mente PL. *Vet Surg* 2004;
33: 191–9

BACKGROUND. This paper examined the biomechanical properties of various suture configurations placed in the muscular process of the arytenoid cartilage. The constructs were tested by statically loading them until failure occurred using both a slow distraction rate (0.83 mm/s) and a rapid distraction rate (36.66 mm/s), the latter designed to mimic coughing or barking by a patient. Various suture configurations that have been described for arytenoid lateralization in the dog were tested, including a double suture, horizontal mattress, locking loop, single suture (placed ventrally or dorsally on the articular surface) and a transverse suture (not penetrating the articular surface).

INTERPRETATION. Hole size had no significant effect on any of the measured or calculated variables. Suture of size 1 had a significantly higher resistance to load and had greater stiffness than other suture types. All sutures failed by pullout from the cartilage. There was a notable trend for sutures to fail from the dorsal surface of the arytenoid first. An anatomical evaluation of the arytenoid cartilage described a longitudinal cartilaginous ridge (arcuate crest) that extends cranially from the apex of the muscular process (Fig. 8.3), and provides a thicker cross-sectional area on the ventral aspect of the articular surface of the arytenoid cartilage. Suture configurations that passed through the arcuate crest were more resistant to pullout than sutures placed solely in the thinner dorsal surface. Suture configurations that traversed both portions of the articular surface provided optimal biomechanical performance. Single suture configurations, particularly those that only traversed the dorsal portion of the articular surface were not recommended.

Comment

Laryngeal paralysis occurs when the vocal folds are unable to abduct (open) in response to exercise or respiratory demands |**13**|. Definitive surgical management of laryngeal paralysis is directed at permanently securing the vocal fold(s) in an abducted position. A risk of cartilage fracture or tearing of the suture from either anchor point is a recognized complication of the surgery |**14**|. In older dogs, mineralization of the laryngeal cartilages may make the tissue less tolerant of handling and suture placement. Although infrequent, suture pullout following arytenoid lateralization can be a frustrating complication of surgery for laryngeal paralysis. The reported incidence of suture failure ranges from 0 to 10%, though the true incidence may actually be higher than this |**14**|. The clinical impact of suture pullout is a failure

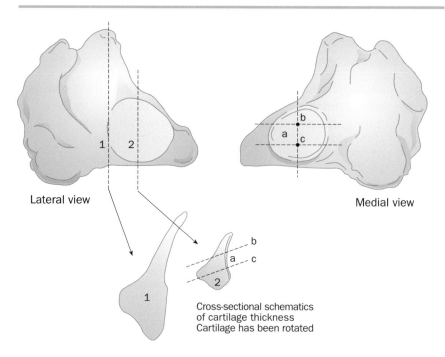

Lateral view

Medial view

Cross-sectional schematics
of cartilage thickness
Cartilage has been rotated

Fig. 8.3 Lateral, cross-sectional and medial diagram of the left arytenoid cartilage with the corniculate and cuneiform processes removed. Lateral view: the dotted circle represents the location of the medially located articular surface. Cross-sectional view: (a) articular surface; (b) dorsally placed sutures pass through the thinner dorsal surface; (c) ventrally placed sutures pass through the arcuate crest. Medial view: (a) articular surface; (b) location of dorsally placed suture; (c) location of ventrally placed sutures. Source: Mathews *et al.* (2004).

of lateralization, with variable redevelopment of the original clinical signs. If failure occurs intra-operatively (due to weak, mineralized cartilage) the surgery may be salvaged by repositioning of the suture (with potential loss of abduction), or by operation on the opposite side. Failure in the immediate post-operative period can result in severe respiratory embarrassment as the dissected arytenoid cartilage may now suck dynamically across the rima glottis, causing complete occlusion of the airways. Because the muscular process only needs to be distracted a few millimetres to achieve full abduction of the vocal fold and arytenoid cartilage, relatively small losses in lateralization (due to suture failure) before fibrosis occurs may result in diminution of the ultimate glottic area, with obvious impact on post-operative function.

This was a cadaveric study, with the breed and age of dogs used in this study not necessarily reflecting those prone to idiopathic laryngeal paralysis. Care is therefore required when extrapolating data from this study to the clinical population. Progressive and variable cartilage mineralization occurs in the older dog, and may be a significant contributor to premature failure in the clinical patient. In addition, the size, shape and orientation of the arytenoid cartilage and articular surfaces can also vary considerably between breeds. Because these variables could not be specifically addressed in this study, it is difficult to assess the clinical relevance of its findings.

Despite these limitations, this was a useful study for providing specific data on the influence of suture placement on ultimate strength and resistance to failure under loading. Double suture configurations, either as two single suture loops or as a horizontal mattress, appear to provide the greatest security against premature failure of the prosthesis. This study has demonstrated that care is essential to ensure the suture passes through the thicker arcuate crest at the ventral third of the articular surface of the arytenoid cartilage (Fig. 8.3). Larger sutures do appear to confer an advantage in terms of resistance to load and stiffness, but can be cumbersome to use and therefore may have negative consequences not revealed in this study. Smaller suture sizes had no significant negative qualities in this paper.

Accessory lung lobe

The accessory lung lobe in thoracic disease: a case series and anatomical review
Lora-Michiels M, Biller DS, Olsen D, Hoskinson JJ, Kraft SL, Jones JC. *J Am Anim Hosp Assoc* 2003; **39**: 452–8

BACKGROUND. Diseases of the accessory lung lobe can be difficult to identify radiographically because it is frequently superimposed on other anatomical structures. This paper nicely reviews the anatomy of the accessory lung lobe and outlines the radiographic appearance of various pathological processes.

INTERPRETATION. Border effacement of the diaphragm was a common finding in dogs with accessory lung disease, making differentiation from diaphragmatic hernia virtually impossible. Contrast or positional radiographs may be very useful. Ultrasonography through the abdomen via a transhepatic window was useful in imaging the caudal mediastinum, and possible abnormalities of the accessory lung lobe. Computed tomography was found to be an extremely useful imaging modality.

Comment

This is a simple paper that addresses the difficulties associated with accurately diagnosing disease affecting the accessory lung lobe of the dog and cat. The accessory lung lobe arises from the right main stem bronchus, and lies between the left and right caudal lung lobes. Radiographically, the accessory lobe is visualized on lateral views as the lucency between the heart and diaphragm, with the caudal lung lobes superimposed. On ventrodorsal or dorsoventral views, the lobe is superimposed on the caudal mediastinum and thoracic spine, making it difficult to evaluate specifically.

Four cases of isolated accessory lung lobe disease are presented, each demonstrating different elements of radiographic interpretation or the use of alternative imaging to attain a diagnosis. In all cases, radiographs showed an increased opacity in the region corresponding to the accessory lung lobe, irrespective of the underlying pathology. Thus, diseases of other mediastinal structures (oesophagus, heart, diaphragm and mediastinum) may mimic accessory lung lobe disease. The use of alternative imaging techniques, particularly computed tomography or ultrasonography, may assist differentiation of pathology.

Clinical experience with thoracodorsal axial pattern flaps

Complications and outcome after thoracodorsal axial pattern flap reconstruction of forelimb skin defects in 10 dogs, 1989–2001
Aper R, Smeak D. *Vet Surg* 2003; **32**: 378–84

BACKGROUND. This paper examined the results of the clinical application of the thoracodorsal axial pattern flap in 10 dogs. Previous experimental studies, and isolated clinical reports, had suggested this flap to be relatively robust.

INTERPRETATION. A high rate of complications were observed in this paper. Only three dogs had complete flap survival. The most serious complication was necrosis of the distal end of the flap, which occurred to a variable extent in seven dogs. The total amount of necrosis ranged from 2 to 53%. Necrosis usually followed a period of oedema and bruising, and was evident 2–6 days after flap transfer. Positive bacterial cultures were obtained from three dogs with distal flap necrosis, but it was not possible to determine whether bacteria were the cause or result of flap necrosis. Partial dehiscence of the flap was also a problem in two dogs. This study highlighted the potential complications that may occur following extensive reconstructive surgery, and advised that owners should be made aware of the likelihood of significant local wound complications.

Comment

Axial pattern flaps are an extremely useful method for reconstructing large tissue defects that may occur following trauma or tumour resection |15|. Axial pattern flaps incorporate a direct cutaneous artery and vein, which supplies a defined angiosome of skin. This arrangement can permit large segments of skin to be raised to cover defects within its arc of rotation. A number of axial pattern flaps have been developed for the dog and cat to reconstruct skin defects about most of the head, trunk and upper limbs. In many cases, creation of an axial pattern flap allows reconstruction of a defect in a single stage procedure, without the need for a delay procedure or extensive open wound management and free skin grafting.

This is the first study to report the results of a large number of clinical cases. The rate of complications reported was higher than anticipated from previous experimental studies and isolated case reports |15,16| but also higher than this author's personal experience with this technique. The high incidence of partial flap necrosis reported in this study is concerning, particularly because it is usually the very tip of the flap that is required for closure of the defect—the remainder of the flap is simply required to facilitate transfer to the wound bed. The cause of necrosis was, however, not specifically investigated in this study, though some vascular compromise to the direct cutaneous artery and vein is likely. Necrosis usually followed a period of oedema and congestion of the distal end of the graft. The thoracodorsal flap is frequently rotated up to 180° from its point of origin behind the shoulder to permit reconstruction of defects about the elbow or below. This rotation may therefore result in some compromise to venous drainage, compounded by the dependant location of the skin flap. Whether these factors influence graft survival was not specifically addressed in this study. It was also unclear whether the flaps were left 'base intact' or rotated as an island. These factors may also influence the degree of vascular compromise that may occur.

Despite the complications reported in the study, successful management of the defect was accomplished in all cases. Some animals required additional procedures to close wound defects, while second intention healing occurred in others. The functional and cosmetic outcome was acceptable to most owners. Where thoracodorsal axial pattern flaps are utilized in wound reconstruction, the owners should be made aware of the higher rate of healing complications that may delay resolution. The need for additional wound care and surgical intervention should be considered. The potential for high rates of distal flap necrosis may also negate the benefits of surgery for some wounds, thus precise application of appropriate surgical technique is essential.

Conclusion

Advances in soft tissue surgery cover a diverse breadth of disease conditions and body systems. The increasing interest and skill in minimally invasive procedures offers promise for successful management for conditions that can be challenging to treat with conventional surgery. However, as with all new techniques, the original implementation can reveal flaws in the methodology or equipment. However, the promise of a simple and effective management for troublesome conditions such as tracheal collapse and PDA is attractive and warrants further investigation and refinement.

Oncological surgery continues to be an area of enormous growth. At times, clinical management of certain tumours is based on accepted clinical dogmas, which sometimes do not correlate with clinical reality. These dogmas may arise from over-interpretation of small case reports comprising only a handful of cases, that may represent a skewed sector of the population. Larger case studies, such as those offered by Williams *et al.* and Polton and Brearley, therefore serve a vital role in challenging some of these dogmas. The work by Murphy *et al.* and Simpson *et al.* has partly addressed this area for mast cell tumours. However, much larger case series are required to completely satisfy the question of margins for this tumour. Therefore, continued clinical judgement and post-operative assessments should continue to form a vital component of oncological management.

Because the ultimate goal of all oncological surgery is curative resection, the assessment of margins and extent of resection is an area of enormous importance. Clinical experience with large resections, as outlined in the paper on thoracodorsal axial pattern flaps, demonstrates that extensive reconstructive surgery does not always proceed as straightforwardly as expected.

References

1. Hedlund CS. Surgery of the perineum, rectum and anus. In: Fossum TW (ed). *Small Animal Surgery*. Missouri: Mosby, 2002: pp 344–8.
2. Thamm DH, Vail DM. Mast cell tumours. In: Withrow SJ, MacEwen EG (eds). *Small Animal Clinical Oncology*, 3rd edn. Philadelphia: WB Saunders, 2001: pp 261–82.
3. Michels GM, Knapp DW, DeNicola DB, Glickman N, Bonney P. Prognosis following surgical excision of canine cutaneous mast cell tumors with histopathologically tumor-free versus nontumor-free margins: a retrospective study of 31 cases. *J Am Anim Hosp Assoc* 2002; **38**: 458–66.
4. Fossum TW, Birchard SJ, Jacobs RM. Chylothorax in 34 dogs. *J Am Vet Med Assoc* 1986; **188**: 1315–18.
5. Kagan KG, Breznock EM. Variations in the canine thoracic duct system and the effects of surgical occlusion demonstrated by rapid aqueous lymphography, using an intestinal lymphatic trunk. *Am J Vet Res* 1979; **40**: 948–58.
6. White RAS, Williams JN. Tracheal collapse in the dog—is there a role for surgery? A survey of 100 cases. *J Small Anim Pract* 1994; **35**: 191–6.
7. White RN. Unilateral arytenoid lateralisation and extraluminal polypropylene ring prostheses for correction of tracheal collapse in the dog. *J Small Anim Pract* 1995; **36**: 151–8.
8. Radlinsky MG, Fossum TW, Walker MA, Aufdemorte TB, Thompson JA. Evaluation of the Palmaz stent in the trachea and mainstem bronchi of normal dogs. *Vet Surg* 1997; **26**: 99–107.
9. Van Israel N, French AT, Dukes-McEwan J. Review of left-to-right shunting patent

ductus arteriosus and short term outcome in 98 dogs. *J Small Anim Pract* 2002; **43**; 395–400.

10. Van Israel N, Dukes-McEwan J, French AT. Long-term follow-up of dogs with patent ductus arteriosus. *J Small Animl Pract* 2003; **44**; 480–90.

11. Hunt GB, Simpson DJ, Beck JA, Goldsmid SE, Lawrence D, Pearson MR, Bellenger CR. Intraoperative hemorrhage during patent ductus arteriosus ligation in dogs. *Vet Surg* 2001; **30**: 58–63.

12. Schneider M, Hildebrandt N, Schweigl T, Schneider I, Hagel KH, Neu H. Transvenous embolization of small patent ductus arteriosus with single detachable coils in dogs. *J Vet Intern Med* 2001; **15**: 222–8.

13. Burbidge HM. A review of laryngeal paralysis in dogs. *Br Vet J* 1995; **151**: 71–82.

14. MacPhail CM, Monnet E. Outcome of and postoperative complications in dogs undergoing surgical treatment of laryngeal paralysis: 140 cases (1985–1998). *J Am Vet Med Assoc* 2001; **218**: 1949–56.

15. Pavletic MM. Canine axial pattern flaps, using the omocervical, thoracodorsal, and deep circumflex iliac direct cutaneous arteries. *Am J Vet Res* 1981; **42**: 391–406.

16. Trevor PB, Smith MM, Waldron DR, Hedlund CS. Clinical evaluation of axial pattern skin flaps in dogs and cats: 19 cases (1981–1990). *Am Vet Med Assoc* 1992; **201**: 608–12.

9

Orthopaedic surgery

KENNETH JOHNSON

Introduction

In recent years there has been a trend for animals with musculoskeletal problems requiring orthopaedic surgery to be afflicted by developmental, inherited or degenerative diseases of joints, rather than being victims of trauma. Accompanying this shift, there has been a growing sophistication in technology, with more routine use of computed tomography (CT) and magnetic resonance imaging of musculoskeletal problems, use of arthroscopy for both diagnosis and surgery, and development of new surgical procedures and implants for stabilizing joints with subluxation as well as prosthetic joint replacement.

These developments have been accompanied by a small revolution in the operative management of fractures. The standard of care for surgical management of fractures in both animals and humans was founded on the principles laid down by the Swiss AO group. Anatomic reduction with rigid internal fixation of articular and shaft fractures permit early return to function, thereby minimizing the problems of fracture disease, including joint stiffness, atrophy and contracture. However, there has recently evolved an increased appreciation for the importance of soft tissue in the process of fracture healing and a realization that development of periosteal callus was usually not a reason for concern, but a positive sign. As such there has been a shift away from the concept of anatomically reconstructing and rigidly fixing every fragment of a fracture, and more to the 'biological approach', allowing nature to do its work |**1,2**|. Such a ground shift has required the development of new implants designed around this philosophy. Two such systems are the interlocking nail and the clamp rod internal fixator (CRIF) for diaphyseal fracture stabilization.

Unfortunately, not all fractures progress to uneventful healing, and the management of non-union can be challenging. Together with some innovations in the surgical handling of non-unions has been the clinical application of recombinant technology. The value of recombinant growth factors in promoting fracture healing seems quite clear, and the problem of economics is the main obstacle to their everyday use in orthopaedic surgery.

The science of evidence-based medicine has not escaped the notice of orthopaedic surgeons, and an exciting new development has been the search for better methods of assessing outcome after orthopaedic surgery and the realization that well-designed prospective randomized studies are needed to provide the highest quality data on which to base recommendations for treatment.

The papers reviewed in this chapter were selected to represent this spectrum of topics in orthopaedic surgery.

Cruciate ligament disease

It is now generally agreed that the events leading to cranial cruciate ligament (CCL) rupture in dogs are related to degeneration and progressive disruption of this structure in most instances, and that acute traumatic rupture, similar to that which occurs in humans is less common in dogs. In dogs, this syndrome of so-called 'cruciate ligament disease' is accompanied by the development of secondary osteoarthritis. Owing to the insidious nature of the ligamentous disruption, secondary osteoarthritis can be well established at the time that the initial diagnosis of CCL rupture has been made. Over the past 50 years innumerable surgical procedures have been devised for the purpose of restoring stability to the femorotibial joint in dogs with CCL rupture. Few have fuelled as much debate and controversy as the tibial plateau levelling osteotomy (TPLO) procedure that was developed by Slocum and Slocum |3|.

Originally, the rationale behind the TPLO procedure was that dogs suffering from cruciate ligament disease had excessive slope of the tibial plateau, and that this deformity subjected the CCL to supraphysiological loading, which eventually resulted in CCL rupture. With ongoing debate about the apparent importance of slope or tibial plateau angle (TPA), it became evident that the accuracy of measurements of TPA could be significantly influenced by factors such as radiographic positioning and observer error |4–6|. After these variables were standardized, it was found that the majority of dogs, whether they have CCL disease or not, have a TPA of 23–26° |7,8|. Certainly, excessive TPA will occasionally be the cause of CCL rupture |9|, but overall other factors such as ageing, intrinsic degeneration, breed predisposition and notch stenosis seem to play more significant roles in the pathogenesis of cruciate ligament disease |10|. Be that as it may, *in vitro* studies found that the cranial thrust in the CCL-deficient canine stifle joint could be neutralized by performance of the TPLO surgery if the TPA was fixed at about 6.5° |11|.

The TPLO is a technically demanding procedure, and precise positioning of the osteotomy is important in obtaining the correct TPA angle |12|. Furthermore, accurate contouring of the plate and alignment of the osteotomy are critical in the prevention of unplanned tibial torsion or axial malalignment |13|. Technical errors during the TPLO procedure can be a significant cause of complications |14,15|. Critics of the TPLO procedure have been quite correct in identifying the lack of well-designed outcome studies that clearly demonstrate superiority of this surgical procedure over others, in terms of return to function.

Progression of osteoarthritis following TPLO surgery: a prospective radiographic study of 40 dogs

Rayward RM, Thomson DG, Davies JV, Innes JF, Whitelock RG. *J Small Anim Pract* 2004; **45**: 92–7

BACKGROUND. Although surgeons have been performing the TPLO procedure for CCL rupture for about 15 years, there are little objective data available on outcome with respect to limb function and progression of osteoarthritis. The aim of this prospective study was to assess the progression of osteoarthritis following TPLO surgery. Osteoarthritis was monitored radiographically by means of an osteophyte scale on entry to the study, and at 6 weeks and 6 months following surgical intervention. Forty dogs were recruited to the study. At each visit, animals were assessed clinically, radiographically, by force platform analysis and by synovial fluid sampling. The radiographic data are the subject of this report.

INTERPRETATION. A significant increase in mean osteophyte score was noted between the entry and 6-month examination time-points (Fig. 9.1). This increase in the mean osteophyte score was due to the increased score recorded in 16 dogs. However, there was no progression of osteophytosis in the majority (60%) of dogs during the course of this study (Fig. 9.2). Dogs with meniscal injury had higher osteophyte scores at entry, but there was no association between degree of osteophyte progression from baseline with meniscal injury, meniscectomy or meniscal release. The authors concluded that their results with the TPLO procedure are comparable with, or superior to, those reported in studies evaluating other surgical techniques for CCL repair.

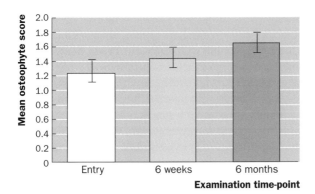

Fig. 9.1 Changes in mean osteophyte scores (±SEM) over a 6-month period following TPLO surgery for the treatment of cranial cruciate ligament deficiency. Source: Rayward *et al.* (2004).

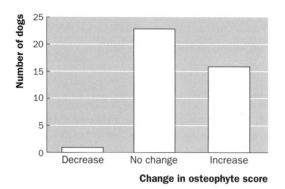

Fig. 9.2 Change in osteophyte score from entry to 6 months. Source: Rayward *et al.*
(2004).

Comment

The TPLO surgery was performed on all 40 dogs by the same surgeon, but as with
most clinical studies, there were numerous other variables. Three dogs had concurrent stifle disease, six only had partial CCL rupture, six had undergone other CCL
surgery prior to TPLO, 21 also had a meniscal injury, and 26 underwent concurrent
meniscal release. Furthermore the follow-up times actually varied over a big range;
32–69 days and 179–307 days. Thus some caution is needed before accepting the
authors' conclusions at face value. Outcome studies of animals and humans with
osteoarthritis are difficult to perform well. While the prospective, randomized
blinded study is the gold standard, the problems with patient compliance and
follow-up are well known. Ideally there should be a panel of outcome measures to
evaluate limb and joint function, as well as clinical, morphological and biochemical
staging of the osteoarthritis. Radiology of joints with osteoarthritis secondary to CCL
rupture can only evaluate joint effusion, intra-articular mineralization, osteophytosis
and alterations in density and contour of subchondral bone. Of these features, osteo-
phytosis shows the greatest degree of change with time |**16**|, but radiographic scoring
of stifle osteoarthritis does not correlate with limb function as measured by force
plate |**17**|. Osteophytes form in response to transforming growth factor β released
from inflamed synovial membrane, but they are probably not a source of joint pain.
Force plate analysis gives a more objective indication of limb function and lameness.
A recent study of force plate data suggested that return of limb function after TPLO
was not significantly better than that following an extracapsular surgery |**18**|. Also a
synovial fluid marker study concluded that neither extracapsular nor intracapsular
stabilization prevented progression of osteoarthritis |**19**|. Thus the analysis of the
remaining forceplate and synovial fluid marker data from this study by Raywood and
colleagues will be of great interest.

Biological fracture management

The interlocking nail and the CRIF described in the following three papers are relatively new devices in veterinary orthopaedics. They have some advantages over other methods of fracture fixation such as bone plating and external fixation, including their utility for biological osteosynthesis. An additional advantage of both systems that will appeal to the practising veterinary surgeon is that they are economical to use.

Use of veterinary interlocking nails for diaphyseal fractures in dogs and cats: 121 cases

Duhautois B. *Vet Surg* 2003; **32**: 8–20

BACKGROUND. The objective of this retrospective study was to report clinical outcome after interlocking nail stabilization of diaphyseal fractures in 78 dogs and 43 cats with fractures of the femur ($n = 96$), tibia ($n = 14$) and humerus ($n = 11$). Interlocking nails (4 mm [$n = 72$], 6 mm [$n = 25$] and 8 mm [$n = 24$] diameter), were used in static ($n = 106$) or dynamic ($n = 15$) fixation modes. Cerclage wires were also used in 63 (52%) cases. Data about the patient (species, breed, weight and age), fracture characteristics, and the surgical and peri-operative complications were recorded. The surgeon evaluated functional outcome, and fracture healing was quantified 6 weeks and 3 months after surgery with a radiographic index.

INTERPRETATION. Twelve fractures had been treated unsuccessfully by another technique, prior to interlocking nailing. Of 106 comminuted fractures, 60 were classified as unstable. Only 112 animals were evaluated at 6 weeks; 86 of 112 (77%) of these had healed without complication and had an excellent ($n = 80$), good ($n = 5$) or fair ($n = 1$) functional outcome. Twenty-six complications were noted; 16 patients did not require any additional surgery and ultimately had a good or excellent outcome, whereas 10 others needed additional surgical intervention to achieve a satisfactory outcome. At the 3-month follow-up, 107 of 112 (96%) of fractures had healed. It was concluded that interlocking nailing can be used to repair diaphyseal fractures of the femur, tibia and humerus in dogs and cats provided the implants are appropriately sized for the fractured bone. The high healing rate (even with unstable fractures), associated with a good functional outcome and low complication rate supports the use of interlocking nailing for these fracture types. However, a period of training and the application of basic principles are necessary to ensure successful results.

Biological osteosynthesis versus traditional anatomic reconstruction of 20 long-bone fractures using an interlocking nail: 1994–2001

Horstman CL, Beale BS, Conzemius MG, Evans R. *Vet Surg* 2004; **33**: 232–7

BACKGROUND. The objective of this retrospective study was to determine surgical and healing times, as well as complication rates in dogs with a comminuted long-bone fracture stabilized with an interlocking nail using either anatomical or biological repair. The medical records of client-owned dogs with comminuted long-bone fractures repaired by interlocking nailing during a 7-year period were reviewed; 20 dogs had had repair with an interlocking nail and radiographic evidence of healing. These 20 dogs where divided into two groups, anatomical (11 dogs) and biological (nine dogs) repair, for statistical evaluation. Surgical times, healing time and complication rates were compared between groups.

INTERPRETATION. Median surgical times for anatomic (110 min) and biological (95 min) repair were similar ($P = 0.06$). Median healing times following anatomic (8 weeks) and biological (6 weeks) reduction were different ($P = 0.04$). There was not a significant difference between groups in the likelihood that a case required a second surgery ($P = 0.58$). Use of a bone graft did not shorten healing times ($P = 0.55$). It was claimed that biological osteosynthesis provides clinical advantages over anatomical reconstruction with respect to a reduction in surgical and healing time without increasing complication rates. Highly comminuted long-bone fractures can be successfully repaired using an interlocking nail without reconstructing the fracture fragments in dogs.

Comment

Complete anatomical reconstruction and rigid plate stabilization of comminuted shaft fractures certainly have an advantage of permitting early weight-bearing; however, there can be long-term problems of delayed union and bone atrophy. 'Bridge plating', in which overall alignment and stability of the proximal and distal fracture fragments are restored without disruption of the fracture haematoma, comminuted fragments or soft tissue attachments, evolved as an interim solution to this problem |20–22|. However, it is now known that interlocking nailing of such fractures provides stability that is equally as good as bridge plating. Being located in the neutral bending axis of the bone, an interlocking nail is also more resistant to cyclic fatigue damage than a buttress or bridge plate |23|. The locking screws or bolts used in conjunction with the interlocking nail control axial shortening and torsional malalignment of the fracture, and thus most of the major problems associated with conventional intramedullary pinning have been eliminated. These two series of fractures managed by interlocking nailing by Duhautois (2003) and Horstman *et al.* (2004) reported comparatively good outcomes that were in accord with those described in earlier publications reporting results of interlocking nailing |24,25|.

For nearly two decades interlocking nailing has been the treatment of choice for stabilization of shaft fractures of the femur and tibia in humans, provided there exists sufficient intact bone in the proximal and distal fragments for interlocking. In humans, interlocking nailing is performed with minimally invasive surgery and indirect reduction techniques, following the philosophy of biological osteosynthesis. The paper by Horstman *et al.* (2004) suggested that this approach is feasible in the management of selected canine fractures as well. Only for the more complex juxta-metaphyseal fractures in humans has there been a return to internal fixation by plating using implants such as the AO locking compression plate |2|.

The clamp rod internal fixator—application and results in 120 small animal fracture patients

Zahn K, Matis U. *Vet Comp Orthop Traumatol* 2004; **17**: 110–20

BACKGROUND. The CRIF, also known as VetFix, consists of clamps that are slid on to a rod and fixed to the bone with screws (Fig. 9.3). The objective of this study was to evaluate the results of using the CRIF in 50 canine and 70 feline patients with closed (*n* = 93) and open (*n* = 10) transverse, oblique and comminuted fractures of the femur, tibia, humerus, acetabulum, radius, scapula and ulna. Fourteen fractures were non-unions. In addition, the CRIF was used to repair three fracture luxations of the spine (*n* = 3). Fracture fixation was performed by application of one or two CRIF devices with 2.0, 2.7 or 3.5 mm cortical screws, using AO osteosynthesis instruments.

INTERPRETATION. Forty-five dogs and 55 cats were re-evaluated clinically and radiographically after an average of 5 months. Uneventful fracture healing occurred in 75 of these patients. In 10 cases, follow-up was only available until 6 weeks post-surgery at which time fracture healing was incomplete. Of the total of 15 complications, five were resolved by exercise restraint only, while the CRIF had to be replaced in six other patients. One cat with a spinal fracture luxation was euthanized due to deterioration of neurological status. Three animals were unavailable for further follow-up. With the inclusion of both uneventful and complicated fracture healing, 86 of 90 patients ultimately achieved complete fracture healing. These results suggested that the CRIF system can be used successfully to treat a variety of fractures in dogs and cats.

Comment

The CRIF was developed for internal fixation of fractures in animals as a simple, economical alternative to the locking compression plate |26,27|. The connecting rod of the CRIF can be readily contoured, and thus it can also be applied to difficult fractures such as supracondylar fractures of the distal humerus and femur. This gives the CRIF an advantage over the interlocking nail for these difficult fractures. However, as with interlocking nailing, accurate reduction of diaphyseal fractures is not essential, and the CRIF can be used with a minimally invasive surgical approach for biological osteosynthesis (Fig. 9.4). If necessary, it can also be applied in combination with a small diameter intramedullary pin used for initial axial alignment of comminuted diaphyseal fractures. Maintenance of the clamp-rod connection relies upon the

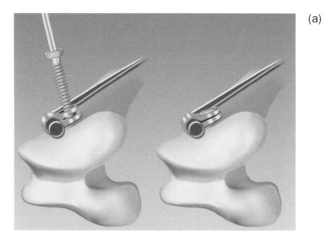

(a)

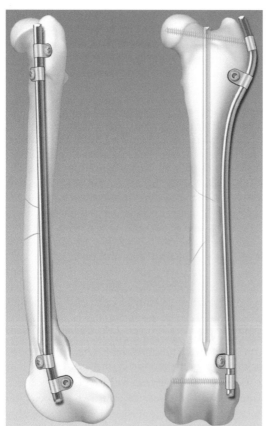

(b)

Fig. 9.3 The CRIF has clamps that are attached to the bone with cortical screws (a). As the screw is tightened, the flanges on the clamp grip the connecting rod. CRIF together with small diameter intramedullary pin stabilizing a femoral fracture (b).

(a)   (b)   (c)   (d)

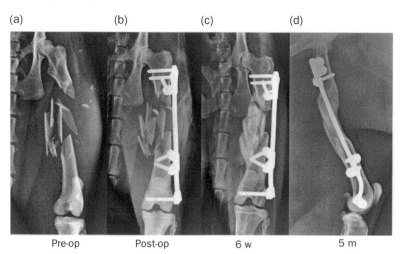

Pre-op   Post-op   6 w   5 m

Fig. 9.4 Comminuted femoral shaft fracture in an 11-month-old, 4 kg cat (a). Radiographs taken immediately after surgery (b), and 6 weeks (c) and 5 months later (d) show biological fixation with a 2.7 CRIF and fracture healing. Source: Zahn and Matis (2004).

fixation being tightly secured by the screw. Therefore it has been recommended that a minimum of three clamps be used in each main fragment, and care be taken with soft bone in young animals. Addition of the end clamp or locking clamp to the CRIF system may overcome this limitation of the CRIF system.

Fracture non-union

A non-union is defined as a fracture that fails to heal during the expected time, and shows no further progression to healing over time. The most common cause of non-union of fractures in small animals is inadequate stability, although the distal radius in toy breed dogs and the tibia of cats seem to be high-risk sites for the development of atrophic non-union. Atrophic non-unions are more challenging to treat because they are biologically inactive. Surgical treatment of these non-unions usually includes some procedure intended to activate the healing process such as shingling, cancellous bone grafting or forage of sclerotic bone. New approaches to this problem described in the following papers include resection of the bone ends and injection of recombinant osteogenic growth factors.

Treatment of biologically inactive non-unions by a limited *en bloc* ostectomy and compression plate fixation: a review of 17 cases

Blaeser LL, Gallagher JG, Boudrieau RJ. *Vet Surg* 2003; **32**: 91–100

BACKGROUND. The objectives of this retrospective study were to describe a surgical technique for the treatment of biologically inactive non-unions using *en bloc* ostectomy and compression plate fixation, and to evaluate clinical outcome in 17 dogs. A transverse ostectomy was performed adjacent and parallel to the non-union to eliminate non-viable tissue and provide new, viable fracture surfaces with a minimum circumferential contact area of 315°. With most of the bony column anatomically reconstructed, compression plate fixation was used to stabilize the fracture. Autogenous cancellous bone grafting was used if a fracture gap was present (<45° of missing circumferential bone contact). Resection of bone was limited so that bone shortening was less than 20% of the overall bone length. Clinical and radiographic follow-up evaluations were obtained whenever possible.

INTERPRETATION. Complete circumferential bone contact and compression plate fixation were achieved after ostectomy in 12 dogs; cancellous bone graft was used in five dogs. *En bloc* ostectomy sites were radiographically healed in a median time of 2.5 months after surgery in 11 dogs that returned for complete in-hospital follow-up, and progressive healing was observed in three other dogs, where in-hospital follow-up was obtained up to 2 months after surgery. These dogs had a median follow-up time of 2 months, at which time six dogs had no lameness, four had minimal lameness, and one had moderate lameness. No complications occurred, and no implants were removed. The authors considered that *en bloc* ostectomy with compression plate fixation was a successful treatment of biologically inactive non-unions. A good to excellent prognosis can be expected with minimal complications.

Comment

Activation of the healing process in atrophic non-unions by resection of the bone ends back to normal bone is a useful strategy, provided that there will be sufficient bone remaining. In toy breed dogs with atrophic non-union of the distal radius, this approach may not be feasible. However, the types of cases included in this series suggest that this could be a useful technique in femoral, tibial and humeral diaphyseal non-union fractures.

Treatment of non-unions with non-glycosylated recombinant human bone morphogenetic protein-2 delivered from a fibrin matrix

Schmökel HG, Weber FE, Seiler G, *et al. Vet Surg* 2004; **33**: 112–18

BACKGROUND. The objectives of this study were to report the results of the treatment of non-unions in animals with non-glycosylated recombinant human bone morphogenetic protein-2 (ngl rhBMP-2) delivered from a designed fibrin matrix. The experimental study was conducted using 20 adult female, albino, Sprague–Dawley rats, and a prospective clinical study used eight client-owned cats and dogs. After development of a fibrin matrix and evaluation of ngl rhBMP-2 in a rodent femoral defect model, eight consecutive long bone non-union fractures (no progression in healing in 3 months or more), in five cats and three dogs were treated using 300 µg ngl rhBMP-2 in a liquid fibrin precursor, injected into the defect gap after fracture revision and stabilization, or through a stab incision into the fracture site. The fibrin matrix was designed to clot in the wound after 60 s and to release the ngl rhBMP-2 continuously over several days.

INTERPRETATION. Using only fibrin gel, 7% of the control rat femoral defect was filled with new formed bone compared with 79% defect filling using 2 µg ngl rhBMP-2 ($P = 0.006$). Five and 10 µg ngl rhBMP in fibrin resulted in union of all femoral defects with complete filling of the gap with new bone. Bony bridging and clinical healing was achieved in seven patients within 24 weeks of administration of ngl rhBMP-2 (Fig. 9.5). The authors concluded that application of ngl rhBMP-2 in a functional matrix can induce bone healing.

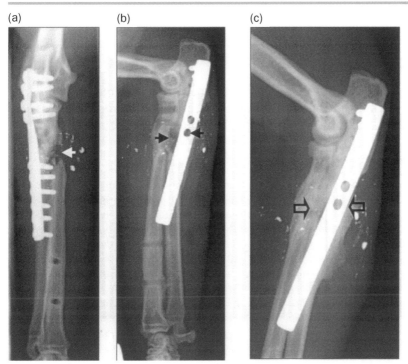

(a)   (b)   (c)

Fig. 9.5 Radiographs of a 3-year-old, 4 kg cat with a comminuted fracture of the radius and ulna that was initially treated with an external skeletal fixator. Three months later the fixation was revised with a plate and screws and 300 µg ngl rhBMP-2 in a fibrin matrix was injected into the fracture gap (a,b). Bony healing (open arrows) is evident 4 months after the ngl rhBMP-2 treatment (c). Source: Schmökel et al. (2004).

Controlled release of ngl rhBMP-2 from a fibrin matrix mimics the natural fracture haematoma. Clinically, ngl rhBMP-2/fibrin can successfully replace a cancellous bone autograft in fracture treatment with an associated reduction in graft donor site morbidity and surgical time.

Comment

Growth factors that have been shown to be potent stimuli of osteogenesis include BMP-2, BMP-7 and platelet-derived growth factor. However, the successful application of any of these growth factors to bone defects requires the concurrent insertion of a suitable carrier that will prevent these small proteins being cleared from the wound too quickly. Schmökel *et al.* used a commercial fibrin gel as the carrier in their studies. The high success rate achieved with ngl rhBMP-2 in treating established non-unions, as well as carpal arthrodeses |28|, clearly indicates that this recombinant protein will be used clinically in the future. The main barrier to everyday application will be expense; however, this needs be weighed against the cost of repeated surgeries and cancellous bone grafting. Delivery of growth factors to a fracture site will not completely replace the need for surgery, because provision of adequate fracture stability is still essential to success.

Percutaneous injection of recombinant human bone morphogenetic protein-2 in a calcium phosphate paste accelerates healing of a canine tibial osteotomy

Edwards RB, Seeherman HJ, Bogdanske JJ, Devitt J, Vanderby R Jr, Markel MD.
J Bone Joint Surg Am 2004; **86A**: 1425–38

BACKGROUND. In this study, we evaluated the capacity of a single percutaneous injection of recombinant human bone morphogenetic protein-2 (rhBMP-2) delivered in a rapidly resorbable calcium phosphate paste (α-BSM) to accelerate bone healing in a canine tibial osteotomy model. We hypothesized that the osteotomy sites would heal faster after percutaneous delivery of rhBMP-2/α-BSM than they would after injection of α-BSM alone or after no treatment. Bilateral tibial osteotomy was performed and the sites were stabilized with external fixators in 16 dogs. Four hours after the surgery, one limb of each dog was treated with a single percutaneous injection of rhBMP-2/α-BSM paste or an equal volume of α-BSM alone. There were eight limbs in each group, and the osteotomy site in the contralateral limb served as an untreated control. The results were evaluated with serial radiography and force-plate analysis at 4 and 8 weeks after surgery and with mechanical testing and histological examination at 8 weeks after the surgery.

INTERPRETATION. At 4 and 8 weeks after the osteotomy and treatment, the scores for radiographic union were significantly greater for the rhBMP-2/α-BSM-treated limbs than they were for the α-BSM-treated or untreated, control limbs (P <0.05). The callus area in the rhBMP-2/α-BSM-treated limbs was significantly greater than that in the α-BSM-treated and untreated, control limbs at 4 and 8 weeks post-injection (P <0.05). The time-integrated vertical force for the rhBMP-2-treated limbs was significantly greater than that for their contralateral controls at 4 weeks and significantly greater than that for the treated and control limbs of the α-BSM-treated dogs at 4 and 8 weeks after the surgery ($P \leq 0.05$). The rhBMP-2-treated limbs were significantly stiffer in bending and in torsion ($P < 0.05$) compared with the α-BSM-treated and control limbs. Histological analysis demonstrated increased bone formation and more mature bone at the osteotomy site in the rhBMP-2-treated limbs compared with that in the α-BSM-treated and control limbs. This study demonstrates the capacity of a single percutaneous injection of rhBMP-2 delivered in a resorbable calcium phosphate paste (α-BSM) 4 h after surgery to accelerate the healing of tibial osteotomy sites in a canine model.

Comment

This is the latest in a series of experimental studies demonstrating the osteogenic effects of BMP-2 in fracture models, in this case using a resorbable calcium phosphate paste as a carrier. As noted previously, expense of these growth factors will be a significant barrier to everyday use, but in the future it seems likely that they will become an integral part of our management of fresh fractures, in conjunction with fracture stabilization. However, I believe that the use of growth factors in orthopaedic surgery will be similar to that of prophylactic antimicrobial drugs administered at the time of surgery; neither will compensate for poor surgical technique.

Primary bone tumour resection defects

Pasteurized tumoral autograft and adjuvant chemotherapy for the treatment of canine distal radial osteosarcoma: 13 cases

Morello E, Vasconi E, Martano M, Peirone B, Buracco P. *Vet Surg* 2003; **32**: 539–44

BACKGROUND. The objective of this prospective study was to report outcome in 13 dogs with distal radial osteosarcoma, without evidence of metastasis, treated by a combination of adjuvant chemotherapy and a pasteurized autograft limb-sparing procedure. Limb-sparing procedure was performed using an autograft from the excised tumoral segment, pasteurized at 65°C for 40 min. Adjuvant chemotherapy (cisplatin or cisplatin and doxorubicin) was administered in all dogs.

INTERPRETATION. Mean and median survival times were 531 and 324 days, respectively (range, 180 to 1868 days). Overall survival was 100% at 6 months, 50% at 12 months, 44% at 18 months, and 22% at 24 months. Lung metastasis occurred in five (38%) dogs. Observed complications were local recurrence (two dogs, 15%), autograft infection (four dogs, 31%) and implant failure (three dogs, 23%). Limb function was good in 12 dogs (92%) and fair in one dog. Pasteurized bone autograft derived from the tumoral bone segment was an effective alternative to cortical bone allograft for limb sparing in canine distal radial osteosarcoma, in terms of feasibility, pattern of healing, complications, and survival. Use of a pasteurized bone autograft eliminates the need for a canine bone allograft bank and has the added advantage of good fit to the recipient site.

Comment

Frozen cortical bone allografts have been used for replacement of large bone defects following trauma and primary bone tumour excision in dogs and humans for more than three decades. However, the problems of incomplete incorporation, implant failure, osteomyelitis and fracture of the allograft continue to be serious complications of this technique. Furthermore, there may also be logistical, ethical and legal barriers associated with harvest of bone allografts in some countries. This paper by Morello *et al.* describes 'pasteurization' as an alternative to using frozen cortical allografts in dogs with radial osteosarcoma. Pasteurization of the resected tumour bone is performed during surgery to kill tumour cells, and then the autograft bone is replaced. The outcome, survival times and complications were similar to that with allografts |**29**|. Fresh cortical autografts contribute to healing of bone defects by acting as a scaffold for new bone formation (osteoconduction) and release of osteogenic growth factors (osteoinduction) such as the bone morphogenetic proteins. While these properties are retained in frozen allografts, it is not known if this is the case following pasteurization. Other methods of bone defect replacement include autologous ulnar transposition |**30**|, Ilizarov bone transport, metallic endoprosthetic replacement and autografting. In the future it seems likely that all these methods will be supplanted by application of a bioengineered matrix scaffold loaded with growth factors and osteogenic cells.

Intra-articular fractures

Radial carpal bone fracture in 13 dogs
Gnudi G, Mortellaro CM, Bertoni G, *et al. Vet Comp Orthop Traumatol* 2003; **16**: 178–83

BACKGROUND. The authors report 13 dogs with radial carpal bone fractures. The lesion was bilateral in six cases and unilateral in seven. Clinical and radiographic examination of both the carpal joints was performed. One or two fracture lines, sagittal oblique and dorsal, of the radial carpal bone were detected. CT examination of two radial carpal bones helped in a better visualization of the fracture lines. A dorsal bone fragment of a fractured radial carpal bone was removed in one dog. Histopathology revealed the presence of fibro-connective tissue on the fracture surface of the bone fragment. The fibro-connective tissue did not seem to be the sequel to acute or chronic diseases, nor to any pathological healing process. The cancellous bone of the fragment was normal as was the bulk of the articular cartilage examined. A CT guided biopsy, including the sagittal oblique fracture surface of the radial carpal bone, was also performed. The specimens revealed the presence of immature cancellous bone with diffuse immature cartilage areas.

INTERPRETATION. The radial carpal bone has three separate centres of ossification: the primitive radial carpal bone, the central and the intermediate carpal bone. The fusion of these centres occurs at 3–4 months of age. Histopathological findings suggest a possible 'incomplete fusion' of the centres of ossification rather than a true fracture of the radial carpal bone or alternatively a 'fatigue fracture'. A similar condition, involving the distal part of the humerus, was originally reported in several cocker spaniel dogs, and more recently in rottweilers and labrador retrievers.

Comment

Fractures of the radial carpal bone are rare and probably pathological in aetiology. These fractures may be unilateral or bilateral, without any history of trauma. Breeds most often affected are the greyhound, boxers, labrador, spaniels, pointers and setters |**31,32**|. These fractures have a characteristic configuration with an oblique sagittal plane fracture, together with a second dorsal plane fracture line. Many dogs have a chronic history of lameness and the diagnosis is often delayed as the fracture may be incomplete initially. It has been hypothesized by Gnudi *et al.* (2003), and others |**31**|, that these fractures are a sequel to incomplete ossification of the radial carpal bone. Gnudi *et al.* (2003) found fibrocartilage, cartilage and woven bone in the fracture lines of two dogs, and suggested that this was evidence for incomplete ossification. These tissues can also be found in non-healed intra-articular fractures, so these findings are somewhat inconclusive.

All dogs developed secondary osteoarthritis. Even though open reduction and internal fixation with lag screws would seem to be the logical treatment of this fracture, progression of osteoarthritis limits recovery |**31**|, and pancarpal arthrodesis was indicated to restore limb function in some cases. This is a poorly understood disorder that could be overlooked without careful attention to historical information, physical examination and good quality radiology. CT should be confirmatory in cases in which radiographic signs are equivocal.

Frequency of post-traumatic osteoarthritis in dogs after repair of a humeral condylar fracture

Gordon WJ, Bescancon MF, Conzemius MG, Miles KG, Kapatkin AS, Culp WTN.
Vet Comp Orthop Traumatol 2003; **16**: 1–5

BACKGROUND. The frequency of post-traumatic osteoarthritis in the dog after repair of a humeral condylar fracture and the relationship of fracture reduction to outcome is unknown. The objectives of this study were to determine the frequency of post-traumatic osteoarthritis in dogs after humeral condylar fracture repair and to

determine the relationship between fracture reduction, limb function and follow-up osteoarthritis score. All dogs were evaluated by physical and radiographic examinations and dogs with unilateral fracture repair were also examined by force platform gait analysis. Initial and follow-up radiographs were also scored for reduction and evidence of osteoarthritis using previously published grading scales. This study evaluated 15 fractures in 13 dogs with a mean follow-up time of 43 months.

INTERPRETATION. Osteoarthritis developed or progressed radiographically in all elbows. Peak vertical force (PVF) was significantly reduced ($P < 0.01$) in the affected limb; however, vertical impulse (VI) did not differ ($P = 0.12$) when compared with the opposite normal limb. Pain-free range of motion was reduced in flexion ($P < 0.01$), but not in extension when compared with the normal limb. Fracture reduction score did not correlate with follow-up osteoarthritis score, PVF, VI, flexion or extension. Owing to the high incidence of post-traumatic osteoarthritis, owners should be warned of the possibility of declining limb function over time despite near anatomic reduction.

Comment

Studies measuring outcome following fracture treatment are difficult to perform well because of the problems of ensuring owner compliance with follow-up visits. Although criticisms of this study of humeral condylar fractures are that it is small and retrospective, it has attempted to evaluate objectively joint mobility and limb function, in addition to the usual radiographic assessment of osteoarthritis. The findings of this study could make us pessimistic about the long-term value of striving for optimal management of articular fractures by open reduction and internal fixation. Although not evaluated in this study, it is safe to assume that the results achieved by surgery will be significantly better than those obtained by conservative management.

Conclusion

In making a selection of just 10 recent papers for inclusion in this chapter on orthopaedic surgery, the omission of other equally significant publications was unavoidable and regrettable. I made a decision to focus directly on operative aspects of orthopaedics, choosing topics that are directly relevant to the daily world of the orthopaedist. This focus also resulted in other notable omissions such as the pathogenesis of musculoskeletal disease, genetics and diagnostic screening of inherited diseases such as hip dysplasia, joint replacement, and new pharmaceuticals for the treatment of osteoarthritis and post-surgical pain.

Cruciate ligament disease has emerged as the most common cause of chronic hind limb lameness in dogs, yet our understanding of the pathogenesis of this disease is in its infancy. It remains be seen if the TPLO procedure will be the answer to this problem long-term, or if it will become another part of orthopaedic history. A much more immediate concern is to develop better solutions for the management and prevention of concurrent meniscal injury in the cruciate-deficient stifle joint. In addition, we look forward to reading more high-quality evidence-based studies in the future that will allow us to make more appropriately informed decisions about the treatment of the entire spectrum of orthopaedic problems.

References

1. Leunig M, Hertel R, Siebenrock KA, Ballmer FT, Mast JW, Ganz R. The evolution of indirect reduction techniques for the treatment of fractures. *Clin Orthop* 2000; **375**: 7–14.

2. Perren SM. Evolution of the internal fixation of long bone fractures. *J Bone Joint Surg* 2002; **84B**: 1093–110.

3. Slocum B, Slocum TD. Tibial plateau leveling osteotomy for repair of cranial cruciate ligament rupture in the canine. *Vet Clin North Am: Small Anim Pract* 1993; **23**: 777–95.

4. Baroni E, Matthias RR, Marcellin-Little DJ, Vezzoni A, Stebbins ME. Comparison of radiographic assessments of the tibial plateau slope in dogs. *Am J Vet Res* 2003; **64**: 586–9.

5. Fettig AA, Rand WM, Sato AF, Solano M, McCarthy RJ, Boudrieau RJ. Observer variability of tibial plateau slope measurement in 40 dogs with cranial cruciate ligament-deficient stifle joints. *Vet Surg* 2003; **32**: 471–8.

6. Reif U, Dejardin LM, Probst CW, Decamp CE, Flo GL, Johnson AL. Influence of limb positioning and measurement method on the magnitude of the tibial plateau angle. *Vet Surg* 2004; **33**: 368–75.

7. Reif U, Probst CW. Comparison of tibial plateau angles in normal and cranial cruciate deficient stifles of Labrador Retrievers. *Vet Surg* 2003; **32**: 385–9.

8. Wilke VL, Conzemius MG, Besancon MF, Evans RB, Ritter M. Comparison of tibial plateau angle between clinically normal greyhounds and Labrador retrievers with and without rupture of the cranial cruciate ligament. *J Am Vet Med Assoc* 2002; **221**: 1426–9.

9. Read RA, Robins GM. Deformity of the proximal tibia in dogs. *Vet Rec* 1982; **111**: 295–8.

10. Comerford EJ, Innes JF, Tarlton JF, Bailey AJ. Investigation of the composition, turnover, and thermal properties of ruptured cranial cruciate ligament of dogs. *Am J Vet Res* 2004; **65**: 1136–41.

11. Warzee CC, Dejardin LM, Arnoczky SP, Perry RL. Effect of tibial plateau leveling on cranial and caudal tibial thrusts in canine cranial cruciate-deficient stifles: an in vitro experimental study. *Vet Surg* 2001; **30**: 278–86.

12. Kowaleski MP, McCarthy RJ. Geometric analysis evaluating the effect of tibial plateau leveling osteotomy position on postoperative tibial plateau slope. *Vet Comp Orthop Traumatol* 2004; **17**: 30–4.

13. Wheeler JL, Cross AR, Gingrich W. In vitro effects of osteotomy angle and osteotomy reduction on tibial angulation and rotation during the tibial plateau-leveling osteotomy procedure. *Vet Surg* 2003; **32**: 371–7.

14. Pacchiana PD, Morris E, Gillings SL, Jessen CR, Lipowitz AJ. Surgical and postoperative complications associated with tibial plateau leveling osteotomy in dogs with cranial cruciate ligament rupture: 397 cases (1998–2001). *J Am Vet Med Assoc* 2003; 222: 184–93.

15. Priddy NH, Tomlinson JL, Dodam JR, Hornbostel JE. Complications with and owner assessment of the outcome of tibial plateau leveling osteotomy for treatment of cranial cruciate ligament rupture in dogs: 193 cases (1997–2001). *J Am Vet Med Assoc* 2003; 222: 1726–32.

16. Innes JF Costello M, Barr FJ, Rudorf H, Barr ARS. Radiographic progression of osteoarthritis of the canine stifle joint: a prospective study. *Vet Radiol Ultrasound* 2004; 45: 143–8.

17. Gordon WJ, Conzemius MG, Riedesel E, Besancon MF, Evans R, Wilke V, Ritter MJ. The relationship between limb function and radiographic osteoarthrosis in dogs with stifle osteoarthritis. *Vet Surg* 2003; 32: 451–4.

18. Evans R, Conzemius M. *Likelihood of clinically significant improvement and probability of normal limb function among surgical techniques for labradors with ruptured cranial cruciate ligament*. Proceedings of Veterinary Orthopedic Society Meeting, 2004; 43.

19. Johnson KA, Hart RC, Chu Q, Kochevar D, Hulse DA. Concentrations of chondroitin sulfate epitopes 3B3 and 7D4 in synovial fluid after intra-articular and extracapsular reconstruction of the cranial cruciate ligament in dogs. *Am J Vet Res* 2001; 62: 581–7.

20. Johnson AJ, Smith CW, Schaeffer DJ. Fragment reconstruction and bone plate fixation versus bridging plate fixation for treating highly comminuted femoral fractures in dogs: 35 cases (1987–1997). *J Am Vet Med Assoc* 1998; 213: 1157–61.

21. Reems MR, Beale BS, Hulse DA. Use of a plate-rod construct and principles of biological osteosynthesis for repair of diaphyseal fractures in dogs and cats: 47 cases (1994–2001). *J Am Vet Med Assoc* 2003; 223: 330–5.

22. Schmökel HG, Hurter K, Schawalder P. Percutaneous plating of tibial fractures in two dogs. *Vet Comp Orthop Traumatol* 2003; 16: 191–5.

23. Bernarde A, Diop A, Maurel N, Viguier E. An *in vitro* biomechanical study of bone plate and interlocking nail in a canine diaphyseal femoral fracture model. *Vet Surg* 2001; 30: 397–408.

24. Dueland RT, Johnson KA, Roe SC, Engen MH, Lesser AS. Interlocking nail treatment of diaphyseal long-bone fractures in dogs. *J Am Vet Med Assoc* 1999; 214: 59–66.

25. Durall I, Diaz MC. Early experience with the use of an interlocking nail for repair of canine femoral shaft fractures. *Vet Surg* 1996; 25: 397–406.

26. Haerdi C, Dalla Costa R, Auer JA, Linke B, Steiner A. Mechanical comparison of 3 different clamp and 2 different rod types of a new veterinary internal fixation system, 4.5/5.5 VetFix. *Vet Surg* 2003; 32: 431–8.

27. Zahn K, Matis U, Frei R, Wunderle D, Linke B, Hehli M, Pohler O. *Biomechanical comparison of the vetfix system and commonly used AO bone plates*. Proceedings of the First World Orthopaedic Veterinary Congress. Munich, 5–8 September 2002; 216.

28. Schmoekel H, Schense JC, Weber FE, Gratz KW, Gnagi D, Muller R, Hubbell JA. Bone healing in the rat and dog with non-glycosylated BMP-2 demonstrating low solubility in fibrin matrices. *J Orthop Res* 2004; 22: 376–81.

29. Morello E, Buracco P, Martano M, Peirone B, Capurro C, Valazza A, Cotto D, Ferracini R, Sora M. Bone allografts and adjuvant cisplatin as treatment of canine appendicular osteosarcoma: 18 dogs (1991–1996). *J Small Anim Pract* 2001; 42: 61–6.

30. Séguin B, Walsh PJ, Mason DR, Wisner ER, Parmenter JL, Dernell WS. Use of an ipsilateral vascularized ulnar transposition autograft for limb-sparing surgery of the distal radius in dogs: an anatomic and clinical study. *Vet Surg* 2003; **32**: 69–79.

31. Li A, Bennett D, Gibbs C, Carmichael S, Gibson N, Owen M, Butterworth SJ, Denny HR. Radial carpal bone fractures in 15 dogs. *J Small Anim Pract* 2000; **41**: 74–9.

32. Tomlin JL, Pead MJ, Langley-Hobbs SJ, Muir P. Radial carpal bone fractures in dogs. *J Am Anim Hosp Assoc* 2001; **37**: 173–8.

10

Gastroenterology

RETO NEIGER

Introduction

While gastrointestinal problems in dogs and cats are the second most important reason for veterinary visits, it is still difficult to diagnose and treat these cases appropriately. As such, research into all aspects of gastrointestinal diseases, including pancreatic and liver abnormalities, are of everyday importance to the practitioner who sees companion animals with more than the usual acute vomiting or diarrhoea.

At initial presentation, veterinarians are faced with an animal with one or more problems needing an appropriate test for finding an aetiopathogenic diagnosis. Unfortunately, with veterinary gastroenterology it is still difficult to carry out cheap and minimally invasive tests with high sensitivity and specificity. Chronic intestinal diseases often require endoscopy with biopsy analysis, hepatopathies rely on liver biopsies, and acute or chronic pancreatitis is even more difficult to diagnose with exact precision. With this in mind, new tests need to be developed and tested under practical conditions.

Despite undertaking a plethora of tests, many organs have only a finite number of ways of responding to a problem. With the World Small Animal Veterinary Association Liver Diseases and Pathology Standardization Research Group, a first step has been taken towards defining unified nomenclature, well-defined histological diagnostic criteria, and precise definition of chronicity stages and grades of diseases. Nonetheless, many aetiopathogenic diseases are still poorly defined and further information is needed.

In experimental settings, the researcher is free to define the exact points for testing and intervention. This is not always the case in a clinical setting where animals are presented at many different stages of the disease. In order to give better prognostic indicators, compare diagnostic tests and therapeutic interventions, we are required to define the stage of the disease process as clearly as possible. This has taken place for many years in human medicine, for example the APACHE (Acute Physiology and Chronic Health Evaluation) scoring system, used to define the stage of acute pancreatitis. Similar scoring systems are clearly needed in companion animal practice and last year saw the beginning of this process.

Finally, it is the intention of every veterinarian to treat an animal with the most appropriate management or drug possible. Unfortunately, for many diseases a specific therapy is not available, the drug is neither approved nor tested for the species, therapy is too expensive or an appropriate medicine has been taken off the market, e.g. cisapride.

With this in mind, 11 papers, pertinent to companion animals, have been selected from peer-reviewed journals of 2003 and have been grouped into the above-mentioned four topics.

Advances in diagnostic testing

An ideal diagnostic test in companion animal gastroenterology is cheap, non-invasive, stable, and easy to perform with almost 100% accuracy. It is clear that no such test exists but several new diagnostic tools have been validated lately and others have undergone a critical reappraisal.

Comparison of direct and indirect tests for small intestinal bacterial overgrowth and antibiotic-responsive diarrhea in dogs

German AJ, Day MJ, Ruaux CG, Steiner JM, Williams DA, Hall EJ. *J Vet Intern Med* 2003; **17**: 33–43

BACKGROUND. It has recently been asked whether a diagnosis of small intestinal bacterial overgrowth (SIBO) does indeed exist or whether the original studies merely used an inadequate cut-off point of intestinal bacterial numbers |1|. At the same time, a critical appraisal of several non-invasive tests for diagnosing SIBO is necessary. This research used the classical approach of drawing upon all available tests in many intestinal diseases for studying the usefulness of each tool.

INTERPRETATION. Thirty pet dogs with chronic gastrointestinal problems underwent a complete medical, including faecal parasitology and culture, routine blood analysis, diagnostic imaging, trypsin-like immunoreactivity (TLI), serum folate, cobalamin and unconjugated bile acid (BA) concentration measurement as well as gastroduodenoscopy. Intestinal histopathology and duodenal juice culture were performed. Dogs were treated with 3 days' fenbendazole and subsequently with 4 weeks' oxytetracycline or tylosin. Non-responders received a 3-week antigen-restricted diet and if clinical signs remained, they were treated with immunosuppressive drugs. A diagnosis of SIBO, as defined previously |1|, was found in 91% of dogs (Fig. 10.1) with no significant difference when dogs with various underlying diseases (e.g. antibiotic-responsive enteropathy, inflammatory bowel disease [IBD], exocrine pancreatic insufficiency [EPI]) were compared. Increases in folate (19 of 29) and decreases in cobalamin (16 of 29) were common, but no pattern was obvious among different disease groups (Fig. 10.2). Similarly, no significant difference was seen in unconjugated BA concentration between disease groups (17% positive based on established reference range) or in comparison with 38 clinically healthy dogs (10% positive). Finally, no significant differences were found in either unconjugated BA concentration or bacterial

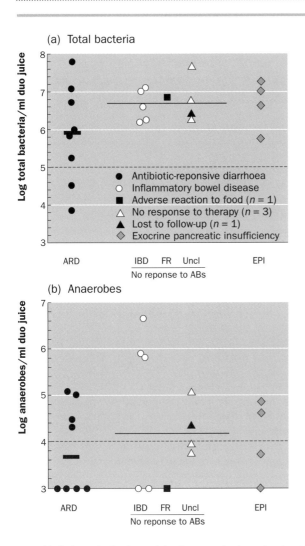

(a) Total bacteria

(b) Anaerobes

Fig. 10.1 Quantitative bacterial culture results from duodenal juice samples collected endoscopically from 22 dogs with chronic gastrointestinal signs. Data are expressed as $\log_{10}$ colony-forming units per millilitre for (a) total bacteria and (b) anaerobes. ARD, antibiotic-responsive diarrhoea (closed circles); IBD, inflammatory bowel disease (open circles); FR, adverse reaction to food ($n = 1$, closed square); Uncl, no response to therapy ($n = 3$, open triangles) and lost to follow-up ($n = 1$, closed triangle); EPI, exocrine pancreatic insufficiency (closed diamonds). The short thick black line represents medians for ARD dogs; the long thin black line represents the median of dogs not responding to the antibiotic trial (e.g. those defined as IBD, FR or unclassified). The dotted lines represent the adopted diagnostic cut-off for a definition of (a) small intestinal bacterial overgrowth, and (b) anaerobic bacterial overgrowth. Source: German et al. (2003).

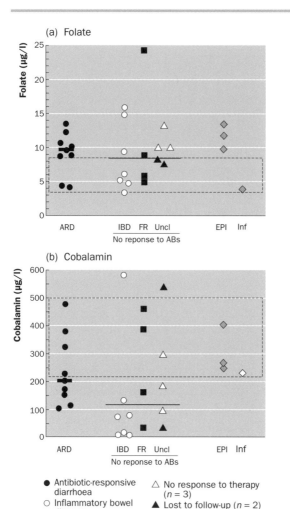

Fig. 10.2 Folate and cobalamin concentrations in serum samples from 29 dogs with chronic gastrointestinal signs. Data are expressed as either (a) folate or (b) cobalamin concentrations in micrograms per litre. ARD, antibiotic-responsive diarrhoea (*closed circles*); IBD, inflammatory bowel disease (*open circles*); FR, adverse reaction to food (*n* = 4, *closed squares*); Uncl, no response to therapy (*n* = 3, *open triangles*) and lost to follow-up (*n* = 2, *closed triangles*); EPI, exocrine pancreatic insufficiency (*closed diamonds*); Inf, infectious diarrhoea (*n* = 1: *open diamond*). The short thick black line represents medians for ARD dogs; the long thin black line represents the median of dogs not responding to the antibiotic trial (e.g. those defined as IBD, FR or unclassified). The dotted lines represent the laboratory reference interval for (a) folate, and (b) cobalamin. Source: German *et al.* (2003).

culture (obligate anaerobes or total bacteria) results between samples taken before and after antibiotic treatment.

Comment

No consensus exists on the definition of SIBO in dogs. Using established cut-off values based on quantified small intestinal microflora seems inappropriate based on this and previous studies. No large-scale investigation has examined duodenal juice culture in healthy pet dogs due to ethical reasons and thus representative numbers are not available. Based on current information, one can duly question the existence of SIBO and it is probably more prudent to speak of an antibiotic-responsive enteropathy in dogs who improve on antimicrobial therapy. However, problems also exist with the definition of this entity. Limitations include the fact that antibiotic therapy is also beneficial in IBD, infectious diarrhoea or secondary SIBO (e.g. due to EPI).

The usefulness of existing non-invasive tools for diagnosing SIBO has been previously shown |2|. Until recently, unconjugated BAs seemed a promising alternative to assessing non-invasively duodenal bacterial numbers |3|. The present study clearly questions the utility of available tests for the diagnosis of SIBO, and given the questionable significance of SIBO altogether, their usefulness is highly debatable. Furthermore, neither bacterial culture of duodenal juice nor non-invasive tests are able to predict response to antibiotics and therefore they cannot be recommended in veterinary gastroenterology.

Relationship between canine mucosal and serum immunoglobulin A (IgA) concentrations: serum IgA does not assess duodenal secretory IgA

Rinkinen M, Teppo A-M, Harmoinen J, Westermarck E. *Microbiol Immunol* 2003; **47**(2): 155–9

BACKGROUND. Most canine IgA is secretory IgA (sIgA) produced by mucosal lymphocytes, transported and released on mucosal surfaces. Especially in the gut, sIgA plays an important defensive role against enteric antigens. Relative IgA deficiency is well known in dogs, especially German shepherd dogs, with an increased susceptibility to intestinal problems. Unfortunately, measuring serum IgA concentrations seem a poor indicator of sIgA |4| and the present study compared the duodenal brush border sample and salivary sIgA with serum IgA.

INTERPRETATION. Four independent cytology brush samples were obtained endoscopically from the duodenal mucosa of 20 healthy dogs. Buccal mucosa swabs and serum samples were taken concurrently. Duodenal, saliva and serum IgA were measured by enzyme-linked immunosorbent assay and to compensate for any disparity in swab sample solutions, concomitant total protein was measured as well and results expressed as sIgA/protein ratio. While a significant negative correlation was found between duodenal sIgA/protein ratio and serum IgA, no correlation could be detected between both duodenal and salivary sIgA/protein ratios.

Comment

Assessment of gut mucosal sIgA is not easy due to the difficulty in accessing the intestine non-invasively. This and previous studies have clearly demonstrated that serum IgA does not reliably assess sIgA levels. While intestinal sIgA production can be estimated by immunohistochemical documentation of IgA-containing cells in the lamina propria, this might be incorrect as these cells are likely to be defective in synthesis or secretion, not in numbers. More recently, humoral gut mucosal IgA production was assessed non-invasively in faecal extracts |5| and these two tests will now need to be compared. Unfortunately, salivary sIgA did not correlate with duodenal sIgA, which would have made sampling a lot easier.

Kinetics and post-mucosal effects on urinary recovery of 5 intravenously administered sugars in healthy cats

Krecic MR, Steiner JM, Kern MR, Williams DA. *Can J Vet Res* 2003; **76**: 88–93

BACKGROUND. Intestinal permeability abnormalities can result in clinical signs, and permeability assessment in dogs has been published. In cats, few studies have looked into the feasibility and accuracy of combined sugar solution protocols |6|. The present investigation tried to assess appropriate marker molecules and kinetics of urinary recovery.

INTERPRETATION. A lactulose–rhamnose–xylose–methylglucose–sucrose solution was given intravenously to 10 healthy cats and urine was collected via a urinary catheter every 2 h for 12 h. High-pressure anion exchange liquid chromatography was used to determine the urinary sugar concentration. For all sugars, the largest percentage urinary recovery occurred during the 0–2 h time period with a strong linear relationship between urine volume and percentage urinary recovery for each sugar. However, cumulative recovery after 24 h was only 42–61%, which is markedly less than in dogs or humans.

Comment

Unfortunately, not many non-invasive diagnostic tests exist in cats with gastrointestinal problems. It is not clear whether a sugar permeability test will help in elucidating any underlying disease processes. Changes in intestinal microflora after antibiotic therapy or dietary changes have not resulted in altered percentage recovery ratios in cats |6|. The cumulative recovery in the present study showed that none of the used sugars is ideal; however, permeability and mucosal function can be assessed and the next step will be to study cats with clinical signs, ideally before and after therapy.

Evaluation of urine sulfated and non-sulfated bile acids as a diagnostic test for liver disease in dogs

Balkman CE, Center SA, Randolph JF, et al. J Am Vet Med Assoc 2003; **222**(10): 1368–75

BACKGROUND. Serum BA analysis is one of the best tests for investigating hepatic function in dogs and many laboratories incorporate it into a routine chemistry panel. It has been shown that inducing the enterohepatic circulation by feeding the patient increases sensitivity; however, dogs should be fasted for routine blood testing. Analysis of BA accumulated over time in urine would obviate this problem. While in health only small amounts of BA are excreted renally, glomerular filtration of water-soluble forms increases with high serum levels. As such, urine BAs are believed to reflect mean serum BA concentration during the urine formation interval. This study evaluated three methods for measuring urine BAs and assessed their accuracy for diagnosing hepatic disorders.

INTERPRETATION. Serum BA, urine sulphated BA, urine non-sulphated BA and urine sulphated plus non-sulphated BA was measured in 15 healthy dogs (to establish reference range), 102 dogs with hepatic disease and nine dogs with non-hepatic disease. Six groups of hepatopathies were formed after routine clinical investigation: portovascular anomaly (27), extrahepatic bile duct obstruction (four), cirrhosis/chronic hepatitis (28), vacuolar hepatopathy (24), neoplasia (10) and miscellaneous disorders (nine). Intra-assay and interassay repeatability of all urinary BAs showed a coefficient of variation percentage of 5.4–21.2%. See Table 10.1 for diagnostic performance of urine and serum BA tests in all dogs with or without hepatic disorders. Urine sulphated BA/creatinine ratio was not significantly elevated in dogs with any single hepatic disorder compared with dogs with non-hepatic disorders. However, all hepatic disorders except neoplasia showed significantly higher values of serum BA, urine non-sulphated BA/creatinine ratio and urine sulphated plus non-sulphated BA/creatinine ratio than non-hepatic disorders.

Table 10.1 Diagnostic performance of urine and serum BA test

	Dog			Cat		
	Sensitivity	Specificity	Accuracy	Sensitivity	Specificity	Accuracy
USBA/Cr	17	100	23	78	94	78
UNSBA/Cr	63	100	66	87	88	87
USBA & UNSBA/Cr	61	100	62	85	88	85
Serum BA	78	67	77	87	88	87

USBA, urine sulphated bile acids; UNSBA, urine non-sulphated bile acids; Cr, creatinine; SBA, serum bile acid.
Source: modified from Balkman et al. (2003) and Trainor et al. (2003) |**8**|.

Comment

This study continues the extensive work of these authors to diagnose hepatopathies with non-invasive tests. Several valid questions have been raised by Steiner *et al.* in a letter to the editor |7|, including why hyperbilirubinaemic dogs were not excluded, as raised bilirubin levels normally make BA analysis unimportant. Furthermore, the cut-off values of serum BA are questioned, leading to a lower than expected specificity. The authors respond adequately showing that even when only dogs with bilirubin concentration <0.5 mg/dl are included, urine and serum BA concentrations remained significantly increased compared with the control group. An important criticism is certainly the low number of dogs with non-hepatic disorders, weakening the calculation of specificity. Further studies are definitely necessary to assess the urine BA under other conditions in dogs.

The same group has reported an almost identical study in the same year on urine BA in 54 cats with liver disease, 17 cats with non-hepatic disease and eight healthy cats |8|. All three urine BAs were significantly elevated in animals with liver disease with urine sulphated BA/creatinine ratio showing the highest specificity (Table 10.1). Interestingly, urine sulphated BA contributed to >10% of urine BA in healthy cats compared with only a very small proportion in dogs suggesting that cats use BA sulphation as an excretory mechanism both in health and when ill.

Development and validation of a radioimmunoassay for the measurement of canine pancreatic lipase immunoreactivity in serum of dogs

Steiner JM, Williams DA. *Am J Vet Res* 2003; **64**(10): 1237–41

BACKGROUND. Diagnosis of canine pancreatitis is difficult as all non-invasive tests have poor sensitivity and specificity. Serum lipase activity has been used for decades; however, as non-pancreatic sources of lipase exist and many other conditions can increase this enzyme, measurement of classical pancreatic lipase would be necessary to evaluate the exocrine portion of the pancreas. These authors have recently purified this substance |9| and the present study validates a new serum test called canine pancreatic lipase immunoreactivity (cPLI).

INTERPRETATION. Polyclonal antibodies against canine pancreatic lipase were raised in two rabbits. Canine pancreatic lipase was iodinated and a radioimmunoassay was established. Assay sensitivity, linearity, accuracy, precision and reproducibility were evaluated. Finally, a reference range for cPLI with 47 sera from clinically healthy dogs was calculated. Overall, the new assay is sensitive, linear, precise and reproducible. The reference range is well within working range.

Comment

This study describes exclusively the validation of a new test for canine pancreatitis. Meanwhile, two preliminary studies have shown conflicting results. One clinical study using abdominal ultrasound as the gold standard calculated in 55 dogs positive and 53 dogs negative for pancreatitis a sensitivity for cPLI of 49% |**10**|. This is similar to measurement of serum lipase or amylase concentrations. Ultrasound has many limitations and thus sensitivity may be incorrectly too low. In a second experimental study, pancreatitis was induced in mild, moderate and severe forms and cPLI measured after various time-points |**11**|. While in control and sham-operated dogs cPLI remained within the reference range at all time-points, cPLI increased above the cut-off value for pancreatitis in four of five dogs with mild pancreatitis and in all five dogs with both the moderate and severe form. Pancreatitis is a dynamic process with release of intracellular content after necrosis early during the acute phase. cPLI will now have to be evaluated in a large group of dogs in which pancreatitis has been reliably diagnosed with several different tests.

New aetiopathogenesis?

It would be nice to be able to pinpoint a given problem in a vast number of specific diseases—unfortunately, this is seldom the case. For example, many icteric animals are still diagnosed with unspecific chronic hepatitis or liver cirrhosis. During the previous decade, many infectious and immune-mediated diseases have been discovered, but most of these publications start with single case reports or case series. They raise the awareness of new pathogenic problems that need further investigation.

Detection of *Bartonella henselae* and *Bartonella clarridgeiae* DNA in hepatic specimens from two dogs with hepatic disease

Gillespie TN, Washabau RJ, Goldschmidt MH, Cullen JM, Rogala AR, Breitschwerdt EB. *J Am Vet Med Assoc* 2003; **222**: 47–51

BACKGROUND. This paper describes the diagnostic procedure and therapy in two dogs with hepatopathy in which *Bartonella* DNA was found.

INTERPRETATION. A 4-year-old basset hound initially diagnosed by liver biopsy with severe pyogranulomatous inflammation and telangiectasia did not respond to antibiotic and supportive therapy. Upon further investigation, microhepatica with mixed echogenicity was found and on a second biopsy granulomatous inflammation was confirmed. No aetiological agent was detected by culture and serology was negative for all agents tested, including *Bartonella vinsonii* (*berkhoffii*), but was positive on Western blot for *Bartonella* organisms. Polymerase chain reaction from hepatic tissue amplified *B. henselae* DNA and the dog was treated with azithromycin on which she improved dramatically. Long-term therapy with azithromycin was given together with supportive medication and the dog survived for 13 months. The other dog was a 6-year-old doberman pinscher that was diagnosed with doberman hepatopathy. This dog's liver tissue was used as a negative control for the first dog's *Bartonella* polymerase chain reaction and was unexpectedly positive, subsequently shown to be 100% identical by DNA sequencing to *B. clarridgeiae*. Beside therapy for doberman hepatopathy, azithromycin was added, resulting in a substantial amelioration of liver enzyme activity.

Comment

This case report was selected to demonstrate the emergence of new infectious diseases that initially were not diagnosed but merely had the histopathological changes described. Pyogranulomatous inflammation is not uncommon and a few years ago the same group reported the first *Bartonella* infection in dogs with this biopsy finding in the lymph node and a nasal mass |**12**|. Liver biopsy sections are usually interpreted histopathologically and sometimes a culture of biopsy specimens is performed. Unfortunately, culture is not often positive and few reports on large numbers of liver or bile bacteriology in domestic animals are available. With advancement in molecular biology, infectious diseases are emerging as a serious cause of hepatic problems. Only recently, *Helicobacter canis* was demonstrated in a 2-month-old puppy with necrotizing hepatitis |**13**|.

Exocrine pancreatic insufficiency as an end-stage of pancreatitis in four dogs
Watson PJ. *J Small Anim Pract* 2003; **44**(7): 306–12

B A C K G R O U N D . EPI is a well-reported entity in dogs, commonly due to pancreatic acinar atrophy, seen mostly in German shepherd dogs. In other species, chronic pancreatitis resulting in loss of exocrine tissue is also well known. However, this cause of EPI in dogs is rarely reported.

I N T E R P R E T A T I O N . During the study period, 13 dogs, seven of which were German shepherd dogs, were diagnosed with EPI by finding low TLI. Two of the remaining six were excluded due to insufficient data, but pancreatitis as the underlying cause seemed most likely. Of the four study dogs, two had diabetes mellitus. One study dog with EPI was diagnosed post mortem, where the pancreas was replaced by fibrous connective tissue with neutrophilic necrosis and adhesions to the liver. In the other three dogs, pancreatitis was diagnosed clinically, on the basis of blood tests and ultrasonographic results. These three dogs responded to pancreatic enzyme supplementation and diet.

Comment

Pancreatitis is not commonly thought to be the cause of EPI in dogs; however, this study showed that at least 36% (46% if the two excluded cases are incorporated) of EPI dogs in one institution might have had an inflammatory background. This seems a surprisingly high incidence considering the paucity of reports but it might reflect the true incidence when excluding breeds with known pancreatic acinar atrophy, such as German shepherd dogs or rough collies.

Diagnosing concomitant EPI and pancreatitis might be difficult as TLI is decreased with EPI but commonly increased with pancreatitis. This was nicely shown in one dog where TLI was subnormal, but during a bout of pancreatitis rose into the normal range. Clinicians need to think of chronic or recurrent pancreatitis in dogs with the triad of EPI—weight loss, polyphagia and steatorrhoea.

Scoring systems

Assessment and comparison among patients is an important tool when evaluating new diagnostic tests or new therapeutic modalities. Generally, patients present in various stages of a disease and only with well-established scoring systems can they be compared. This is of course most important when considering high cost, for example, in a national publicly-funded health system; however, veterinary medicine doctors also need to be able to give accurate prognosis and owners expect to know the expected cost. Again, scoring systems for each disease need to be established.

A scoring index for disease activity in canine inflammatory bowel disease
Jergens A, Schreiner CA, Frank DE, *et al. J Vet Intern Med* 2003; **17**(3): 291–7

BACKGROUND. IBD has highly variable clinical signs, histopathological findings and may differ considerably between dogs. The pathogenesis is still mostly unclear and many causes are discussed. Furthermore, this mixture of signs makes assessments between patients in terms of medical or dietary therapy very difficult. This study describes a possible scoring index to be used in all future research on this disease.

INTERPRETATION. Fifty-eight dogs with IBD according to well-established criteria and nine healthy control dogs had their clinical signs scored by a simple numeric scoring system termed 'canine IBD activity index' (CIBDAI) (Fig. 10.3). Endoscopic biopsies were graded and a histological lesion severity score assigned for each dog. Before and after therapy, C-reactive protein, haptoglobin, α_1-acid glycoprotein and serum amyloid A were measured in serum to assess the acute phase proteins. Only serum amyloid A was significantly different between control and all IBD dogs. However, IBD dogs with a CIBDAI score >5 had significantly higher C-reactive protein concentration than control dogs. Dietary therapy and immunomodulation resulted in significantly decreased CIBDAI and C-reactive protein concentration and significantly increased haptoglobin concentration.

Comment

Several histological grading systems based on immunohistochemical staining have been reported but this is the first simple yet practical scoring system for the assessment of dynamic changes in the clinical picture of dogs with IBD. At present, patient assessment is markedly hampered by virtually non-existent standardized histological systems. It is hoped that the new World Small Animal Veterinary Association Gastro-

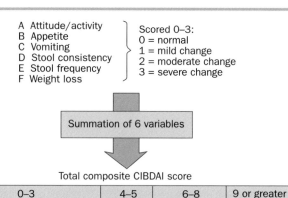

Fig. 10.3 Criteria for assessment of the canine inflammatory bowel disease activity index (CIBDAI). Source: Jergens et al. (2003).

enterology Standardization Group will be able to devise an easy-to-use standardization system for biopsy specimens. The present paper has started this in the clinical setting. Of course, it is highly desirable that all future studies on IBD use the CIBDAI.

The increased C-reactive protein concentration in dogs with moderate to severe IBD, which decreases significantly post-therapy, gives the clinician a tool with which the severity of the clinical signs can be objectively quantified. Most recently, two new serum markers, namely perinuclear antineutrophilic cytoplasmic antibodies and antibodies to *Saccharomyces cervisiae* have been reported and both have reasonable sensitivity and specificity for diagnosing IBD |14|. It would of course now be interesting to have a study combining all available markers and scoring systems before and after therapy in IBD dogs.

Assessing the severity of canine pancreatitis
Mansfield CS, Jones BR, Spillmann T. *Res Vet Sci* 2003; **74**: 137–44

BACKGROUND. Acute pancreatitis is a severe clinical disease with high mortality, both in humans and in dogs. Complications are common, possibly resulting in disseminated intravascular coagulation and multiple organ failure. In human medicine, considerable efforts have been directed towards early identification of patients at risk. Clinical scoring systems, serum markers and diagnostic imaging are used concomitantly. The results are then combined to guide treatment decisions, monitoring intensity and help in giving a prognosis. Some risk factors have been reported in dogs previously, but no study has used as many variables as this present one.

INTERPRETATION. Pancreatitis in dogs was classified as severe or mild based on the occurrence of at least two of five specified criteria, among them histopathology. Dogs with clinical signs had a multitude of markers for pancreatitis analysed, such as amylase, lipase, TLI, trypsin activation peptide (TAP) and pancreas biopsies. Severe pancreatitis was found in 12 dogs while 10 dogs had mild pancreatitis. Neither TLI nor serum TAP was able to distinguish between both forms. However, urine TAP/creatinine ratio was significantly different and had a sensitivity and specificity of 85.7% and 100%, respectively, to distinguish between mild and severe pancreatitis.

Comment

Besides urine TAP/creatinine ratio some other parameters were significantly different in dogs with severe and mild forms of pancreatitis, such as serum lipase, creatinine, phosphate and urine specific gravity; however, their diagnostic accuracy is too low to be of any clinical significance. Similar to a previous report, TLI cannot differentiate between the two forms and neither can α-macroglobulins |15|. Unfortunately, a good number of dogs did not have the full set of markers analysed thus making valid statistical interpretation difficult. Furthermore, the study number in each group was small. However, the inclusion of pancreatic histology helped to strengthen the classification. By using a two-graph receiver operating curve giving sensitivity, specificity and values for a given parameter, it would have been possible to set individual cut-off points and define a 'grey zone'.

Advances in therapy

Treatment of gastrointestinal diseases involves various drugs, some of them well established, others new and still hardly known. As the dog is frequently used as an animal model to investigate gastrointestinal physiology and therapeutics, veterinarians can benefit from this, and new drugs intended for human use are often tested in dogs. Over the years, many reports on new drugs, often in the developing stage, have been publicized in this respect. I have selected just two interesting new compounds that might eventually hit the market. However, besides medical interventions, several problems of the gastrointestinal tract are best managed with dietary interventions. This might be with novel ingredients and many publications have appeared with nutritional aspects. However, just the pure act of feeding severely sick animals may make the difference, as shown in one study.

Effect of early enteral nutrition on intestinal permeability, intestinal protein loss, and outcome in dogs with severe parvoviral enteritis

Mohr AJ, Leisewitz AL, Jacobson LS, Steiner JM, Ruaux CG, Williams DA. *J Vet Intern Med* 2003; **17**(6): 791–8

BACKGROUND. General belief is that in patients with severe gastrointestinal disturbance the 'gut should rest'. This is surprising as it is now well known that early enteral nutrition in critical illness is vastly superior to fasting or even total parenteral nutrition. Enteral nutrition has a plethora of beneficial effects on the gut, including reduced intestinal mucosal permeability, increased motility, reduced bacteraemia and many others. This present study investigated in a prospective, randomized trial outcome and objective intestinal parameters (permeability and protein loss) in dogs with severe parvoviral enteritis treated with early enteral nutrition.

INTERPRETATION. Thirty puppies (8–24 weeks old) with naturally occurring parvovirus infection necessitating hospitalization were included. All dogs received standard therapy for 6 days consisting of intravenous fluid, supplemented with appropriate electrolytes if necessary, intravenous antimicrobial therapy and – depending on albumin levels – plasma transfusion. Fifteen dogs were starved until vomiting had ceased after which small amounts of a diet were offered six times daily. The other 15 dogs received enteral nutrition 12 h after admission via nasogastric feeding tube and the diet was offered after the dog stopped vomiting. All dogs underwent a daily clinical scoring system taking into account attitude, appetite, vomiting and faecal consistency. Intestinal permeability was assessed every other day by lactulose/rhamnose sugar recovery. Faecal protein loss was assessed on days 1, 2, 4 and 6 by evaluating faecal α1-proteinase inhibitor concentration. At admission there was no difference between both groups in any parameter evaluated. The enteral nutrition group showed significant improvement over time compared with the fasting group in the following parameters: composite clinical score, weight gain (Fig. 10.4) and urinary lactulose recovery. Serum albumin, urinary lactulose/rhamnose ratio, and faecal α1-proteinase inhibitor concentration were not different between both groups; nor was survival where 13 dogs survived in the fasting group and all survived in the early feeding group.

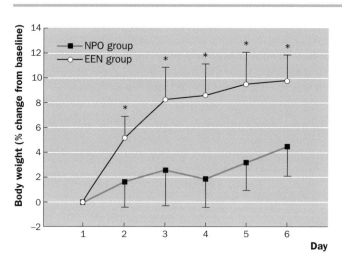

Fig. 10.4 Body weight changes presented as percentage change from baseline values for 30 dogs with parvoviral enteritis. Data are presented as mean with standard error. *Significant differences from baseline; NPO, nothing PO; EEN, early enteral nutrition. Source: Mohr et al. (2003).

Comment

Severe parvovirus infection in puppies is frequently fatal and even though no statistical significance was reached, a 100% survival after early nutrition is quite astonishing. Furthermore, dogs in the early feeding group had consistently 1 day earlier normalization of all clinical scoring parameters. Unfortunately, the more objective assessment of gut function did not show a significant improvement with early feeding. This could be either due to the small group size, as some trends were evident. Just as likely is that these parameters are not well enough established to assess amelioration of digestion and absorption in a markedly disrupted mucosa after a parvovirus infection. As such, just because these tests were not clear-cut, one should not overlook the clear improvement in clinical scores in this randomized, prospective study. No other study has shown so well the benefit of the dictum 'when the gut works—use it'. I can only add to this '… and use it early'.

Two new peptides to improve post-operative gastric ileus in dog

Trudel L, Bouin M, Tomasetto C, *et al. Peptides* 2003; **24**: 531–4

BACKGROUND. Gastrointestinal motility disorders are well recognized in dogs despite the difficulty of assessing this problem. In some diseases, such as the paralytic ileus, the pathophysiological background is unknown; however, they are encountered with various underlying problems, i.e. metabolic derangements or post-operatively. Until recently, the prokinetic benzamide cisapride was used to propagate gastrointestinal motility, but this compound has been removed from the market. It is therefore important that new drugs which could be used to treat such conditions are investigated. The present study tested two new peptides on gastric emptying function in dogs shortly after laparotomy.

INTERPRETATION. Eleven dogs undergoing surgery to implant devices intragastrically and intraduodenally for other experiments were used. Gastric emptying was assessed by measuring plasma increases of acetaminophen ingested with a meal on days 1–4 post-operatively as well as at day 7 pre-operatively and at day 14 post-operatively. Saline as negative control and the two peptides CGRP receptor antagonist 8-37 and MLT-RP/Ghrelin were studied. The gastric emptying function decreased post-operatively quite drastically (day 1 post-operatively: 31% of normal capacity). Both peptides increased total emptying significantly (Figs. 10.5 and 10.6) and no side effects were noted after intravenous infusion.

Comment

This study did not investigate the mode of action of either peptide in increasing gastric emptying in dogs. However, it showed nicely that post-operative delayed emptying can be reversed by intravenous infusion with either of these peptides. There are several drawbacks of the study protocol. First, anaesthesia was solely induced with pentobarbital and no analgesic was utilized. This should not be used

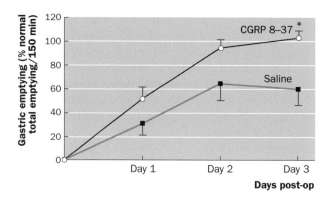

Fig. 10.5 Gastric emptying rate of a solid meal in dogs submitted to a laparotomy on post-operative days 1, 2 or 3 while under treatment with CGRP antagonist 8-37 ($n = 3$) or with saline ($n = 5$). The results are expressed as a percentage of ingested acetaminophen emptied during 150 min post-prandially in control normal condition (here defined as 100%). Data are expressed as mean ± SEM. *$P < 0.05$. Source: Trudel et al. (2003).

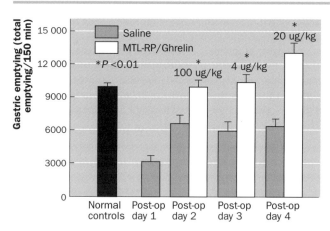

Fig. 10.6 Gastric emptying (total emptying of ingested acetaminophen emptied over 150 min post-prandially) in normal control animals or during the post-operative period (days 1–4) in dogs treated with saline or with MTL-RP/Ghrelin given at various doses. Data are expressed as mean ± SEM. Source: Trudel et al. (2003).

due to ethical reasons but also due to the negative effect on gastrointestinal motility in animals devoid of pain management. Secondly, implanting devices into the stomach and duodenum will undoubtedly have some deleterious effect on motility shortly after the operation, which was not addressed. Finally, assessing gastric emptying with the acetaminophen absorption test has many drawbacks and better means have been published recently, such as ^{13}C-octanoic acid breath tests or scintigraphy |16|. Nonetheless, both compounds seem promising to ameliorate gastric emptying in dogs and hopefully one of these peptides or another with similar effects will become available in the near future for veterinary use.

Conclusion

There is no better time than now to be involved in companion animal gastroenterology. New techniques are constantly developed and can be utilized to investigate new or improved diagnostic tests, discover new diseases or invent new drugs. Molecular biology and advances in diagnostic imaging open up a completely new perspective not only to our colleagues in human medicine but also to veterinary researchers. This of course will undoubtedly help the private practitioner with many of the dogs or cats presented with vomiting, diarrhoea and all the other signs of gastrointestinal abnormality. The 11 studies presented here are just a small portion of the many published reports in companion animal gastroenterology and important others, such as all the dietary and nutritional aspects, had to be left out. The dog is used as an animal model in a huge number of gastrointestinal problems but I decided to omit most of these papers as more research is necessary before their information will be useful in private practice. Nonetheless, the selection of these articles gives a nice overview of what has been published in 2003.

References

1. Johnston KL. Small intestinal bacterial overgrowth. *Vet Clin North Am Small Anim Pract* 1999; **29**: 523–50 (Review).
2. Neiger R, Simpson J. Accuracy of folate, cobalamin and the hydrogen breath test to diagnose small intestinal bacterial overgrowth in dogs. *J Vet Intern Med* 2000; **14**: 376 (Abstract).
3. Melgarejo T, Williams DA, O'Connell, Setchell KDR. Serum unconjugated bile acids as a test for intestinal bacterial overgrowth in dogs. *Dig Dis Sci* 2000; **45**: 407–14.
4. German AJ, Hall EJ, Day MJ. Measurement of IgG, IgM and IgA concentrations in canine serum, saliva, tears and bile. *Vet Immunol Immunopathol* 1998; **64**: 107–21.
5. Little RM. Gut mucosal immunoglobulin A deficiency in the German shepherd dog. *J Vet Intern Med* 2004; **18**: 423 (Abstract).
6. Johnston KL, Ballèvre OP, Batt RM. Use of an orally administered combined sugar solution to evaluate intestinal absorption and permeability in cats. *Am J Vet Res* 2001; **62**: 111–18.

7. Steiner JM, Williams DA, Bunch SE. Bile acid diagnostic test believed to contain limitations. *J Am Vet Med Assoc* 2003; **223**: 429 (Letter).

8. Trainor D, Center SA, Randolph F, Balkman CE, Warner KL, Crawford MA, Adachi K, Erb HN. Urine sulfated and non-sulfated bile acids as a diagnostic test for liver disease in cats. *J Vet Intern Med* 2003; **17**: 145–53.

9. Steiner JM, Williams DA. Purification of classical pancreatic lipase from dog pancreas. *Biochimie* 2002; **84**: 1245–53.

10. Walker J, Watson PJ, Herrtage ME. Sensitivity of canine pancreatic lipase immunoreactivity, compared with other diagnostic tests in the diagnosis of pancreatitis in dogs. *Proceedings of the 14th ECVIM-CA Congress, Barcelona* 2004; 216 (Abstract).

11. Steiner JM, Simpson KW, Teague SR, Williams DA. Serum pancreatic lipase immunoreactivity concentration in dogs with experimentally induced pancreatitis. *Proceedings of the 14th ECVIM-CA Congress, Barcelona* 2004; 199 (Abstract).

12. Pappalardo BL, Brown T, Gookin JL, Morrill CL, Breitschwerdt EB. Granulomatous disease associated with *Bartonella* infection in 2 dogs. *J Vet Int Med* 2000; **14**: 37–42.

13. Fox JG, Drolet R, Higgins R, Messier S, Yan L, Coleman BE, Paster BJ, Dewhirst FE. *Helicobacter canis* isolated from a dog liver with multifocal necrotizing hepatitis. *J Clin Microbiol* 1996; **34**: 2479–82.

14. Allenspach K, Luckschander N, Styner M, Seibold F, Doherr M, Aeschbach D, Gaschen F. Evaluation of assays for perinuclear antineutrophilic cytoplasmic antibodies and antibodies to *Saccharomyces cerevisiae* in dogs with inflammatory bowel disease. *Am J Vet Res* 2004; **65**: 1279–83.

15. Ruaux CG, Atwell RB. Levels of total α-macroglobulin and trypsin-like immunoreactivity are poor indicators of clinical severity in spontaneous canine acute pancreatitis. *Res Vet Sci* 1999; **67**: 83–7.

16. Wyse CA, McLellan J, Dickie AM, Sutton DGM, Preston T, Yam PS. A review of methods for assessment of the rate of gastric emptying in the dog and cat: 1898–2002. *J Vet Int Med* 2003; **17**: 609–21.

11

Veterinary ophthalmology

DAVID WILLIAMS

Introduction

Publications in veterinary ophthalmology can generally be divided into two groups: those developing new techniques and identifying new diseases, and those evaluating old techniques or common diseases in either a novel manner or at greater depth than before. This is certainly true over the recent past as will be shown here, particularly with regard to corneal ulceration and canine cataract. Work in veterinary ophthalmology covers all areas of the subject from eyelids to optic nerve; however, we have concentrated on corneal ulceration and canine cataract in this review as they are such commonly encountered problems in veterinary practice and ones in which research has been undertaken (ranging from epidemiological investigations showing the prevalence of age-related cataract to ultrastructural studies investigating the aetiopathogenesis of recurrent corneal ulceration).

Corneal ulceration

Treatment of corneal erosion and ulceration encompasses a large number of different therapeutic strategies well recognized and used for many years. Yet for many of these a full understanding of the ultrastructural changes in the disease of recurrent erosion and thus the mechanisms by which the treatment has its effects still require further work as detailed below. Other techniques simply have not been subject to a case review process and recently a number of studies have provided more in-depth evaluation of their application and efficacy.

Recurrent and persistent ulceration has been recognized in the boxer dog and some other breeds for many years—treatments ranging from debridement of devitalized epithelium, through grid keratotomy to superficial keratectomy are widely used. Yet detailed investigation of the mechanisms of ulcer formation and reasons for lack of epithelial adhesion, with subsequent failure to heal have not been investigated in depth until now. To understand the pathology of recurrent erosion, we must first understand the normal microscopic anatomy of the corneal epithelium and then the ultrastructural changes in both the disease and after treatment. Chris Murphy and his co-workers have studied the corneas in these dogs with chronic and recurrent

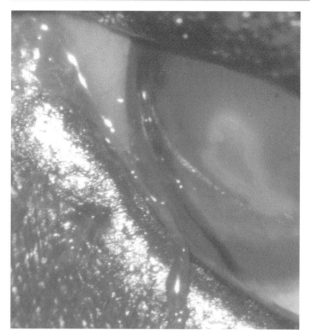

Fig. 11.1 Persistent recurrent canine corneal erosion showing the characteristic devitalized annulus of tissue at its margin.

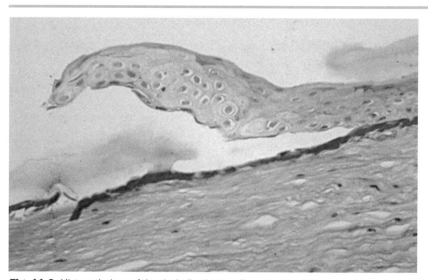

Fig. 11.2 Histopathology of the devitalized non-adherent epithelial tissue at the ulcer edge together with thickened abnormal basement corneal epithelial membrane.

corneal epithelial erosions in great detail and, over the last couple of years, provided us with exactly the information needed to understand this disease and what is happening when we treat the condition.

The effect of chronic corneal epithelial debridement on epithelial and stromal morphology in dogs

Bentley E, Campbell S, Woo HM, Murphy CJ. *Invest Ophthalmol Vis Sci* 2002; **43**(7): 2136–42

BACKGROUND. Two previous reports from Murphy's group have detailed ultrastructural findings of the epithelial basement membrane in normal cornea showing (i) the intricacy of the basement membrane, which provides the set of filaments anchoring the epithelium to the stroma |1|, and (ii) in chronic non-healing epithelial defects where reductions in laminin, collagen IV and collagen VII are critical in destabilizing the critical adhesive complex, which anchors the epithelium to the underlying stroma |2|. The recommended treatment for persistent corneal superficial ulceration is debridement of devitalized epithelium. It is presumed that this removes the perilesional ring of dead tissue, which prevents epithelial healing, but to date no microscopic work has confirmed this hypothesis. This study determines the effect of corneal epithelial debridement on epithelial and stromal morphology and extracellular matrix components in an experimental corneal injury.

INTERPRETATION. Ten-millimetre diameter corneal epithelial wounds were created weekly for 8 weeks in five normal adult laboratory beagles. Three days after the last debridement the dogs were killed humanely, and corneas were processed for light and electron microscopy and immunohistochemistry for collagen IV, collagen VII, fibronectin and laminin. All samples demonstrated epithelial dysmaturation adjacent to the wound edge, and, in four of five, a narrow zone of non-adherent epithelium formed adjacent to the exposed stroma. All samples had a stromal acellular zone in the area of the defect and continuing for a short distance under the adjacent attached epithelium. Experimentally wounded dogs did not form the superficial hyaline acellular lamina found in most dogs with persistent non-healing epithelial defects. Laminin, collagen IV, and fibronectin were present on the stromal surface in all samples, and collagen VII was present in four of five samples. Transmission electron microscopy demonstrated the presence of basement membrane on the surface of the exposed stroma.

Comment

While epithelial changes in this experimental study were similar to those seen in dogs with recurrent persistent corneal erosions, the stromal acellular zone forming in experimentally wounded dogs was distinct from the hyaline lamina observed in dogs with naturally occurring persistent corneal epithelial ulceration. The difference in the acellular stromal layers between chronically wounded dogs and dogs with recurrent persistent epithelial erosions may be of relevance to our understanding of the pathophysiology of persistent epithelial defects.

Another treatment regimen for these persistent corneal ulcers is the use of topical cyanoacrylate glue. Cyanoacrylate adhesive has been used in corneal ulceration for many years in human ophthalmology |3,4| and anecdotally in veterinary medicine as well; however, only in the last 2 years have detailed surveys of the use of these rapidly acting glues been reported in veterinary literature.

Clinical experience with butyl-2-cyanoacrylate adhesive in the management of canine and feline corneal disease

Watte CM, Elks R, Moore DL, McLellan GJ. *Vet Ophthalmol* 2004; **7**(5): 319–26

BACKGROUND. As noted above, butyl 2-cyanoacrylate adhesive has been used for the management of ulcerative keratitis in humans and animals but without a detailed survey of outcome in non-human patients. This report, and one other from the previous year document successes and failure of cyanoacrylate use in corneal ulcers in small animal patients.

INTERPRETATION. This retrospective survey documented 37 animals in which corneal disease was managed by the application of butyl 2-cyanoacrylate. Indications for application, complicating factors prior to gluing, glue retention time, post-operative comfort, and extent of subsequent corneal reaction and scarring were noted for each case. Indications for corneal gluing in this series included: stromal ulceration (26 of 39 eyes), descemetocoele (four of 39 eyes), corneal laceration/foreign body (five of 39 eyes), lamellar keratectomy (three of 39 eyes) and superficial ulceration (one of 39 eyes). Cyanoacrylate was generally well tolerated by patients with only eight of 34 eyes demonstrating transient blepharospasm and increased lacrimation post-operatively. Retention time of cyanoacrylate varied widely from less than 1 week to approximately 6 months, but was less than 2 months in the majority (89%) of eyes. Exaggerated corneal vascularization was an infrequent post-operative complication, noted in only six canine eyes, and did not appear to be related to initial corneal disease, glue retention time or breed.

Comment

This report and Bromberg's study from 2002 detailing glue use in 19 animals |5|, show butyl 2-cyanoacrylate to offer a convenient, economical and effective alternative to other treatment modalities, such as conjunctival grafts, in the management of corneal defects in canine and feline patients.

A number of chronic persistent corneal ulcerative conditions are associated not with epithelial basement membrane abnormalities but with corneal stromal oedema. Such corneal erosions are difficult to treat, but for some time anecdotal evidence has suggested that thermocautery may give sufficient superficial scarring to ameliorate this ulcerative keratopathy. Opinion still appears divided on whether such a technique reduces corneal oedema, but thankfully in the last year reports detailing clinical results from this treatment have been published, as discussed below.

Thermal cautery of the cornea for treatment of spontaneous chronic corneal epithelial defects in dogs and horses

Bentley E, Murphy CJ. *J Am Vet Med Assoc* 2004; **224**(2): 250–3

BACKGROUND. Dogs with corneal oedema can develop fluid-filled bullous excresences of their corneal epithelium and these can lead to painful non-healing ulcers when they rupture. Treatment of these can be difficult—the standard debridement and grid keratotomy as discussed above does not lead to epithelial healing and while thermal cautery has been suggested, evidence from substantial studies has been lacking until now.

INTERPRETATION. In this study a handheld thermal cautery unit was used to make multiple, small (≤ 1 mm in diameter), superficial burns throughout the affected area of ulcerated cornea together with treatment of a rim of epithelium that extended approximately 1 mm around the denuded ulcer bed. Following surgery, a contact lens was placed in the eye and was treated with broad-spectrum antimicrobial ophthalmic solutions. Defects in all eyes healed with minimal scarring; mean time to healing in dogs was 2.1 weeks (range 2–3 weeks).

Comment

While this is clearly not a controlled study, in that time to healing was not compared with that observed in similar ulcers with other treatments (e.g. simple debridement and anterior stromal puncture afforded by grid keratotomy), the rapid healing and long-term lack of re-ulceration suggest that this is a useful technique for this taxing condition. A retrospective study of 13 dogs similarly treated over an 8-year period demonstrated healing of ulcers in 2.2 ± 1.1 weeks, which is a significantly shorter period than for debridement and grid keratotomy in the same eyes prior to the thermokeratoplasty |6|.

A big problem in corneal ulceration is knowing whether the use of topical antibiotics, anti-inflammatories and analgesics will impede ulcer healing. A number of recent papers have investigated this as shown below.

Effect of topical administration of 1% morphine sulfate solution (MSS) on signs of pain and corneal wound healing in dogs

Stiles J, Honda CN, Krohne SG, Kazacos EA. *Am J Vet Res* 2003; **64**: 813–18

BACKGROUND. Animals with corneal ulceration commonly exhibit signs of ocular discomfort. A topical analgesic would be ideal in such circumstances but toxicity of these drugs in prolonged use is a significant problem |7,8|. Some years ago topical morphine was suggested as a valuable topical ocular surface anaesthetic and here this technique is successfully applied to the canine cornea.

INTERPRETATION. The researchers evaluated the effect of topical application of a 1% morphine sulphate solution on signs of pain and wound healing in 12 dogs with surgically created corneal ulcers and examined normal corneas immunohistochemically for the presence of μ and δ opioid receptors. Blepharospasm, tearing, conjunctival hyperaemia, aqueous flare, aesthesiometer readings, and pupil size were recorded before and 30 min after treatment in all dogs. Ulcer size and days to completion of healing were recorded. Normal canine corneas were evaluated immunohistochemically for the presence of μ and δ opioid receptors. Dogs treated with morphine sulphate solution had significantly less blepharospasm and lower aesthesiometer readings than did control dogs. Duration of ulcer healing and findings of histological evaluation of corneas did not differ between groups. Numerous δ and infrequent μ opioid receptors were identified in the corneal epithelium and anterior stroma of normal corneas.

Comment

Topical use of 1% morphine sulphate solution in dogs with corneal ulcers provided analgesia and did not interfere with normal wound healing. Both μ and δ opioid receptors were identified in normal corneas of dogs, although the μ receptors were present only in small numbers. This technique of topical analgesia should be used more widely in dogs with irritation caused by corneal erosions or ulcers.

Effects of antibiotics on morphologic characteristics and migration of canine corneal epithelial cells in tissue culture

Hendrix DV, Ward DA, Barnhill MA. *Am J Vet Res* 2001; **62**(10): 1664–9

BACKGROUND. A significant conundrum in the treatment of corneal ulceration is whether topical antibiotic solutions should be used. They will clearly reduce the risk of infection but may also retard corneal epithelial healing. Several studies of human corneal tissue *in vitro* have addressed this but until now no canine-centred work has been published.

INTERPRETATION. The effects of several commonly used ophthalmic antibiotics on cellular morphological characteristics and migration of canine corneal epithelium in cell culture were observed. Cells were treated with various antibiotics after a defect was created in the monolayer. Cellular morphological characteristics and closure of the defect were compared between antibiotic-treated and control cells. Cells treated with ciprofloxacin and cefazolin had the greatest degree of rounding, shrinkage and detachment from plates. Cells treated with neomycin–polymyxin B–gramicidin and gentamicin sulphate had rounding and shrinkage but with less detachment. Cells treated with tobramycin and chloramphenicol grew similarly to control cells. On the basis of comparisons of defect circumference between control cells and cells exposed to antibiotics, tobramycin affected cellular migration the least. Of the antibiotics tested that have a primarily Gram-negative spectrum of coverage, gentamicin inhibited corneal epithelial cell migration and had greater cytopathological effects than did tobramycin. For antibiotics with a Gram-positive coverage, chloramphenicol had no cytopathological effects on cells in comparison with cefazolin, which caused most of the cells to shrink and detach from the plate. The effects of polymyxin B–neomycin–gramicidin on cellular morphological characteristics and migration were midway between chloramphenicol and cefazolin.

Comment

The effects of antibiotics on corneal epithelial morphology, survival and migration should be taken into account before the drugs are used in cases of corneal ulceration. While gentamicin has generally been regarded as epitheliotoxic, its effects here were less marked than some other drugs, while chloramphenicol showed least toxic effects.

Cataracts

Published research on canine cataract through 2003 and 2004 has ranged from analysis of inherited cataracts in specific breeds through evaluation of antioxidant status of cataractous and normal dogs to population-based epidemiology of age-related cataract in the dog. We will begin with an epidemiological study of cataracts occurring in all ageing dogs.

Prevalence of canine cataract: preliminary results of a cross-sectional study
Williams DL, Heath MF, Wallis C. *Vet Ophthalmol* 2004; **7**: 29–35

BACKGROUND. A major problem is that, while in human ophthalmology several large cross-sectional and longitudinal surveys have been undertaken to determine the prevalence and incidence of cataract in defined populations |9–11|, in veterinary ophthalmology no such studies have been undertaken. It is widely accepted that older dogs have some degree of cataract, with comments in recent literature such as 'cataracts are commonly seen in older dogs' |12| and 'senile cataracts are common in dogs and most animals presenting for cataract surgery are middle aged and older' |13|, but there are no firm data on which to base such anecdotal suggestions. The other problem is that, as ophthalmologists, any attempt to gain information on a specific condition from animals referred with the disease or lesion will necessarily result in a biased population. We set out, therefore, to examine 2000 dogs with no history of eye disease and determine the prevalence of cataract in different breeds at different ages, publishing the results of the survey in early 2004.

INTERPRETATION. Animals were accessed from hospital populations both referral and first opinion, while excluding animals referred for ocular conditions and those with cataractogenic systemic disease such as diabetes. The results showed that by the age of 13.5 every dog has some degree of lens opacification. A more interesting finding was that when results were broken down into age of cataract onset in different breeds, excluding breeds with inherited late-onset cataract such as retriever breeds with posterior polar

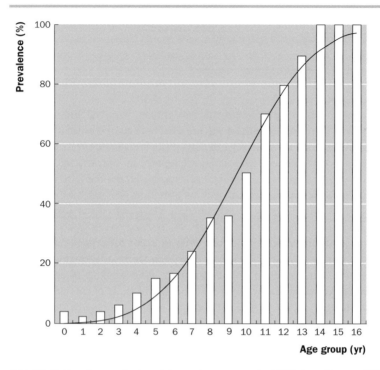

Fig. 11.3 Prevalence of cataract for each year group in 2000 dogs. Source: Williams *et al.* (2004).

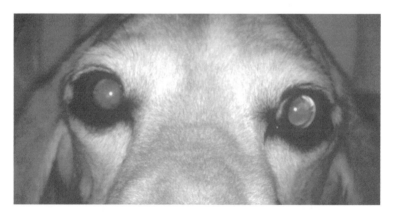

Fig. 11.4 Ophthalmoscopy of a 13-year-old beagle showing both nuclear sclerosis and cataract. Source: Williams *et al.* (2004).

subcapsular cataracts, animals with a longer life expectancy, as detailed previously by Michell |14|, developed cataracts at a later age. While this may not seem particularly surprising, it leads to the question of what difference in the lens of a German shepherd dog causes it to have an earlier onset cataract than a West Highland white terrier, inherited early onset cataracts in the breeds naturally being excluded.

Comment

This paper is the first large-scale study of the prevalence of cataract across different breeds of dog at different ages. It does not indicate the incidence of cataract, however; that is to say, the number of dogs developing cataract over a given time, nor the speed of progression of lens opacities after incipient cataract has been detected. The influence of cataract on visual acuity is unclear in this study; both incidence and influence of lens opacification in older dogs are areas to be included in future work.

Cataracts have been attributed to oxidative injury affecting lenticular proteins and lipids. Primary defences that directly protect the lens against oxidative damage include small molecule antioxidants (vitamin C, vitamin E, glutathione and carotenoids) and antioxidant enzymes (superoxide dismutase, catalase, and the glutathione enzyme systems—glutathione peroxidase, glutathione reductase and glucose-6-phosphate dehydrogenase). In humans, low plasmatic levels of vitamin C, vitamin E and carotenoids have been associated with a high risk of senile cataracts. A decrease in antioxidant defences could be responsible for increased lens oxidation and cataract development in both humans and dogs. A number of different genes coding for enzymes in the system protecting from antioxidant stress may be involved, as may differences in the lenticular chaperone molecular α crystallin that protects other lens proteins damaged accumulated through oxidative stress. While such comparisons are arduous with the limited lens material available in age-matched dogs of different breeds, some very interesting work on systemic and ocular antioxidant profile has been undertaken by Barros and colleagues in specific breeds (see below).

Blood and aqueous humour antioxidants in cataractous poodles

Barros PS, Safatle AM, Queiroz L, Silva VV, Barros SB. Can J Ophthalmol 2004;
39: 19–24

BACKGROUND. Barros et al.'s work on miniature poodles mirrors previous studies on oxidative profiles in cocker spaniels |15|. One might question the value of repeating a study undertaken in one breed on the same problem in another, but Barros et al.'s research shows the potential benefit of such comparisons.

INTERPRETATION. In the cocker spaniel, first investigated in the late 1990s, plasma ascorbic acid concentrations were consistently lower in cataractous when compared with normal dogs. Yet in miniature poodles there was no difference in mean plasma ascorbic acid concentration between cataractous and non-cataractous poodles nor between these and non-cataractous mixed-breed dogs, all these having about 25 μg/ml. The activity of superoxide dismutase, glucose-6-phosphate dehydrogenase and catalase was, however, significantly higher in non-cataractous poodles than in cataractous poodles (*P* <0.05). The activity of glutathione peroxidase was lower in non-cataractous poodles than in cataractous poodles, but not significantly so.

Comment

The significance of these differences between cocker spaniels and poodles is unclear but this study points to the need for further research on oxidative stress in the genesis of canine cataract, and thus the possibility of treatment with supplemental dietary antioxidants, which is being investigated by a number of human ophthalmic groups.

Lens morphometry determined by B-mode ultrasonography of the normal and cataractous canine lens

Williams DL. *Vet Ophthalmol* 2004; **7**(2): 91–5

BACKGROUND. It is widely accepted that in diabetic cataracts lens opacification occurs through the osmotic attraction of water into the lens when the insoluble sugar sorbitol builds up in the lens. This results in intumescence where the lens increases in size. Similar, although less pronounced, effects may be occurring in mature cataracts in non-diabetic animals. However, such changes have not been documented *in vivo* until this work measuring lens thickness in normal and cataractous canine lenses by B-mode ultrasonographic biometry.

INTERPRETATION. Axial B-mode ultrasonograms were used to determine lens thickness, anterior chamber depth and globe diameter in normal dogs and in dogs with cataract at various stages. Axial globe lengths were not statistically significantly different between groups apart from the smaller globes in younger dogs with congenital cataract. Axial lens thickness in diabetics (8.4 ± 0.9 mm) was statistically significantly different from lens thickness in normal eyes (6.7 ± 1.0 mm), eyes with immature cataract (6.4 ± 0.8 mm) and eyes with mature cataract (7.4 ± 0.9 mm). Anterior chamber depth was statistically significantly reduced in eyes with diabetic cataract (2.9 ± 0.1 mm) from that in normal eyes (3.8 ± 0.1 mm), eyes with immature cataract (3.5 ± 0.1 mm) and eyes with mature cataract (3.2 ± 0.6 mm).

Comment

While previous studies on cataract pathobiology have suggested a reduction in lens thickness in immature cataract through lens protein loss and an increase in thickness in mature cataracts and in diabetic cataracts through intumescence, this study is the first to document these changes in the canine lens. The reduction in anterior chamber depth in diabetic cataract suggests that in such dogs care should be taken to assess whether phacomorphic angle-closure glaucoma may occur.

Cataract surgery

The superiority of phacoemulsification over extracapsular extraction has been well recognized for some years, yet even phacoemulsification has its failures. To overcome the problems leading to these failures, both clinical and histopathological assessment of globes lost from problems arising after cataract extraction is needed. Recently, reports on both pathological findings of failed globes and abnormalities in eyes after phacoemulsification have been published. These will aid in combating these problems in the future. First, what does a study of enucleated and eviscerated globes tell us?

A study of the morphology of canine eyes enucleated or eviscerated due to complications following phacoemulsification

Moore DL, McLellan GJ, Dubielzig RR. *Vet Ophthalmol* 2003; **6**(3): 219–26

BACKGROUND. It is widely recognized that post-operative glaucoma and uveitis are problems leading to vision loss and in some cases the need for globe removal. This study sought to: describe the histopathological abnormalities observed in canine eyes enucleated or eviscerated due to complications following phacoemulsification; correlate these findings with the clinical abnormalities reported; and suggest, if apparent, likely causes and effects of these abnormalities.

INTERPRETATION. Sixty-six canine globes or evisceration samples received for histopathological interpretation over a 10-year period were studied. Clinical information obtained from the pathology submission form was reviewed in all cases, and obtained from questionnaires completed and returned by an ophthalmologist for the majority of cases. The most frequent histopathological diagnoses were glaucoma (76%) and retinal detachment (64%). Five problem areas were identified that appear to make a significant contribution to the failure of canine cataract surgery and merit further investigation: pre-iridal fibrovascular membranes; lens fibre regrowth; lens epithelial membranes; endophthalmitis; and the health of the corneal surgical incision.

Comment

It might be assumed that evisceration of a globe as opposed to its enucleation would preclude histopathological examination of the contents to ascertain the pathogenesis of the lesions necessitating removal of the eye. Yet here Moore *et al.* demonstrated that careful examination of fixed tissues from an eviscerated globe can be used to determine cause of ocular disease. They demonstrated the high prevalence of pre-iridal fibrovascular membranes as a complicating feature of post-phacoemulsification surgery failure together with the number of eyes in which lens fibre regrowth plays an important part in subsequent operative failure.

Intraocular pressure development after cataract surgery: a prospective study in 50 dogs (1998–2000)

Chahory S, Clerc B, Guez J, Sanaa M. *Vet Ophthalmol* 2003; **6**: 105–12

BACKGROUND. Elevated intraocular pressure is another significant problem leading to failure of phacoemulsification cataract surgery. Several reports have detailed retrospective surveys of post-operative glaucoma |16–18|; however, this is a prospective study of post-operative intraocular pressure.

INTERPRETATION. Fifty dogs without pre-operative ocular hypertension were selected for cataract surgery, 25 by manual extracapsular extraction and 25 by phacoemulsification. For each dog, intraocular pressure was measured before surgery, and at intervals after surgery. No significant difference in mean intraocular pressure between the two surgical methods was observed for each time measurement. Nine dogs had post-operative hypertension (intraocular pressure >25 mmHg) during the first 5 h post-surgery. Incidence of post-operative hypertension was not significantly different between the two surgical techniques. A decrease of mean intraocular pressure was observed immediately after surgery but there was an increase 3 and 5 h post-surgery.

Comment

In this study incidence of post-operative ocular hypertensive was not high; however, even the nine cases in which it occurred show that measurement of intraocular pressure in the first hours after cataract surgery is required to allow administration of hypotensive treatment, such as carbachol, if necessary.

Conclusion

In the wide field of veterinary ophthalmology from eyelids to optic nerve, we have only examined two areas, corneal ulceration and canine cataract. Yet in general practice these are two of the most common and important areas. It is hoped that the mixture of paraclinical papers investigating the pathogenesis and epidemiology of these two conditions and clinical papers evaluating treatment regimens, successes and failures, will have been valuable to veterinarians in a general practice setting as well as those with a more academic interest in the subject.

References

1. Abrams GA, Bentley E, Nealey PF, Murphy CJ. Electron microscopy of the canine corneal basement membranes. *Cells Tissues Organs* 2002; **170**: 251–7.

2. Bentley E, Abrams GA, Covitz D, Cook CS, Fischer CA, Hacker D, Stuhr CM, Reid TW, Murphy CJ. Morphology and immunohistochemistry of spontaneous chronic corneal epithelial defects (SCCED) in dogs. *Invest Ophthalmol Vis Sci* 2001; **42**(10): 2262–9.

3. Golubovic S, Parunovic A. Cyanoacrylate glue in the treatment of corneal ulcerations. *Fortschr Ophthalmol* 1990; **87**(4): 378–81.

4. Prause JU, Jensen OA. Studies on human corneal ulcers treated with histoacrylic glue. Morphological studies of a successful and unsuccessful membrane. *Acta Ophthalmol (Copenh)* 1982; **60**(4): 547–56.

5. Bromberg NM. Cyanoacrylate tissue adhesive for treatment of refractory corneal ulceration. *Vet Ophthalmol* 2002; **5**: 55–60.

6. Michau TM, Gilger BC, Maggio F, Davidson MG. Use of thermokeratoplasty for treatment of ulcerative keratitis and bullous keratopathy secondary to corneal endothelial disease in dogs: 13 cases (1994–2001). *J Am Vet Med Assoc* 2003; **222**(5): 607–12.

7. Liu JC, Steinemann TL, McDonald MB, Thompson HW, Beuerman RW. Topical bupivacaine and proparacaine: a comparison of toxicity, onset of action, and duration of action. *Cornea* 1993; **12**(3): 228–32.

8. Bisla K, Tanelian DL. Concentration-dependent effects of lidocaine on corneal epithelial wound healing. *Invest Ophthalmol Vis Sci* 1992; **33**(11): 3029–33.

9. Klein BE, Klein R, Lee KE. Incidence of age-related cataract over a 10-year interval: the Beaver Dam Eye Study. *Ophthalmology* 2002; **109**: 2052–7.

10. Klein BE, Klein R, Linton KL. Prevalence of age-related lens opacities in a population. The Beaver Dam Eye Study. *Ophthalmology* 1992; **99**: 546–52.

11. Mitchell P, Cumming RG, Attebo K, Panchapakesan J. Prevalence of cataract in Australia: the Blue Mountains eye study. *Ophthalmology* 1997; **104**: 581–8.

12. Petersen-Jones S. The lens. In: Crispin SM, Petersen Jones S (eds). *BSAVA Manual of Small Animal Ophthalmology*, Shurdington: BSAVA, 2002.

13. Davidson MG, Nelms SR. Diseases of the lens and cataract formation. In: Gelatt KN (ed). *Veterinary Ophthalmology*, 3rd edn. Philadelphia: Lippincott/Williams & Wilkins, 1999: 797–825.

14. Michell AR. Longevity of British breeds of dog and its relationships with sex, size, cardiovascular variables and disease. *Vet Rec* 1999; **145**: 625–9.

15. Barros PS, Angelotti AC, Nobre F, Morales A, Fantoni DT, Barros SB. Antioxidant profile of cataractous English Cocker Spaniels. *Vet Ophthalmol* 1999; **2**(2): 83–6.

16. Smith PJ, Brooks DE, Lazarus JA, Kubilis PS, Gelatt KN. Ocular hypertension following cataract surgery in dogs: 139 cases (1992–1993). *J Am Vet Med Assoc* 1996; **209**: 105–11.

17. Lannek EB, Miller PE. Development of glaucoma after phacoemulsification for removal of cataracts in dogs: 22 cases (1987–1997). *J Am Vet Med Assoc* 2001; **218**(1): 70–6.

18. Biros DJ, Gelatt KN, Brooks DE, Kubilis PS, Andrew SE, Strubbe DT, Whigham HM. Development of glaucoma after cataract surgery in dogs: 220 cases (1987–1998). *J Am Vet Med Assoc* 2000; **216**(11): 1780–6.

12

Nephrology

DENNIS CHEW, PATRICIA SCHENK

Introduction

Many papers have been published within the last several years addressing various aspects of renal disease. This review focuses on studies within three main categories: methodology, parasitic/infectious diseases and chronic renal failure (CRF). This is not meant to be an all-inclusive review; papers were chosen on the basis of importance of findings, contribution to the literature, and clinical relevance within these three areas of focus.

Methodology

A number of papers have evaluated different methods used in the study of renal disease. Some reviewed standard techniques such as urinalysis or biochemical parameters of renal disease and some reviewed relatively newer techniques.

Comparison of plasma/serum urea and creatinine concentrations in the dog: a 5-year retrospective study in a commercial veterinary clinical pathology laboratory

Medaille C, Trumel C, Concordet D, Vergez F, Braun JP. *J Vet Med A Physiol Pathol Clin Med* 2004; **51**(3): 119–23

BACKGROUND. Renal function evaluation is based on urinalysis, and serum or plasma urea (S/P urea) and creatinine (S/P creatinine). S/P urea and S/P creatinine provide an estimate of glomerular filtration rate (GFR) and, typically, both are measured. The objectives of this study were to determine the correlation between S/P urea and S/P creatinine, and to examine the possible effects of sex, age and body size on these measurements.

INTERPRETATION. This paper examines the relationships between urea nitrogen and creatinine in either plasma or serum from nearly 5000 canine samples submitted for analysis to a commercial veterinary laboratory in France. Urea nitrogen and creatinine were measured by standard automated methods using an enzymatic method for urea nitrogen and the Jaffe reaction for creatinine. Specific diagnoses were not available in association with these samples, and accuracy of prediction of renal disease was not attempted. It also was not determined if fasted samples were collected as recommended.

There was significant correlation between urea nitrogen and creatinine concentrations ($R = 0.795$), which is similar to previous reports. There was concordance in 70.9% of cases, where both analytes were either normal or both were elevated (>120 µmol/l for creatinine, or >8 µmol/l urea nitrogen) (Table 12.1). Discordance between analytes was more common when increased urea nitrogen was associated with normal creatinine concentration (27.5% of cases). Elevated creatinine was increased in association with normal urea nitrogen in far fewer cases (1.6% of cases). Urea nitrogen or creatinine concentrations were not affected by sex or age.

An effect of body weight on creatinine concentrations was found when comparing those breeds of dogs with the lowest body weights compared with those with the highest body weights. In dogs with a normal urea concentration, creatinine concentration increased significantly with the size of the dog. The upper limit of creatinine in those with normal urea concentrations was 106 µmol/l for very small dogs, 124 µmol/l for small and medium-sized dogs, and 133 µmol/l for large and very large dogs. The percentage of dogs with normal creatinine but high urea nitrogen concentration was much higher in small dogs (54.4%) than medium-sized dogs (36.9%), or large dogs (28.8%).

Comment

A limitation of this study is that the number of normal dogs or those with substantial liver or kidney disease included is not known. Despite this, the large number of samples analysed still provides valuable information about changes in urea nitrogen and creatinine concentration in dogs from a primary veterinary care population. Urea nitrogen and creatinine concentrations in blood or plasma are used most often to estimate GFR. Neither is very good for estimation of GFR, as at least 75% of nephron mass is lost prior to the development of elevated urea nitrogen or creatinine concentrations. Thus, normal urea and creatinine concentrations do not exclude the presence of renal disease. Increased concentrations of urea or creatinine in serum or plasma could indicate primary renal failure, or may be pre-renal or post-renal in origin. Urea concentration involves more non-renal factors in its physiology than for creatinine, which is why creatinine concentration is most often preferred for the evaluation of renal disease. When azotaemia is present, both may be better indicators

Table 12.1 Distribution of S/P urea and S/P creatinine concentrations in 4799 dogs

	S/P urea normal (%)	S/P urea elevated (%)	Total (%)
S/P creatinine normal (%)	45.0	27.5	72.5
S/P creatinine elevated (%)	1.6	25.9	27.5
Total (%)	46.6	53.4	100

Source: Medaille et al. (2004).

of GFR as they change more readily with either further loss or reclamation of renal function (explained by the exponential relationship between creatinine or urea nitrogen and GFR).

The increased urea nitrogen concentration in those with normal creatinine concentrations could be explained by postprandial effects following protein ingestion and digestion in dogs that were not fasting prior to collection of blood samples. This commonly occurs in general practice in which the client may not follow directions or fasting prior to blood sampling, the veterinarian may not have recommended fasting, or it may be an emergent condition in which there was no opportunity to recommend fasting. When fasting status is not certain, and only the urea concentration is increased, another sample should be submitted after fasting is verified. Gastrointestinal haemorrhage may also be associated with increased urea and normal creatinine concentration, as blood is high in protein. In addition, increased urea nitrogen may occur with normal creatinine concentration by any process that increases passive tubular reabsorption of urea, such as mild dehydration or early effects of urinary obstruction. Early in the course of uroabdomen, urea is more readily reabsorbed across peritoneal membranes than creatinine and could account for the discrepancy. Severe loss of lean muscle mass may account for lack of expected increase in creatinine concentration at times of increased urea concentration during renal disease as muscles are the source of creatinine in the blood.

Liver disease with resulting decreased hepatic synthesis of urea is a consideration when creatinine is increased and urea concentration is normal. Though rare, increased creatinine with normal urea concentration may also occur during acute myopathy with accelerated release of creatinine.

A similar relationship between creatinine concentrations and body mass has been previously reported in dogs [1,2]. Puppies normally have much lower serum creatinine concentrations than do adult dogs. In a puppy, observation of a serum creatinine concentration within the adult reference range may be incorrectly interpreted as 'normal' when, in reality, early renal failure may exist.

This paper confirms that urea and creatinine concentrations usually are either both normal, or are both increased. In the event that one is increased and not the other, consideration must be given to non-renal factors for those with increased urea but not creatinine concentrations. We agree with the authors that normal ranges for serum or plasma creatinine concentrations should be established for breed, or at least for body size. A recent study demonstrated that greyhounds had higher normal serum creatinine concentrations than non-greyhounds [3]. Ideally, lean body mass should be used as an estimator of the source of creatinine in the blood stream. Body condition score should always be considered during the evaluation of creatinine, as those with low muscle mass will typically have a lower concentration of serum creatinine.

Effects of storage time and temperature on pH, specific gravity, and crystal formation in urine samples from dogs and cats

Albasan H, Lulich JP, Osborne CA, Lekcharoensuk C, Ulrich LK, Carpenter KA.
J Am Vet Med Assoc 2003; **222**(2): 176–9

BACKGROUND. It is a general observation in the veterinary urological community that *in vitro* formation of crystals in urine is common, especially when examining urine sediment from refrigerated samples. The presence of crystalluria is important in further evaluation of stone-forming patients, as persistent crystalluria in fresh samples is a risk factor for future stone formation and growth, and for recurrent urethral plug formation in male cats. This study was designed to determine how often *in vitro* formation of crystals occurs in stored urine samples compared with fresh samples. If crystals form during storage of urine samples that were not present at the time of collection, erroneous conclusions about the risks of crystalluria will be made when evaluating results from stored urine.

INTERPRETATION. Urine samples were stored either at room temperature or under refrigeration, and examined microscopically after 6 and 24 h of storage. A fresh urine sample was defined as one that was analysed within 60 min of collection; no attempt was made to store this fresh sample at body temperature. Crystals were counted in quantitative wells and their dimensions measured with an ocular micrometer. Thirty-one samples were of urine from dogs and eight were from cats. Crystals formed *in vitro* in 11 of 39 (28%) samples during storage for 24 h under refrigeration that were not present in the analysis of fresh urine. Eight of 31 dogs had crystalluria detected from fresh urine samples; three of these samples developed calcium oxalate crystals *in vitro* (two dogs had amorphous phosphates and one had magnesium ammonium phosphate (MAP) in the sediment from fresh urine).

Of the 11 samples that developed *in vitro* crystal formation, calcium oxalate crystalluria developed in one cat and eight dogs. Of these nine samples, oxalate crystals were detected at 6 h of room temperature storage in one of nine and in two of nine at 24 h of storage. During storage at refrigeration temperature, four of nine developed calcium oxalate crystalluria at 6 h, and nine of nine at 24 h. MAP crystals developed *in vitro* from the urine of two dogs in samples at 6 and 24 h with both room temperature and refrigeration. Overall, crystal formation increased over time and during refrigeration. The number of calcium oxalate crystals that formed was greater during refrigeration and at 24 h compared with those analysed at room temperature and at 6 h. The magnitude of MAP crystalluria was increased over fresh samples, but did not differ between 6 and 24 h nor between room temperature and refrigeration. The mean length of crystals formed *in vitro* was greater in refrigerated samples compared with those stored at room temperature. *In vitro* formation of calcium oxalate crystals resulted in longer crystals during refrigeration compared with room temperature, but no effect of temperature was found on the length of MAP crystals. The mean pH of samples associated with *in vitro* MAP crystal formation was 6.83, and was 6.09 in those associated with *in vitro* formation of calcium oxalate crystals.

Urine samples stored prior to analysis of urine sediment increases the number and size of crystals *in vitro*. This effect is greater in samples stored at refrigeration temperatures.

Previous reports of *in vitro* crystal formation have only been noted in association with MAP crystals; however, *in vitro* formation of calcium oxalate crystalluria was more common in this study. Reports of crystalluria on stored urine may not correlate with those from fresh samples. As *in vitro* formation of crystals is less common at room temperature, the authors recommend collection of a large enough urine sample so that one aliquot can be refrigerated and one stored at room temperature. If crystals are present in the refrigerated but not the room temperature sample, then crystals seen in the refrigerated sample were an artefact.

Comment

Six of 41 (15%) initial samples from normal cats eating a wet and dry food mixture in another study had MAP crystalluria, and cats fed exclusively wet foods had 0% crystalluria |4|. The magnitude of crystalluria increased dramatically during all methods of storage. Ninety-two per cent of urine samples had MAP crystalluria in at least one sample that was stored, compared with 24% of fresh samples. Compared with fresh urine, samples stored at room temperature for 4 h increased the level of crystalluria by more than twofold, and those that were stored in the refrigerator for 4 h or simulated postal transport for 24 h by about threefold. Fresh urine in this study was evaluated within 15 min.

The actual frequency of *in vitro* formation of crystals may be considerably higher than reported in this study as they compared crystal formation at 6 and 24 h of storage to so-called 'fresh' urine. As the urine may have set for up to 60 min before analysis of the fresh sample, it is conceivable that the temperature of the urine sample dropped below body temperature allowing precipitation of crystals, which were previously in solution at the animal's body temperature. Temporary storage of urine samples at body temperature (38°C) and examination of urinary sediment on microscope slides that have been pre-warmed may be needed to distinguish further between *in vivo* and *in vitro* crystal formation. Attempts to rewarm and mix urine to dissolve crystals that formed *in vitro* have not been successful in our experience and in one report of cats with MAP *in vitro* crystal formation |4|.

The interpretation of crystalluria in urine that has been stored, especially if refrigerated, may lead to erroneous conclusions. Crystals noted during examination of stored urine may not actually be present in urine when initially collected, and treatment based on these findings may not be warranted. When crystals are discovered in urine samples that have been stored and there is concern about their potential pathophysiological role in urinary tract disease, a new urine sample should be collected and analysed within 15 min to minimize the likelihood of *in vitro* crystal formation. Many normal animals have crystalluria without risk of developing urinary tract disease. In those with urolithiasis or urethral plug formation, the presence of 'real' crystalluria is an important finding as treatment interventions to reduce their presence are warranted. The size of crystals and their tendency to aggregate are other morphological properties of crystals that are important in recurrent urolithiasis. In order to assess the true risks of crystalluria, standard methods of reporting quantity, type and habitat of crystals must be developed among veterinary laboratories.

Diagnostic relevance of qualitative proteinuria evaluated by use of sodium dodecyl sulfate-agarose gel electrophoresis and comparison with renal histologic findings in dogs

Zini E, Bonfanti U, Zatelli A. *Am J Vet Res* 2004; **65**(7): 964–71

BACKGROUND. Electrophoresis allows for the separation of proteins based on charge and molecular mass. Sodium dodecyl sulphate–agarose gel electrophoresis (SDS–AGE) allows detection of proteins with a molecular mass from 9 kDa to 900 kDa. In urine, proteins of different molecular mass may be detected using SDS–AGE. Theoretically, proteins with a molecular mass ≥69 kDa (that of albumin) represent the existence of glomerular lesions. Proteins with a molecular mass <69 kDa may be consistent with tubular damage. The purpose of this study was to evaluate the correlation between urinary proteins identified using SDS–AGE to histological lesions noted with renal biopsy.

INTERPRETATION. A total of 49 dogs with an increase in serum creatinine concentration and/or abnormal urinary protein loss were studied. Dogs with polycystic kidney disease, end-stage renal disease, renal agenesis, abdominal masses, urinary neoplasia, or urinary tract infections were excluded. Dogs with abnormal coagulation test results were also excluded. Ultrasound-guided renal biopsy was performed on each dog using a semiautomatic true-cut device. Urine from each dog was collected via ultrasound-guided cystocentesis for SDS–AGE.

Biopsy samples were fixed in formalin, sectioned and stained with haematoxylin and eosin, periodic acid-Schiff, Goldner's trichrome, methenamine and Congo red. Tubulointerstitial lesions were categorized as: 0, no lesions; 1, focal lymphoplasmacytic infiltration; 2, focal lymphoplasmacytic infiltration and corresponding tubular ectasia or atrophy; 3, focal lymphoplasmacytic infiltration, corresponding tubular ectasia or atrophy, and focal fibrosis; and 4, vascular lesions, acute tubular necrosis, or lesions observed in categories 2 or 3 but with a diffuse pattern.

Urinary proteins were classified as high molecular weight (HMW, ≥69 kDa) or low molecular weight (LMW, <69 kDa). HMW proteins were considered indicative of glomerular lesions, and LMW proteins were of tubular origin. As there is controversy as to the significance of a 69 kDa band (albumin) alone, the presence of an albumin band alone was considered pathological only if the urinary protein-to-creatinine ratio was >0.5. The limit of sensitivity for each protein fraction was 15 mg/l.

Histological examination of biopsy samples revealed isolated glomerular disease in 8 dogs (16.3%), isolated tubulointerstitial lesions in 5 dogs (10.2%), and a mixture of both glomerular and tubulointerstitial lesions in 36 dogs (73.5%). In the dogs with glomerular lesions, 11 dogs had membranous glomerulonephritis (GN), 2 had membranoproliferative GN, 14 had mesangial GN, 8 had focal segmental glomerulosclerosis, 2 had amyloidosis, 5 had pyelonephritis, and 2 had ischaemic disease. Categories of tubulointerstitial disease in all dogs were: category 0, 8 dogs; category 1, 7 dogs; category 2, 14 dogs; category 3, 10 dogs; and category 4, 3 dogs. Dogs with tubulointerstitial lesions in categories 1 and 2 were combined as indicative of mild to moderate disease, and dogs in categories 3 and 4 were combined as indicative of more severe disease. Tubulointerstitial lesions in dogs infected with leishmaniosis, ehrlichiosis or babesiosis were distributed among all categories, with no relationship between infected dogs and tubulointerstitial lesions.

Sensitivity of SDS–AGE for the detection of glomerular lesions and tubulointerstitial lesions was 100% and 92.6%, indicating a low rate of false negatives. Specificity of SDS–AGE for the detection of glomerular lesions and tubulointerstitial lesions was 40% and 62.5%, indicating the presence of false positives. Fewer false positives were seen in cases of tubulointerstitial lesions.

On SDS–AGE of urine, HMW proteins were identified at 69, 80 and 155 kDa. Of the HMW proteins, seven of 44 dogs had bands at 69 and 80 kDa, 13 dogs had bands at 69 and 155 kDa, and 24 dogs had bands at 69, 80 and 155 kDa. These patterns were equally represented among the different histological glomerular lesions, indicating that SDS–AGE was useful for determining that glomerular lesions were present, but not helpful in the definitive histological diagnosis.

On SDS–AGE of urine, LMW proteins were identified at 12, 15, 21, 25, 33 and 50 kDa. Proteins presumably of tubulointerstitial origin were identified in three dogs with no histological evidence of tubulointerstitial lesions (Table 12.2). These dogs may represent false positives with SDS–AGE, or it could be that SDS–AGE is able to identify tubulointerstitial proteins prior to the microscopic detection of lesions. Future studies could be directed at chronologically following these patients with repeated renal biopsy at a later date. The presence of LMW protein bands at 12, 15 and/or 21 kDa were noted in a significantly higher number of dogs with severe tubulointerstitial disease (categories 3 and 4), indicating that SDS–AGE can be a useful tool in the determination of severity of tubulointerstitial disease. In addition, dogs with leishmaniosis, ehrlichiosis or babesiosis had a significantly higher chance of having a 25 kDa urinary protein compared with those not affected by these conditions.

SDS–AGE of urinary proteins may result in confusing interpretation if other existing renal conditions are present. Urine from dogs with inflammation or neoplasia of the urinary tract may have HMW and LMW protein bands that could appear to be glomerular or tubulointerstitial lesions. Therefore urine sediment should be non-inflammatory before SDS–AGE of urine.

Table 12.2 Distribution of low molecular weight urinary proteins in dogs with renal tubulointerstitial lesions (% of dogs with protein band)

Protein molecular weight	Normal interstitium	Mild to moderate tubulointerstitial damage	Severe tubulointerstitial damage
12	0	0	54
15	0	0	69
21	0	25	100
25	38	89	100
33	0	25	15
50	0	46	31
No bands	62	11	0

Source: Zini et al. (2004).

Comment

Overall, SDS–AGE of urinary proteins is able to differentiate dogs with glomerular lesions from those with tubulointerstitial lesions. Severity of tubulointerstitial lesions may be suggested by the presence of specific LMW protein bands, but specific types of glomerular lesions cannot be determined by HMW protein patterns.

Echo-assisted percutaneous renal biopsy in dogs. A retrospective study of 229 cases

Zatelli A, Bonfanti U, Santilli R, Borgarelli M, Bussadori C. *Vet J* 2003a; **166**: 257–64

BACKGROUND. Renal biopsy is an integral part of diagnostic nephrology, and has been attempted since 1944. Refinements in technique have led to increased acceptance of renal biopsy. Definitive diagnosis of glomerular pathology cannot be based on biochemical parameters alone and, in human patients, the use of renal biopsy altered the diagnosis and therapy in approximately 40% of cases |5|, which altered clinical prognosis |6|. In this retrospective study, renal biopsies were reviewed for adequacy of samples obtained, accuracy of diagnosis and complications following biopsy.

INTERPRETATION. Echo-assisted renal biopsy was performed in 229 dogs, all of which presented with hyperazotaemia or nephrotic syndrome, haematuria and/or proteinuria. Biopsies were not performed if hydronephrosis, suspected renal infection, polycystic kidney disease or end-stage kidney disease was evident. Renal biopsy was also not performed in patients with uncontrolled hypertension or alterations in blood coagulation. Biopsies were performed under sedation after a 12 h fast using a Tru-cut semiautomatic instrument (TEMNO biopsy device T 189, 18 gauge × 9 cm biopsy needle), samples fixed in 10% buffered formalin, and stained with haematoxylin–eosin, periodic acid-Schiff, Goldner's trichrome, methenamine silver, and in some cases, Congo red.

Histological samples with five or more glomeruli per section were included in the analysis, and five or more glomeruli per section were observed in 96% of biopsies. Samples that were more peripheral (pericapsular) had smaller numbers of glomeruli; samples taken from the internal two-thirds of the cortex appeared most suitable. Diagnosis based on histology (Table 12.3) was: mesangial GN, 89 dogs; membranous GN, 13 dogs; membranoproliferative GN, 24 dogs; exudative proliferative GN, 3 dogs; ischaemic GN, 18 dogs; focal segmental GN, 3 dogs; glomerular immaturity, 5 dogs; amyloidosis, 14 dogs; diabetic glomerulopathy, 3 dogs; acute interstitial nephritis, 5 dogs; chronic interstitial nephritis, 6 dogs; tubular necrosis, 16 dogs; neoplasia, 6 dogs; end-stage kidney disease, 15 dogs; normal histopathology, 9 dogs. Hyperechogenicity was correlated to lesions involving the tubulointerstitial compartment.

Few complications were noted in these dogs undergoing renal biopsy. Two dogs developed subcapsular haematoma, and three exhibited macrohaematuria. These complications resolved without surgery or transfusion. No post-biopsy infections were noted.

In these cases, renal biopsy made an histological diagnosis possible, which has an impact on selection of appropriate therapy. In addition, end-stage kidney disease was observed using renal biopsy prior to evidence on ultrasound examination.

Table 12.3 Summary of canine renal biopsy histopathology

Histopathological diagnosis	No. of cases	% of cases
Mesangial glomerulonephritis (GN)	89	38.9
Membranous GN	13	5.7
Membrane-proliferative GN	24	10.5
Exudative proliferative GN	3	1.3
Ischaemic GN	18	7.9
Focal segmental glomerulosclerosis	3	1.3
Glomerular immaturity	5	2.2
Amyloidosis	14	6.1
Diabetic glomerulopathy	3	1.3
Acute interstitial nephritis	5	2.2
Chronic interstitial nephritis	6	2.6
Tubular necrosis	16	7.0
Neoplasia	6	2.6
End-stage kidney disease	15	6.6
Normal histopathology	9	3.9

Source: Zatelli *et al.* (2003a).

Comment

Echo-assisted renal biopsy using a semi-automatic method requires skill and experience, but provides an accurate diagnosis. Renal biopsy is associated with few complications in dogs that do not have hypertension or coagulation defects.

Antegrade pyelography for suspected ureteral obstruction in cats: 11 cases (1995–2001)
Adin CA, Herrgesell EJ, Nyland TG, *et al*. *J Am Vet Med Assoc* 2003; **222**(11): 1576–81

BACKGROUND. Ureteral obstruction from calcium oxalate urolithiasis is a relatively new syndrome over the past decade and appears to be increasing in cats of North America. Ureteral stones may be obstructive or non-obstructive. Cats rarely display signs of pain related to the passage of ureteral stones or when stones are lodged in the ureter. Ureteral stones may occur only in the ureter or in some combination with stones in the kidneys, bladder and urethra. Many times ureteral stones are fortuitously discovered in cats with a diagnosis of chronic intrinsic renal failure. If the ureteral stone is obstructive (causing ureteral dilatation, pyelectasia or hydronephrosis) in cats with CRF, an element of post-renal azotaemia is added to azotaemia from intrinsic CRF. Some cats present with what initially appears to be acute intrinsic renal failure when in reality it is acute post-renal failure due to obstruction in addition to the previously existing CRF. After initial stabilization the question is whether or not the ureter is obstructed, and whether the cat should undergo surgery. If surgery is chosen to relieve the obstruction, detailed planning of the surgery depends on an accurate assessment of the obstruction and its location.

INTERPRETATION. This study evaluated the usefulness of methods for detection of suspected ureteral obstruction in 11 cats with relatively severe azotaemia. Obstruction was confirmed by the inability to pass a 5-0 polypropylene suture up the ureter at the time of surgery or autopsy. These results were compared with those found on antegrade pyelography, ultrasonography and survey radiography. Intravenous urography was not performed in most cats due to concerns about radiocontrast injury to already injured kidneys.

Survey radiographs revealed asymmetry of renal size in 6 of 11 cats, and radiopaque calculi were identified in 9 of 15 ureters determined to be obstructed at surgery or autopsy (Table 12.4). The location of the obstruction was correctly assigned in 9 of 15 ureters; three of six ureters were correctly identified as non-obstructed.

Ultrasonography identified mild to severe dilatation of the renal pelvis in 17 of 18 kidneys. All 15 obstructed ureters were correctly identified with ultrasonography, but only one of three non-obstructed ureters was correctly identified. Distal ureteral dilatation of the ureter was not detected in any cat. Ureteral calculi were identified in 5 of 10 ureters (focal hyperechoic shadowing) determined to have calculi at surgery or autopsy. Location of the ureteral obstruction was properly assigned in 9 of 15 obstructed ureters.

Antegrade pyelography was performed under anaesthesia. Contrast agent was injected through a 25-gauge spinal needle placed into the renal pelvis under ultrasound guidance. This procedure was performed in 18 kidneys (unilateral in four cats and bilateral in seven cats), but interpretation was only possible in 13 of 18 due to leakage of contrast agent. Antegrade pyelography in these 13 correctly identified the obstruction and its site in 12 instances, and also correctly identified one ureter as non-obstructed. Complications of this procedure included contrast leakage in eight of 18, and subcapsular haemorrhage in six of 18 kidneys. Contrast leakage resolved in seven of eight without specific treatment, but surgery was required in one cat to repair an iatrogenic tear of the renal pelvis. Haemorrhage into the renal pelvis (contrast filling defect) developed in one cat during the procedure and resolved without event.

Surgery or autopsy was performed on all 11 cats. Causes of ureteral obstruction were unilateral calcium oxalate urolithiasis in four cats, bilateral calcium oxalate urolithiasis in three cats, bilateral mucus plug in one cat, bilateral ligation of ureter in one cat, and allograft ureteral stenosis in one cat. In one cat sent to surgery, obstruction was not confirmed as a 5-0 polypropylene suture passed from the bladder to the renal pelvis.

Comment

This paper confirms that the most common cause of ureteral obstruction in cats of North America is either unilateral or bilateral calcium oxalate urolithiasis. When there was no leakage of contrast material, antegrade pyelography was an excellent tool to confirm or rule out ureteral obstruction and to determine accurately its location. This technique is more invasive than more familiar imaging techniques of survey radiography and ultrasonography, and would not be considered for use in primary care practices due to the level of technical expertise required.

Table 12.4 Summary of methodology used for identification of obstructive lesions (% of cases)

	Survey radiographs	Ultrasound	Antegrade pyelography
Correct identification			
Obstructed	60	100	100
Non-obstructed	50	33	100
Correct location of obstruction	60	60	100
Complications			
Contrast leakage	0	0	44
Subcapsular haemorrhage	0	0	33

Source: Adin *et al.* (2003).

Survey radiography underestimated and ultrasonography overestimated the numbers of obstructed ureters. Ultrasonography found fewer ureteral stones than survey radiography.

Though the presence of a radiopaque ureterolith can be associated with obstruction, it may not be obstructive and in some cases ureteral stones are observed to pass the ureter into the bladder. All cats with CRF should have an abdominal radiograph taken to assess renal mass and renal symmetry, and to check for the presence of renal and ureteral urolithiasis. The assumption should be made that the presence of a radiopaque ureteral stone could be obstructive and that further imaging studies are needed. Usually the next step would be to perform ultrasonography to see if there is hydroureter or hydronephrosis. If the stone is not causing dilatation of the ureter or renal pelvis, conventional wisdom has been to give the cat more time to see if the stone will pass or if obstruction will develop. Some cats with CRF and obstructive ureteral stones are desperately ill and may benefit from tube nephrostomy to enhance stabilization before any surgical interventions. Antegrade pyelography through the nephrostomy tube provides the same anatomical information as described in this paper; however, leakage of contrast material is a still a problem with this method.

Though not discussed in this paper, CT of the urinary tract can provide detailed anatomical information of the ureters without need for injection of contrast material and should receive future imaging considerations. Ureteroscopy is being used at the time of surgery to further define the cause and site of ureteral obstruction in some specialty practices and institutions. Lithotripsy has been successfully employed to treat some cats with ureteral urolithiasis.

Parasitic/infectious diseases

Glomerular lesions in dogs infected with Leishmania organisms

Zatelli A, Borgarelli M, Santilli R, *et al. Am J Vet Res* 2003b; **64**(5): 558–61

BACKGROUND. Leishmaniosis is caused by infection with the protozoa *Leishmania donovani infantum*, and is endemic in the Mediterranean area. Renal pathology is often the cause of death in *Leishmania* infections. The objectives were to identify histopathological glomerular lesions in dogs infected with *Leishmania*, and to determine the correlation with patterns of urinary proteinuria as determined by SDS–AGE.

INTERPRETATION. The presence of *Leishmania* organisms was confirmed in 41 dogs with a positive indirect fluorescent antibody (IFA) test for leishmaniosis. Renal biopsies were obtained from each dog using ultrasound-assisted biopsy. Urine collected by cystocentesis prior to renal biopsy was qualitatively evaluated for proteinuria using SDS–AGE. The following histopathological lesions were identified in renal biopsy samples: mesangial GN, 9 dogs; membranous GN, 11 dogs; membranoproliferative GN, 12 dogs; focal segmental GN, 9 dogs (Table 12.5). Most of the dogs (95.1%) had non-selective glomerular proteinuria, with presence of albumin, transferrin and IgG. Mixed proteinuria (both glomerular and tubular) was present in 4.9% of dogs.

Comment

There was no correlation of type of proteinuria with different types of glomerular lesions, as almost all dogs showed the same pattern of non-selective glomerular proteinuria. SDS–AGE did allow for the identification of a glomerular pattern of proteinuria, which would not be possible with a urinary total protein concentration alone. Detection of glomerular proteinuria followed by subsequent renal biopsy may provide for the early identification of renal lesions.

Table 12.5 Summary of renal biopsy histopathological findings in leishmaniosis

Histopathological finding	No. of cases	% of cases
Mesangial GN	9	21.9
Membranous GN	11	26.8
Membranoproliferative GN	12	29.3
Focal segmental GN	9	19.5

Source: Zatelli *et al.* (2003b)

Table 12.6 Reservoir hosts for *Leptospira* serovars

Serovar	Reservoir host
L. icterohaemorrhagiae	Rat, dog
L. canicola	Dog
L. pomona	Cattle, pig, deer
L. hardjo	Cattle
L. grippotyphosa	Cattle, wildlife (raccoon, opossum)
L. autumnalis	Mice
L. bratislava	Horse, swine, rat, raccoon, opossum

Canine leptospirosis

Leptospirosis is caused by a number of different serovars of *Leptospira*. When a bivalent vaccine against *Leptospira interrogans* serovars canicola and icterohaemorrhagiae was introduced in the 1970s, the incidence of canine leptospirosis decreased in the United States. The incidence of leptospirosis is once again increasing, and this may be due to disease caused by serovars other than those included in the bivalent vaccine. At least one primary host acts as the reservoir for each serovar (Table 12.6), and *Leptospira* organisms that are shed in the urine of infected animals may survive for long periods in surface water. Other animals become infected through contact of mucous membranes or damaged skin with contaminated water. Several papers have been published in the past year investigating prevalence and risk factors for canine leptospirosis.

Serovar-specific prevalence and risk factors for leptospirosis among dogs: 90 cases (1997–2002)

Ward MP, Guptill LF, Prahl A, Wu CC. *J Am Vet Med Assoc* 2004a; **224**(12): 1958–63

BACKGROUND. There are recent reports of leptospirosis caused by *L. interrogans* serovars bratislava and pomona and *L. kirschneri* serovar grippotyphosa for which livestock and wildlife serve as the reservoir. Thus increased contact between dogs and livestock or wildlife may account for some of the increase in cases of leptospirosis. The objective of this study was to estimate the serovar prevalence of leptospirosis at a Midwestern diagnostic laboratory, and to identify risk factors and seasonal patterns of leptospirosis.

INTERPRETATION. Dogs were diagnosed with leptospirosis based on clinical signs supported by a positive microscopic agglutination test (MAT; reciprocal titre ≥800) or visual identification of *Leptospira*-like organisms seen on silver stain of liver or kidney tissue. Cases were identified both from dogs presented to the veterinary hospital, and from serum submitted to the diagnostic laboratory. MAT titres against *Leptospira* last only a few months, and vaccination titres rarely are >100–400, so a serum sample with an observed reciprocal titre ≥800 was assumed to be submitted due to clinical signs of leptospirosis.

Over a 6-year period, 39 dogs were hospitalized with leptospirosis (0.25% of admissions). During this same time period, a total of 51 samples (11% of samples submitted for leptospirosis testing) submitted from practitioners in Indiana, Illinois and Michigan were positive for leptospirosis. Most of the hospitalized cases of leptospirosis occurred during the fall, whereas the majority of positive cases from diagnostic laboratory submissions occurred during the summer. The highest prevalence of leptospirosis among hospitalized patients was in 2000, whereas the highest prevalence of leptospirosis among samples submitted to the diagnostic laboratory was in 1998. In both hospitalized patients and submitted samples, *L. kirschneri* serovar grippotyphosa showed the highest prevalence. Both *L. kirschneri* serovar grippotyphosa and *L. interrogans* serovar bratislava were detected in every year of the study, and *L. interrogans* serovar pomona was detected in every year except 2002 (Table 12.7). Leptospirosis was 5.7 times more likely in dogs between the ages of 4 and 6.9 years, as compared with dogs <1 year old, and was 4.2 times more likely in sexually intact male dogs as compared with intact females. No breed associations were noted.

Comment

In the Midwest region, the increase in incidence of leptospirosis is at least partly caused by the increase in prevalence of *L. kirschneri* serovar grippotyphosa. Several wildlife species are reservoir hosts for *L. kirschneri* serovar grippotyphosa, and the racoon population is endemically infected in parts of the Midwestern and southern United States. This is the first study of a seroprevalence survey of leptospirosis in the United States. Comparison with previous studies is difficult due to different MAT cut-off titres among studies, and different study designs. *L. interrogans* serovar autumnalis was not included in this panel of MAT serovars, which could possibly have underestimated the prevalence of leptospirosis. However, it is not believed that this serovar is present in the Midwest. Also as MAT results may be negative within

Table 12.7 Prevalence (%) of serovars of *Leptospira* in sera samples submitted to the Purdue University Animal Disease Diagnostic Laboratory from 1997 to 2002

Serovar	Year						
	1997	1998	1999	2000	2001	2002	1997–2002
L. kirschneri serovar grippotyphosa	7.5	14.6	2.7	3.6	4.2	5.9	6.4
L. interrogans serovar bratislava	2.5	6.1	1.4	1.8	3.4	1.0	2.8
L. interrogans serovar icterohaemorrhagiae	0	0	1.4	7.1	0	2.0	1.5
L. interrogans serovar pomona	2.5	4.9	1.4	3.6	1.7	0	2.1
L. interrogans serovar canicola	0	0	0	0	0	0	0
L. borgpetersenii serovar hardjo	0	0	1.4	0	0	0	0.2
All serovars	12.5	25.6	8.3	16.1	9.3	8.9	10.9

Source: Ward et al. (2004a).

the first several weeks of leptospirosis infection, prevalence of leptospirosis may be underestimated. Previous studies have identified breed-associated risk for leptospirosis; however, this risk was not observed in this study. There may be regional breed-associated risks, and future studies should examine breed and environment. With the increase in prevalence of *L. kirschneri* serovar grippotyphosa, it may be prudent to vaccinate dogs with exposure to racoons in their environment to this serovar.

Evaluation of environmental risk factors for leptospirosis in dogs: 36 cases (1997–2002)
Ward MP, Guptill LF, Wu CC. *J Am Vet Med Assoc* 2004b; **225**: 72–7

BACKGROUND. Environmental risk factors for canine leptospirosis were determined in 36 cases from 1997 to 2002. Dogs included in the study were presented to the Purdue University Veterinary Teaching Hospital (Indiana) and diagnosed with leptospirosis on the basis of history, clinical signs, laboratory evaluation, response to treatment, and either a positive MAT titre, or the visualization of leptospires in silver-stained liver or kidney tissue specimens. Cases seronegative for *Leptospira* serovars were considered controls for comparison. A number of geographical and environmental factors were investigated in association with the incidence of leptospirosis.

INTERPRETATION. In 19 of 30 dogs in which a serovar could be identified, leptospirosis was associated with *L. kirschneri* serovar grippotyphosa (Table 12.8). With age and sex adjustment, a dog living within 1000 m of an area urbanized between 1990 and 2000 was 26 times more likely to have leptospirosis (of any serovar), and was 11.5 times more likely to be infected with *L. kirschneri* serovar grippotyphosa.

Table 12.8 Significant associations of canine leptospirosis caused by *L kirschneri* serovar grippotyphosa and environmental factors

	Odds ratio
Increased risk of infection	
Urbanized areas 1990–2000	15.46
Rural areas	2.22
School with recreation facility	2.51
Decreased risk of infection	
Areas frequently flooded	0.19
Areas with poor drainage	0.45
County dairy cattle density > median	0.52
County forest density > median	0.48

Source: Ward *et al.* (2004b)

Comment

Unfortunately, wildlife survey data were unavailable for analysis in conjunction with this study. With recent urbanization of rural areas, small periurban areas of forest may remain with a high concentration of wildlife. This increased population in newly urbanized areas may provide a high level of exposure to wildlife within a relatively small area. With the increased risk of leptospirosis in dogs living in a newly urbanized area, vaccination against *Leptospira* serovars may be recommended.

 ## Leptospirosis in dogs: a serologic survey and case series 1996 to 2001

Boutilier P, Carr A, Schulman RL. *Vet Ther* 2003; **4**(4): 387–96

BACKGROUND. Of 1260 canine serum samples submitted to the University of Illinois diagnostic laboratory, 364 (29%) were considered positive for one of more serovars of *Leptospira* using MAT. A positive titre was considered to be any titre greater than 1:100, and six serovars were included: *L. icterohaemorrhagiae*, *L. canicola*, *L. pomona*, *L. hardjo*, *L. bratislava* and *L. grippotyphosa*. In addition, cases that were positive from the University of Illinois Veterinary Teaching Hospital were reviewed, and a clinical diagnosis of leptospirosis was made if the titre was ≥1:800, clinical signs of leptospirosis were present, and the dog had not recently been vaccinated.

INTERPRETATION. A majority (66%) of the positive cases submitted to the diagnostic laboratory had low titres. The remaining positive samples had titres ≥1:800. Of the positive samples, 54% had titres to more than one serovar. The predominant serovar in the group with low titres was *L. canicola* (38%), followed by *L. icterohaemorrhagiae* (34%), *L. bratislava* (25%), *L. grippotyphosa* (14%) and *L. pomona* (8%). In the group with high titres (≥1:800), the predominant serovar was *L. grippotyphosa* (72%), followed by *L. bratislava* (31%), *L. canicola* (10%), *L. icterohaemorrhagiae* (8%) and *L. pomona* (6%) (Table 12.9).

A total of 87 of the 364 positive samples were from patients admitted to the University of Illinois Veterinary Teaching Hospital. Predominant serovars in this subpopulation with low titres were to *L. icterohaemorrhagiae* and *L. canicola*. Serovars *L. bratislava* and *L. grippotyphosa* were the most common serovars in this subpopulation with high titres.

In 15 hospital cases, clinical leptospirosis was the final diagnosis. All cases had a titre ≥1:800, and the predominant serovar was *L. grippotyphosa*. Three dogs had an equal titre to *L. bratislava*. The majority of these cases had titres to more than one serovar. Clinically, 67% of these dogs had signs of renal disease with no hepatic involvement, 20% had clinical signs of hepatic disease with no renal involvement, and 13% had signs of both renal and hepatic involvement. There was no apparent breed predilection, and all cases had been previously vaccinated with a bivalent vaccine for *L. canicola* and *L. icterohaemorrhagiae*. Fifty-three per cent of cases presented during the summer, and 40% presented in the fall. Clinical signs included: anorexia (67%), vomiting (53%), polyuria/polydipsia (33%), lethargy (13%), fever (13%) and weight loss (7%).

The predominance of *L. grippotyphosa* in clinical cases may be the result of contact of dogs with racoons. In a wildlife survey, 48% of wild racoons in Illinois were positive for

Table 12.9 Incidence of serovar (%) in all cases testing positive for leptospirosis

Serovar	High titre (≥1:800)	Low titre	Clinical cases
L. grippotyphosa	72	14	100
L. bratislava	31	25	20
L. canicola	10	38	0
L. icterohaemorrhagiae	8	24	0
L. pomona	6	8	0
L. hardjo	0	0	0

Source: Boutilier et al. (2003).

leptospirosis, and *L. grippotyphosa* was the predominant serovar in 99% of seropositive racoons |7|. Farm-captured racoons had a higher seropositive rate than did park-captured racoons.

Comment

This study confirms the serovar *L. grippotyphosa* as a major cause of leptospirosis in Midwest US, causing both renal and hepatic disease. Vaccination with new vaccines containing this serovar may decrease the incidence of leptospirosis. However, other serovars may also be present that were not included in the testing regimen. *L. autumnalis* has been reported in association with hepatic disease, and it would be interesting to determine if this serovar is also present within this population.

Epidemiology of leptospirosis: observations on serological data obtained by a 'diagnostic laboratory for leptospirosis' from 1995 to 2001
Cerri D, Ebani VV, Fratini F, Pinzauti P, Andreani E. *New Microbiol* 2003; **26**: 383–9

BACKGROUND. Over a 7-year period, 9885 serum samples from domestic and wild animals and humans living in northern and central Italy were examined by the MAT test. Sera was collected from those with clinical symptoms consistent with leptospirosis, and sera with titres ≥1:400 were considered positive for leptospirosis.

INTERPRETATION. Percentages of seropositivity were: 12.13% of sheep, 11.40% of horses, 9.46% of swine, 6.36% of dogs, 2.39% of wild boars, 1.39% of deer and 5.60% of humans (Table 12.10). *L. interrogans* serovar bratislava was the most widespread serovar, infecting 97% of swine, 81% of horses and 55% of dogs. *L. interrogans* serovar icterrohaemorrhagiae infected a large percentage of dogs (45%), horses (18%) and humans (85%). All infections (100%) in sheep were caused by *L. borgpetersenii* serovar hardjo.

Table 12.10 Incidence of *Leptospira* serovars in serum samples from 1995 to 2001 in Italy

Serovar	Cattle	Swine	Equine	Ovine	Canine	Buffalo	Deer	Wild boar	Man	Total
Bratislava	33%	97%	81%	0	55%	0	50%	100%	15%	55%
Balum arboreae	0	0	0	0	0	0	0	0	0	0
Canicola	0	0	0	0	0	0	0	0	0	0
Grippotyphosa	0	0	0	0	0	0	0	0	0	0
Icterohaemorrhagiae	33%	<1%	18%	0	45%	0	0	0	85%	22%
Pomona	0	3%	<1%	0	0	0	0	0	0	<1%
Hardjo	33%	0	0	100%	0	100%	50%	0	0	22%
Tarassovi	0	0	0	0	0	0	0	0	0	0
Total infection in species	<1%	9%	11%	12%	6%	22%	1%	2%	6%	7%

Source: Cerri *et al.* (2003).

The highest incidence of leptospirosis in canines occurred in 1995, with a decreased incidence in 1996 through 2001. The highest incidence of leptospirosis in both swine and horses occurred in 1998. In general, a decrease of infections with icterohaemorrhagiae and an increase of infections with bratislava was observed from 1995 to 2001.

Comment

Unfortunately at this time, there is no vaccine available against *L. interrogans* serovar bratislava. This study demonstrates the geographical differences in serovars of *Leptospira*. No canine cases of *L. grippotyphosa* were seen in this population, yet the grippotyphosa serovar was the most common serovar noted in Midwest United States. This may be due to differences in exposure to reservoir hosts.

Chronic renal failure

Clinical efficacy and safety of recombinant canine erythropoietin in dogs with anemia of chronic renal failure and dogs with recombinant human erythropoietin-induced red cell aplasia

Randolph JF, Scarlett J, Stokol T, MacLeod JN. *J Vet Int Med* 2004; **18**: 81–91

BACKGROUND. Erythropoietin (EPO) is necessary for erythrocyte production, and is produced in the renal cortex. In CRF, a decrease in EPO production is the main cause of non-regenerative anaemia. This anaemia contributes to the weakness, lethargy and anorexia observed in dogs with CRF. Recombinant human EPO (rhEPO) is effectively used in human patients with CRF, and is also used in dogs with CRF to stimulate erythrocyte production. Unfortunately, many dogs treated with rhEPO develop antibodies against rhEPO that block the bioactivity of rhEPO and may neutralize residual endogenous canine EPO leading to red cell aplasia. Recombinant canine EPO (rcEPO) has been produced but is not commercially available. The purpose of this study was to evaluate the efficacy and safety of rcEPO in dogs with CRF, and to determine if treatment with rcEPO could restore erythrocyte production in dogs with red cell aplasia caused by previous rhEPO treatment.

INTERPRETATION. A total of 25 dogs with naturally occurring CRF were identified; 19 dogs had not been previously treated with rhEPO (group 1), and six dogs had red cell aplasia as a consequence of rhEPO treatment (group 2) (Table 12.11). All dogs received rcEPO (subcutaneously) for up to 52 weeks. Only 2 of 19 dogs in group 1 survived for 52 weeks, and only one dog in group 2 survived for 24 weeks.

Mean haematocrit (Ht, %) in all dogs at the start of the study was approximately 16 (target range 35–45). Dogs that had not been previously treated with rhEPO (group 1) showed a steady increase in Ht during the first 8 weeks of treatment. After 1 week of treatment with rcEPO, Ht was significantly higher than the pretreatment value. Eighteen of these 19 dogs responded to rcEPO treatment. In group 1, 74% of the dogs showed a significant increase in Ht by week 3, and 90% had responded by week 5. None of the dogs in group 1 developed anaemia refractory to rcEPO treatment. Dogs in group 1 that survived for 8–16 weeks showed a significant weight gain, and subjective evaluation indicated that appetite increased in 53% and energy level increased in 74% of dogs in group 1. Dogs in group 1 survived significantly longer than dogs in group 2, with 50% of dogs in group 1 and <17% in group 2 surviving to day 53.

Dogs that had red cell aplasia due to rhEPO treatment never showed a significant increase in mean Ht, despite five of the six dogs receiving blood transfusions. Only two of these six dogs responded to rcEPO treatment. Two dogs in group 2 survived to week 8 of the study, and only one survived to week 24.

Adverse effects of rcEPO administration appeared minimal. Pain at injection sites were noted in four dogs; however, three of these four dogs were also receiving subcutaneous

Table 12.11 Selected parameters in dogs receiving rcEPO

	CRF dogs that had not received rhEPO ($n = 19$)	CRF dogs with rhEPO-induced red cell aplasia ($n = 6$)
Survival time (% surviving)		
24 weeks	32	17
52 weeks	11	0
Haematocrit (%)		
Week 0	16.2	15.1
Week 2	23.9	14.0
Week 8	46.0	19.8

Source: Randolph et al. (2004).

fluids, and pain resolved even though injections with rcEPO was continued. One dog developed a fever and anorexia after the first injection of rcEPO, which resolved when treatment was discontinued, and did not return when rcEPO therapy was reinstituted. This same dog developed elevations in serum alanine transaminase activity and serum alkaline phosphatase activity after 3 weeks of rcEPO therapy. When rcEPO therapy was discontinued, alanine transaminase and alkaline phosphatase activities returned to normal. Episodic vomiting and poor appetite developed in many dogs, but this was attributed to uraemia.

Comment

Results of this study showed that red blood cell production was stimulated in group 1 dogs treated with rcEPO without development of red cell aplasia as noted with rhEPO treatment. However, rcEPO treatment was not as effective at restoring red blood cell production in dogs with red cell aplasia due to prior rhEPO treatment. Treatment with rcEPO may be instituted earlier in the course of CRF, and may provide a longer period of increased quality of life.

Association between initial systolic blood pressure and risk of developing a uremic crisis or of dying in dogs with chronic renal failure

Jacob F, Polzin DJ, Osborne CA, et al. *J Am Vet Med Assoc* 2003; **222**(3): 322–9

BACKGROUND. Systemic hypertension is a known risk factor for the progression of CRF in humans and in experimental models of renal failure in dogs and cats. Systemic hypertension is also suspected to be a factor in the progression of clinical CRF in dogs and cats. Systemic hypertension occurs in as many as 50% of dogs with CRF, depending on definition of normal blood pressure, and whether the evaluation is from a first opinion or referral specialist evaluation. Serious systemic hypertension is often first suspected in dogs or cats that have retinal lesions (vascular congestion, vascular tortuosity, retinal detachment) and visual deficits.

INTERPRETATION. This study examines the effect of systemic systolic blood pressure in 45 dogs with CRF. Thirty-eight of these dogs were described previously in a study demonstrating a salutary effect of a renal diet on CRF; seven dogs were excluded from the initial study due to systolic blood pressure >180 mmHg, but are now included in this study. Nearly all the blood pressure measurements were made with use of oscillometric methods; Doppler methods were used in a few dogs in which heart rate was not accurately measured by the oscillometric machine. Though the 38 dogs were assigned to either a maintenance diet or a veterinary renal diet, the effects of hypertension were found to be independent of diet, so all dogs were grouped together for statistical analysis. Treatment with antihypertensive medication was recommended if systolic blood pressure was >180 mmHg on two consecutive visits.

Blood pressure groups were assigned based on either blood pressure value recorded on first visit or the average of the first and 1 month visits. Results were similar regardless of which assignment method of blood pressure groups was used. High blood pressure was defined as 161–201 mmHg on the first visit or 161–217 on the averaged two visits. Intermediate blood pressure was defined as 144–160 or 147–163, and low pressure as 107–143 or 109–145. Because of high mortality in the high blood pressure group, data were analysed for only 12 months in this study (compared with 2 years in the diet study).

Baseline data were not different among groups, with the exception that dogs in the high pressure group had significantly higher urinary protein to urinary creatinine ratios. Fourteen dogs were candidates for antihypertensive therapy with persistent increases of systolic pressure to ≥180 mmHg; seven were found at these pressures during initial evaluation and seven developed later for an incidence of 30% of dogs in this series. Three of these 14 dogs did not receive medication due to decisions of the owner. The remaining 11 dogs were treated with a variety of drugs commonly used in veterinary medicine to lower systemic blood pressure, but a decrease to <160 mmHg as the desired target range for blood pressure was achieved in only one dog.

Risks for a uraemic crisis, death from a renal cause, or death from any cause were significantly increased to at least threefold in dogs of the high pressure group compared with those with intermediate or low systolic pressure (Table 12.12). Dogs in the high pressure group developed a uraemic crisis, and death due to renal or any cause occurred much more quickly than those in the intermediate and lower pressure groups. Median days of survival were less than half for dogs of the high blood pressure group. Renal function as estimated by the reciprocal of serum creatinine declined much more rapidly in the high blood pressure group; the slope of this line did not change significantly in those with intermediate or lower blood pressures.

Retinal lesions suggestive of hypertension were found in only three dogs of this study and in those the systolic pressures were 191–201 mmHg. In the additional 11 dogs of the high blood pressure group, no retinal lesions were detected. Obviously, the presence of ocular lesions in dogs with CRF can be associated with systemic hypertension but the absence of such lesions does not exclude the presence of high blood pressure.

Comment

This paper provides compelling evidence that high blood pressure during initial evaluation of CRF in dogs is a major risk factor for more rapid progression of the loss of renal functions, uraemic crises and death. As only one dog with high blood pres-

Table 12.12 Association between development of uraemic crisis or death and initial systolic blood pressure (SBP) in dogs with CRF

	Low SBP		Intermediate SBP		High SBP	
	% of dogs	Days to event	% of dogs	Days to event	% of dogs	Days to event
Development of uraemic crisis	44	599	40	624	57	289
Death from renal causes	44	599	53	624	57	281
Death from any cause	62	425	73	348	79	154

Source: Jacob et al. (2003).

sure actually achieved some degree of control of hypertension with medication, it could be argued that much of the progression continued at a rapid rate due to failure to control the systemic blood pressure. The results of this study are important in that systemic hypertension in the higher ranges is a risk factor if the blood pressure cannot be controlled. Will conversion of high blood pressure group dogs with CRF to those with intermediate or low blood pressure groups provide protection for the progression of CRF? We hypothesize that the answer is yes, but evidence-based outcomes of this treatment remain to be reported.

Assessment of acid-base status of cats with naturally occurring chronic renal failure

Elliott J, Syme HM, Reubens E, Markwell PJ. *J Small Anim Pract* 2003a; **44**(2): 65–70

Acid-base balance of cats with chronic renal failure: effect of deterioration in renal function

Elliott J, Syme HM, Markwell PJ. *J Small Anim Pract* 2003b; **44**(6): 261–8

BACKGROUND. The presence of metabolic acidosis may activate the catabolic process in muscle that would be adverse in patients with CRF. Metabolic acidosis is known to potentiate renal osteodystrophy in humans and contribute to progression of CRF is some rodent models. Some consider metabolic acidosis a uraemic toxin. Based on previous reports from teaching hospitals in North America, the occurrence of metabolic acidosis in cats with CRF has been considered common.

INTERPRETATION. In the first paper, samples from 59 cats with CRF and 27 normal control cats from a first opinion clinic in London (UK) were analysed to determine how frequently acid–base disturbances occurred. Only cats that had stable CRF at initial evaluation were recruited into this study. No cat had evidence for severe dehydration and none were considered for hospitalization at the first visit. Cats with mild or moderate CRF were recruited into the study if they had not been treated with any diet or drug therapy. Some of the severe CRF cats had been on long-term dietary treatment and antihypertensive medication; they were studied when their renal function deteriorated. Mild CRF was defined as those cats with serum creatinine from 155 to 249 μmol/l, mild CRF as those with serum creatinine from 250 to 399 μmol/l, and severe CRF as those with serum creatinine over 400 μmol/l. It is interesting that the urinary specific gravity decreased as the magnitude of the azotaemia increased in this study. Packed cell volume (PCV) was progressively less than control cats in those with mild azotaemia and in those with either moderate or severe azotaemia.

Mean venous pH and bicarbonate concentration was significantly decreased only in the group of cats with severe CRF (Table 12.13). The anion gap was increased in cats with mild CRF and more so in cats with severe CRF. Ten of 19 cats with severe CRF had venous pH less than the lower limit of the reference range of 7.27. Interestingly, only 6 of these 10 cats had bicarbonate values less than the reference range of 14 mmol/l. P_{CO2} did not differ among groups. No cat in the mild CRF group had venous pH <7.27, but three cats in the moderate CRF group did have venous pH <7.27. Plasma chloride was significantly less in the severe CRF cats than in other groups of cats.

Urine pH decreased progressively as the degree of severity of the CRF became more severe. All cats with metabolic acidosis had a urinary pH <6.1.

Most cats of this study with mild (100%) or moderate CRF (85%) maintained normal venous pH and bicarbonate concentration. Over 50% of cats with severe CRF in this study had decreased venous pH and bicarbonate concentrations. It is likely that cats of previous reports had advanced renal failure similar to that of cats in the category of severe CRF in this report. Hypokalaemia or potassium depletion has been associated with the development of metabolic acidosis in cats. Though hypokalaemia was documented in 14 of 59 cats with CRF, only 4 of these 14 had metabolic acidosis; it would appear that this is not a major mechanism in cats of this study.

The second study was designed to determine if metabolic acidosis preceded an increase in severity of CRF or only happened after CRF deteriorated. Fifty-five cats were studied serially to assess renal function and acid–base status with blood gas analysis; no data were included for analysis from times of uraemic crisis. Cats were assigned as follows: group 1 had no trend of increasing serum creatinine ($n = 34$), group 2 had cats with sudden increases in serum creatinine ($n = 14$), and group 3 cats had gradual increases in serum creatinine concentration ($n = 7$). All cats were prescribed a diet restricted in protein and phosphate; antibiotics, oral potassium supplementation and antihypertensive medications were prescribed as needed.

Group 1 cats were followed for a median of 327 days. Metabolic acidosis was identified in only one of the cats in this group despite lack of increase in serum creatinine concentration (Table 12.14). This cat lost over 10% of its body mass and was euthanized due to poor quality of life. Two of the remaining 33 cats that did not develop acidosis or increased serum creatinine were euthanized due to weight loss and poor quality of life.

Three of 14 cats in group 2 progressed from mild to moderate CRF, and four cats progressed within the mild or moderate CRF categories as described in the first study. Six of 14 cats progressed from mild or moderate CRF to severe CRF, and one progressed within the severe category of CRF. Cats in group 2 that progressed to severe CRF had substantial weight loss. There were no detected changes in acid–base status in group 2 cats that progressed from mild to moderate CRF. Cats that progressed to or within severe CRF had lower mean pH and bicarbonate values but did not achieve statistical significance. The prognosis for survival

Table 12.13 Selected acid–base parameters in cats with CRF

	Normal cats	Mild renal failure	Moderate renal failure	Severe renal failure
Venous pH	7.353[a]	7.355[a]	7.341[a]	7.275[b]
Blood HCO_3 (mmol/l)	17.67[a]	18.20[a]	18.35[a]	15.89[b]
Anion gap (mmol/l)	13.91[a]	17.23[b]	16.00[a]	22.53[c]
Urine pH	6.08[a]	6.00[a,b]	5.79[b,c]	5.72[c]
Ammonium/creatinine ratio	5.15[a]	4.21[a,b]	2.41[b]	3.33[b]

Values within a row with a different superscript are significantly different. Source: Elliott et al. (2003a).

Table 12.14 Metabolic acidosis development in cats with CRF

	Group 1: no increase in creatinine	Group 2: sudden increase in creatinine	Group 3: gradual increase in creatinine
Developed metabolic acidosis (%)	3	0	14
Euthanized due to poor quality of life (%)	9	86	86

Source: Elliott et al. (2003b).

was poor overall in group 2 cats as 12 of the 14 cats were euthanized within about 2 months due to poor quality of life or uraemic crises.

One of seven cats in group 3 progressed within mild CRF but no acidosis was detected in this cat. Six of seven cats progressed to or within the severe CRF category; only one of these cats developed venous pH <7.249.

Comment

It is possible that the metabolic acidosis encountered in cats with severe CRF may have been worse than documented in the first study, as many of the cats were eating veterinary foods designed to help correct metabolic acidosis. Cats with mild to moderate CRF are not expected to have metabolic acidosis, a situation more likely to be encountered in first opinion clinics rather than specialty referral or teaching hospitals.

Results from the second study suggest that metabolic acidosis is rare in cats with stable CRF (prior to further deterioration in renal function). Even in cats that transformed from milder to more severe CRF, acidosis was uncommon until severe CRF was encountered. Metabolic acidosis was more common in cats that had stepwise reduction in renal function rather than in cats with gradual reductions.

It is important to remember that progressive decreases in excretory renal function may not be reflected in an increasing concentration of serum creatinine especially if muscle mass (the origin of creatinine) declines substantially. Four of the 34 cats in group 1 lost over 10% of their body weight without an increase in serum creatinine.

The degree of metabolic acidosis is expected to be substantially higher in cats that are in an uraemic crisis but is relatively uncommon otherwise.

Conclusion

Many exciting papers regarding veterinary nephrology have recently emerged. We selected 12 papers with international appeal to review in detail from more than 100 papers under consideration.

Exciting advancements have been made in methodology and diagnostics. The clinical utility for the measurement of serum or plasma urea nitrogen and creatinine concentrations has wide implications for private practitioners. An increase in urea nitrogen alone may be due to a non-fasting state, and should not necessarily cause alarm prior to repeating the analysis with a fasting sample. The finding that serum creatinine varies with body weight is important and suggests that body weight needs to be factored into the interpretation of serum creatinine concentration, despite laboratory normal ranges that presently incorporate all sizes of dogs. The development of weight based normal ranges for serum creatinine concentration is encouraged. Urinary crystals must be interpreted with caution, especially if urine has been refrigerated. This has important implications in that crystals observed in laboratory observation of stored urine may not have been present in the urine when collected. When crystals are detected in urine from stored samples, a second urine sample should be obtained and urinary sediment analysed within 15 min to determine if the crystals are pathologically present. Urinary protein electrophoresis is a relatively new technique, and is able to differentiate dogs with glomerular lesions from those with tubulointerstitial lesions. Severity of tubulointerstitial lesions can be determined by the presence of specific patterns of LMW urinary proteins. Renal biopsy performed with ultrasonographic guidance was shown to provide diagnostic samples without complications in most dogs, though it was noted that proper training in this technique is essential. Antegrade pyelography can be a highly accurate tool for the localization of ureteral stones in cats but this methodology is mostly limited to tertiary referral centres. The largest limitation for use of antegrade pyelography is leakage of contrast materials, which renders the imaging study non-diagnostic in some instances.

Several studies focused on parasitic diseases. Leishmaniosis is often associated with glomerular lesions as shown by renal biopsy, but a specific glomerular lesion could not be predicted by the type of proteinuria, as non-selective proteinuria occurs with all renal lesions. Clinical leptospirosis is usually associated with some form of renal and or liver involvement, though it appears that renal involvement is more common. Disease is usually due to serovars for which dogs are not vaccinated, and varies by geographic location. It appears that encroachment of wildlife on living spaces for people and their pets may provide exposure to serovars that have not been recognized previously. Dogs living in newly urbanized areas of Midwest United States appear to be at increased risk especially for *L. kirshneri* serovar grippotyphosa. Interestingly no cases attributed to this serovar were noted in Italy, as infections with serovar bratislava and icterohaemorrhagiae were most common.

A number of studies focused on the diagnosis and treatment of CRF. Dogs with CRF and anaemia treated with rcEPO responded well by increasing Ht without apparent development of anti-EPO antibodies. Unfortunately, dogs that had developed red cell hypoplasia as a result of previous treatment with rhEPO did not respond to treatment with rcEPO. Treatment with rcEPO is obviously superior to the use of rhEPO for treatment of anaemia associated with CRF as it is not associated with the development of anti-EPO antibodies. Unfortunately, there is presently no commercially available formulation of rcEPO, which dampens our enthusiasm about the effectiveness of this treatment. Control of hypertension may be important in the prognosis of CRF. Risks for an uraemic crisis or death increased by at least threefold in dogs with high blood pressure and CRF. Discovery of high systolic blood pressure at the time of diagnosis of CRF is a factor that needs to be considered when discussing the prognosis for a particular dog. It remains to be determined what the risks would be if the hypertension were adequately controlled, as unfortunately nearly none of the dogs in this study achieved targeted levels of blood pressure considered adequate for control of hypertension. Concerns about the presence of metabolic acidosis may be over-rated in cats with CRF, at least in those with compensated forms of CRF. Metabolic acidosis does not appear to precede decrements in renal function especially if the decrements are gradual in nature.

This is an exciting time in veterinary nephrology as we continue to advance in our understanding of renal diseases and our ability to provide accurate diagnoses and treatment. We anticipate that next year will continue this trend, especially with drugs that may countervail chronic inflammation and scarring in damaged kidneys with use of angiotensin-converting enzyme inhibitors and possibly with use of other new generation drugs designed to limit renal fibrosis (spironolactone, eplerenone, BMP-7).

References

1. Riviere JE, Coppoc GL. Pharmacokinetics of gentamicin in the juvenile dog. *Am J Vet Res* 1981; **42**(9): 1621–3.
2. van den Brom WE, Biewenga WJ. Assessment of glomerular filtration rate in normal dog: analysis of the 51Cr-EDTA clearance and its relation to several endogenous parameters of glomerular filtration. *Res Vet Sci* 1981; **30**(2): 152–7.
3. Feeman WE 3rd, Couto CG, Gray TL. Serum creatinine concentrations in retired racing Greyhounds. *Vet Clin Pathol* 2003; **32**: 40–2.
4. Sturgess CP, Hesford A, Owen H, Privett R. An investigation into the effects of storage on the diagnosis of crystalluria in cats. *J Feline Med Surg* 2001; **3**(2): 81–5.
5. Richards NT, Darby S, Howie AJ, Adu D, Michael J. Knowledge of renal histology alters patient management in over 40% of cases. *Nephrol Dial Transpl* 1994; **9**: 1255–9.
6. Turner MW, Hutchinson TA, Barre PE, Prichard S, Jothy S. A prospective study on the impact of the renal biopsy in clinical management. *Clin Nephrol* 1986; **26**: 217–21.
7. Mitchell MA, Hungeford LL, Nixon C, Esker T, Sullivan J, Koerkenmeier R, Dubey JP. Serologic survey for selected infectious disease agents in raccoons from Illinois. *J Wildl Dis* 1999; **35**(2): 347–55.

13

Cardiology

ADRIAN BOSWOOD

Introduction

In recent years some fundamental shifts in our understanding of cardiac diseases and their treatment have occurred. These shifts have taken place in a number of areas affecting the diagnosis, treatment and prognosis of the animals that we treat. Many of the trends developing in the field of human cardiology are reflected in the trends emerging in the veterinary arena. It is easy in this rapidly altering environment to lose one's bearings. This chapter will try to review some of the areas in which small animal cardiology appears to be developing most rapidly. I will also try to make some sense of and provide a structure for the way in which these recent studies should be interpreted. Finally, and perhaps most challenging, I will try to indicate the directions in which these changes may take us in future.

It is impossible to review all of the literature that has been published in the last 18 months in the field of small animal cardiology and, therefore, I will try to choose themes and a few key publications that I think illustrate the way in which these themes are developing. The main areas can roughly be summarized as the development and use of biomarkers in small animal cardiology, the diagnosis and classification of myocardial diseases of the dog and cat, interventional techniques in congenital heart disease and, finally, developments in our understanding of therapy for heart disease and failure.

Biomarkers in heart disease

A biomarker is 'a characteristic that is objectively measured and evaluated as an indicator of normal biologic processes, pathogenic processes, or pharmacologic responses to a therapeutic intervention' [1]. A very wide array of characteristics can be considered as biomarkers of cardiac disease and failure. A number of circulating markers of cardiac disease have been established. Numerous recent studies have evaluated the utility of these substances in the veterinary field. Among the many circulating markers that have been evaluated, the two most promising markers appear to be the natriuretic peptides and the cardiac troponins. These substances increase in the circulation for different reasons and give us quite different information about the type of heart disease present.

The natriuretic peptides were first discovered in the early 1980s |2|, and it is now established that an array of natriuretic peptides are present in the body |3|. These are present in varying concentrations in the circulation in both their active form and as precursor molecules and breakdown products. Broadly speaking, as the filling pressures of the cardiac chambers increase, the levels of these peptides increase. Increases in atrial pressure, or more specifically atrial wall stretch result in the release of increased amounts of atrial natriuretic peptide (ANP) and its precursor molecule proANP. Increases in left ventricular end diastolic pressure increase the manufacture and release of B-type natriuretic peptide (BNP) into the circulation. Numerous studies of these natriuretic peptides in veterinary patients have been performed and the results published. An excellent review of the activation of this system in canine patients with myxomatous mitral valve disease has also been published |4|. Recent publications have added further to our understanding in this area and the potential use of these in the diagnosis of cardiac disease and the prognostication for patients with cardiac disease. I will consider two of these papers as a basis for a more general discussion of this area.

Brain natriuretic peptide concentration in dogs with heart disease and congestive heart failure

MacDonald KA, Kittleson MD, Munro C, Kass P. *J Vet Intern Med* 2003; **17**(2): 172–7

BACKGROUND. Of the natriuretic peptides that have been discovered, BNP is widely thought to be the most accurate for the diagnosis of heart failure in human patients with cardiac disease. Until recently, BNP has received proportionately less attention than ANP in veterinary patients for two practical reasons. First, ANP was the first natriuretic peptide discovered and characterized and, secondly, ANP has a sequence that is conserved across many species, whereas BNP differs between species in both sequence and number of peptides. The latter point therefore means that assays developed for the measurement of BNP in human patients will not necessarily be effective in canine patients. This paper is among a number of emerging studies looking at the assessment of BNP in veterinary patients with cardiac disease.

INTERPRETATION. In this study the authors evaluate BNP concentrations in 34 dogs, 9 control dogs and 25 dogs affected by mitral valve disease. The assay used was a radioimmunoassay specific for canine BNP. The concentrations of BNP were then analysed to look for differences according to the presence and severity of heart disease or failure. The BNP concentrations were also analysed to see whether there was any predictive value, i.e. whether those dogs with higher BNP concentrations had different outcomes to those dogs with lower BNP concentrations.

There were a number of interesting findings. First, there was a significantly higher mean concentration of BNP in the group with heart disease but without heart failure compared with the controls. Secondly, there was an apparently progressively greater concentration of BNP as the signs of heart failure became worse. Finally, there was evidence that animals with higher concentrations of BNP did not survive as long as those with lower concentrations.

The implications of this study are interesting. The fact that dogs with signs of heart disease, but not heart failure (i.e. modified NYHA class I animals), have elevated concentrations of BNP suggests that these animals already have neurohumoral activation despite their apparent outward compensation for their disease. The related finding, that the BNP concentration increased as the class of heart failure worsened, suggests that there is a graded response and that progressively worsening cardiac function is associated with progressive upregulation of BNP production. This might mean that improvement in class of heart failure associated with therapy may result in a reduction of the BNP concentration. Thus, it might prove to be something that we could monitor as an indicator of success of therapy in future.

Finally, the finding that BNP concentrations have prognostic significance is an important one. Currently, our ability to prognosticate accurately in patients with cardiac disease is poor and any tool that may help us in this respect should be welcomed.

Comment

This study shares with many other veterinary studies a common weakness in that it is based on a relatively limited population of animals with only nine normal animals included, and only two animals in class IV heart failure. Despite the limited numbers, there are clear statistically significant differences between groups. This underlines the magnitude of the alterations in BNP concentrations that appear to be occurring.

What are the likely implications of these findings? If one can extrapolate from the human field, BNP and potentially other markers can be used in various ways. First, they may be used as a diagnostic indicator of the presence of heart failure. In this respect, however, one must ask what the evaluation of BNP brings to our assessment of the patient that other tests cannot, or do not, already provide? The second way in which BNP concentrations may be utilized is as a guide to the necessity for and success of therapy. Finally, as mentioned above, they may be of significance in prognostication.

In order to fulfil some of these roles, the assessment of BNP must be easy and relatively fast, particularly from the point of view of utility in rapid diagnosis and indication of success of therapy. This perhaps allows us to see some of the future directions in which research efforts might be channelled. A rapid, convenient and accessible assay, coupled with more detailed evaluation of the longitudinal effects of disease and natural fluctuations on BNP concentrations is required before the true value of BNP assessment can be realized; however, we can at least speculate about some of the potential uses of this marker in light of the information presented in this paper.

Measurement of plasma atrial natriuretic peptide as an indicator of prognosis in dogs with cardiac disease

Greco DS, Biller B, Van Liew CH. *Can Vet J* 2003; **44**(4): 293–7

B A C K G R O U N D. ANP was the first natriuretic peptide to be discovered and characterized. There are probably a greater number of publications studying this

peptide in the veterinary literature than there are concerned with BNP. This paper
studies the value of ANP concentrations from a slightly different perspective to the
publications that have gone before.

INTERPRETATION. In this study 10 control animals and 23 animals with cardiac disease
were studied. Those that had cardiac failure were further divided into those that had mild to
moderate signs of heart failure and those that had advanced heart failure. The assay used
was a radioimmunoassay that had previously been validated for use in the dog. In contrast to
the above paper, those animals with mild to moderate heart failure did not have detectable
elevations of the ANP concentrations. Those with advanced heart failure had marked
elevations. The most interesting finding was the predictive value of an ANP concentration
above or below 92 pg/ml. Those animals with an ANP concentration below 92 pg/ml had a
much better outcome than those with a concentration above that level.

Figure 13.1 shows survival curves for these two populations demonstrating that there were
significantly different median survival times for the two populations.

Comment

Again this study is hampered by the relatively low numbers of animals in each of the
groups. The significant difference in outcome is striking and again gives some idea of
the potential utility of assessment of this biomarker in future.

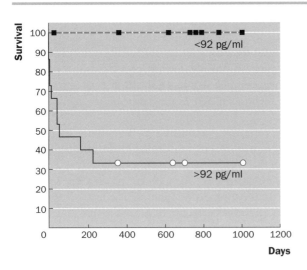

Fig. 13.1 Survival curves for two groups of dogs with plasma ANP concentrations greater or
less than 92 pg/ml. Source: Greco *et al*. (2003).

Cardiac troponin I in cats with hypertrophic cardiomyopathy

Connolly DJ, Cannata J, Boswood A, Archer J, Groves EA, Neiger R. *J Feline Med Surg* 2003; **5**(4): 209–16

BACKGROUND. Cardiac troponin I is another biomarker that has been studied extensively in recent years in both human and veterinary patients with cardiac disease |5–9|. It is such a successful marker of myocardial injury in human patients that an elevation of troponin is now a necessary finding for the ante mortem diagnosis of an acute myocardial infarct |10|. Troponins are intracellular myofibrillar proteins that are only released into the circulation when there is active breakdown of cardiac myocytes. The myocardial troponins I and T are sufficiently distinct from their skeletal muscle counterparts to be specific in their indication that cardiac, rather than skeletal, myocyte breakdown is occurring. Hypertrophic cardiomyopathy of cats is a disease state characterized by gradual loss of cardiac myocytes, and the idea behind this and similar studies was that there may be detectable levels of troponin I in the serum of cats affected by this disease process.

INTERPRETATION. The authors looked at troponin I concentrations in a population consisting of 16 cats with hypertrophic (or hypertrophic obstructive) cardiomyopathy and 18 normal cats. They demonstrate that, compared with the normal cats, cats with hypertrophic cardiomyopathy had significant elevations of circulating troponin I. The degree of elevation was sufficient to be able to discriminate the two populations with reasonable accuracy: elevated troponin I had a specificity and sensitivity of approximately 85% for discriminating the two groups. There was also a weak correlation between the degree of hypertrophy evidenced by the thickness of the left ventricular free wall, and the degree of elevation of the troponin I concentration.

Comment

This study is further demonstration of the potential utility of assessment of troponin concentrations in animals with heart disease. If anything the problem with troponin lies in its tendency to be elevated in almost every cardiac disease and its inability therefore to distinguish between cardiac diseases. The question with which clinicians are often faced is 'Which cardiac disease does this patient have?' and not 'Does this patient have cardiac disease?' Therefore tests that discriminate between diseases rather than simply demonstrate the presence of a cardiac disease may be more useful.

Conclusion

The three papers described above are drawn from a widening pool of information on various biomarkers in veterinary patients with cardiac disease. It is only with further refinement of our knowledge of these markers and the ways in which they behave in response to cardiac diseases and their treatment that we are likely to be able to optimize their utility. As with many studies, the questions that are ultimately posed often outnumber the questions that have been answered. Future directions for further research are suggested by these studies and include longitudinal studies looking at the variability of and alterations to levels of these markers in disease states. Only after collection and analysis of these data will we be able to clarify their true value as diagnostic, prognostic and therapeutic tools in individuals affected by disease.

Myocardial diseases of dogs and cats

Primary myocardial diseases are some of the most common diseases encountered by veterinary cardiologists. Dilated cardiomyopathy is the second most common acquired cardiac disease of dogs, and cardiomyopathies represent the most common group of cardiac diseases in feline patients. Despite the frequency with which they are diagnosed there is much confusion over their aetiology, classification and diagnosis. Over the last year a series of papers has appeared in the *Journal of Veterinary Cardiology* – a journal started by the European Society of Veterinary Cardiology – attempting to address some of the controversies with respect to diagnosis and classification of these diseases. These are bold and brave attempts to provide a navigable path through the various controversies surrounding myocardial disease in small animals and I will consider some of the papers here.

Proposed guidelines for the diagnosis of canine idiopathic dilated cardiomyopathy
Dukes-McEwan J, Borgarelli M, Tidholm A, Vollmar AC, Häggström J; the ESVC Taskforce for Canine Dilated Cardiomyopathy. *J Vet Cardiol* 2003: **5**(2): 7–19

BACKGROUND. The description 'idiopathic dilated cardiomyopathy' is applied to a variety of disease states affecting a number of different breeds of dog. It is a disease state that is characterized by primary systolic failure of the myocardium and usually manifests with gradual contractile failure leading ultimately to the development of signs of heart failure. It is a condition that is often accompanied by cardiac rhythm disturbances. What has become apparent over the years is that in some breeds of dog the syndrome has a characteristic presentation that differs slightly from other breeds. Distinct cardiomyopathic syndromes have been described in dobermans |11|, Irish wolfhounds |12|, newfoundlands |13| and boxers |14|, to name but a few. This article is an attempt to draw together criteria for the diagnosis of cardiomyopathy in various different breeds of dog and provide a classification system that will enable a more definite diagnosis of dilated cardiomyopathy to be made. It is illustrative of the type of article that appears relatively frequently regarding cardiac diseases in human patients where a consensus is reached about how such diseases should be diagnosed |10|.

INTERPRETATION. The article begins with an excellent review of the clinical and research literature on dilated cardiomyopathy in the dog. It goes on to suggest a series of major and minor criteria that might be used to reach a diagnosis of dilated cardiomyopathy. The three major criteria are: abnormal left ventricular M-mode measures; increased sphericity of the left ventricle; and evidence of depressed systolic function either through depression of the fractional shortening of the myocardium or decreased ejection fraction (by Simpson's rule). The minor criteria are: presence of an arrhythmia (particularly in breeds where these are characteristic of the condition); atrial fibrillation; increased E point to septal separation; abnormal ratio of the systolic time intervals; pre-ejection period and left ventricular ejection time (PEP:LVET); equivocal fractional shortening; and left or bi-atrial enlargement. The authors also stress that these criteria can only be applied once a diagnosis of predisposing primary cardiac conditions has been ruled out. It is proposed that a scoring system should be applied with major criteria receiving a score of three points and minor criteria a single point. Finally, it is proposed that an aggregate score of more than 6 should allow a diagnosis of dilated cardiomyopathy to be made.

The authors are aware of both the ambitious nature of these proposals and also the likely problems associated with their application. They state 'we welcome critical review from colleagues so the guidelines may be refined or adapted for different, specific breeds'.

Comment

I think this paper represents a brave attempt at harmonizing what is meant by the term 'dilated cardiomyopathy' in canine patients. It analyses a wealth of different sources and attempts to give us criteria that can, to some extent, be applied irrespective of breed. We must accept that the necessity for such a system is imposed upon us by our attempts to strive for a less equivocal and subjective method of diagnosis of early or pre-clinical cases of dilated cardiomyopathy. This necessity is to some extent self-imposed as we try to diagnose the disease earlier and earlier. It is also to some extent imposed upon us by the wish of breeders to know whether animals are affected from the point of view of breeding programmes that attempt to eradicate the disease. In a disease that undergoes a gradual transition from normality to an overtly affected phenotype what we are trying to do, by tightening up the criteria we apply in making a diagnosis, is improve our ability to be sure of the presence of disease at an earlier stage. This shifts the 'equivocal zone' (that period of time when the disease is suspected but not definitely present) of the disease to earlier in its course. The new classification system is helpful but we will still agonize over whether a dog with a score of 5 is affected or going to become more overtly affected.

It is a widely held belief that this condition is, in many cases, due to specific genetic abnormalities in particular breeds. If this turns out to be true then in years to come such stringent echocardiographic rules may no longer be necessary. If genetic abnormalities are identified and can be screened for it may no longer be necessary to diagnose pre-clinical cases on the basis of echocardiographic and clinical findings. At the moment echocardiography is our 'most gold' standard and, therefore, any attempt to standardize and harmonize the criteria we use to diagnose this condition should be applauded.

Hypertrophic cardiomyopathy: clinical and pathologic correlates
Fox PR. *J Vet Cardiol* 2003; **5**(2): 39–45

Endomyocardial fibrosis and restrictive cardiomyopathy: pathologic and clinical features
Fox PR. *J Vet Cardiol* 2004; **6**: 25–31

BACKGROUND. The feline cardiomyopathies represent a group of well recognized but poorly characterized diseases. Cardiomyopathies are the single most common group of acquired diseases in cats. There have been numerous attempts to classify the cardiomyopathies over recent years. The most widely adhered to system of classification is that proposed by the World Health Organization |15| subdividing cardiomyopathies into four types with a final category for those that still defy categorization. The four currently acceptable terms to describe primary cardiomyopathies are as follows: (i) dilated cardiomyopathy; (ii) hypertrophic cardiomyopathy; (iii) arrhythmogenic right ventricular cardiomyopathy; and (iv) restrictive cardiomyopathy. The category 'unclassified' cardiomyopathy is used for those cases that 'do not fit readily into any group'.

Using this classification of cardiomyopathies in cats the most common forms we encounter are hypertrophic cardiomyopathy (with the subform hypertrophic obstructive cardiomyopathy) and restrictive cardiomyopathy. There is still confusion and disagreement over exactly what is meant when these terms are applied. This is reflected by the numerous slightly different categorizations of restrictive cardiomyopathy that can be found in standard texts on the subject. For some time a clear account of the two conditions in cats and how they may be recognized and distinguished has been needed.

INTERPRETATION. These two articles (also published in the new *Journal of Veterinary Cardiology*) are both written by Phil Fox and describe in a simple, lucid, comprehensible and complete manner the clinical findings characteristic of these conditions and how these correlate with the post mortem findings of gross pathological and histopathological examination of the heart.

Hypertrophic cardiomyopathy is characterized by a non-dilated hypertrophied left ventricle. There is substantial variation in the nature and location of the hypertrophy that occurs leading to various phenotypic presentations. The main histopathological features are summarized as myofibre disorganization, intramural arteriosclerosis and pathological fibrosis.

Restrictive cardiomyopathy is characterized by a lack of marked hypertrophy. Ventricular function is impaired by the development of myocardial or endomyocardial fibrosis. The fibrosis particularly impairs diastolic function. This results in elevated filling pressures and significant enlargement of the atria.

Although, as is pointed out in the article 'restrictive cardiomyopathy is uncommon and embodies not one but several idiopathic disorders', there are two main forms of the condition that are characterized by either endomyocardial or myocardial fibrosis. The ante mortem and post mortem findings in these cases are illustrated and described.

Comment

These articles serve to remind us that sometimes, in an effort to resolve confusion, one should return to basic considerations rather than delve deeper into complicated and arcane means of classification. The combination of ante mortem and post mortem illustrations serve to clearly illustrate the disease processes and show how these relate to the microscopic changes occurring within the heart itself. It also reminds us that extensive studies correlating ante mortem findings with pathological findings in a large population of affected cats are still to be performed. In an era when the emphasis of research is at the molecular level, one should not lose sight of the fact that there are still considerable gaps in our knowledge at the gross and microscopic level.

Arrhythmogenic right ventricular cardiomyopathy causing sudden cardiac death in boxer dogs: a new animal model of human disease

Basso C, Fox PR, Meurs KM, et al. Circulation 2004; **109**(9): 1180–5

BACKGROUND. Over many years boxers have been recognized as suffering from a fairly distinct form of myocardial disease. Many publications have described the clinical features recognized in this breed, including their proclivity to develop ventricular arrhythmias and experience sudden death |14,16,17|. What has not been clear in the past is the pathological nature of the condition leading to the observed syndrome, or the name that we should use to refer to it. Previously, the terms 'boxer cardiomyopathy' and 'familial ventricular arrhythmias' have been used (among others).

INTERPRETATION. This paper describes the findings, including detailed pathological evaluation, of 23 cases from a cohort of 239 dogs studied at the Ohio State University College of Veterinary Medicine. In all of the animals studied there was evidence of change similar to that described in human patients with arrhythmogenic right ventricular cardiomyopathy. This is characterized by two main findings: (i) fatty or fibrofatty replacement of right ventricular myocardium, and (ii) myocarditis. Apoptosis was also identified in some of the cases. Interestingly, despite the histopathological similarity to arrhythmogenic right ventricular cardiomyopathy in humans, only eight (35%) of the dogs showed evidence of right ventricular chamber dilation. The weight of the hearts in the affected dogs did not differ significantly from the weight of the hearts of a group of normal mongrel dogs, suggesting that, although diseased, the hearts from affected dogs were not hypertrophied. These findings contrast with those described in cats with right ventricular cardiomyopathy |18| where right ventricular dilatation was one of the predominant features.

Comment

This paper has helped to characterize further the nature of this well recognized condition in boxer dogs. It also provides us with clues as to the likely nature of this disease. There are specific genetic mutations in people that are known to result in the development of this condition. The finding of the histopathological similarity between the canine and human forms of the disease begs the question: Are similar genetic mutations responsible for the development of the syndrome in dogs? With this, as with many other familial or hereditary cardiac conditions affecting dogs, one suspects that active research is ongoing in this area and will hopefully bring forth fruit in the future that may enable us to identify more effectively individuals affected by this condition at an earlier stage.

Interventional techniques for the management of congenital heart disease

Congenital heart diseases, although not as common as acquired diseases, are still frequently encountered in small animal patients. Over the last decade and longer, a considerable body of literature has built up to demonstrate the effectiveness of minimally invasive interventional techniques in the management of cardiac disease. Conditions that can clearly be improved in the short term by the use of interventional techniques are pulmonic stenosis, through balloon valvuloplasty, and patent ductus arteriosus, through various occlusion techniques. As more cases have undergone a particular intervention and more time since the development of the particular intervention elapses, medium- and long-term follow-up on these cases becomes available. Interesting developments in the last 12 months have been publications addressing the use of these techniques in considerable numbers of cases and reports of the long-term outcomes related to the use of these techniques.

Interventional and surgical management of aortic stenosis has waned in popularity as studies demonstrating disappointing medium- and long-term effects of such therapies have been published |19|. It is on the basis of rigorous evaluation of the effects of interventional techniques that we will be able to make future judgements as to whether they should be more widely utilized.

Results of balloon valvuloplasty in 40 dogs with pulmonic stenosis
Johnson MS, Martin M. *J Small Anim Pract* 2004; **45**: 148–53

Pulmonic stenosis in dogs: balloon dilation improves clinical outcome

Johnson MS, Martin M, Edwards D, French A, Henley W. *J Vet Intern Med* 2004; **18**: 656–62

BACKGROUND. Balloon valvuloplasty was first used for the management of congenital pulmonic stenosis in a dog more than two decades ago |20|. Since that time the technique has been widely used in increasingly greater numbers of dogs. Despite the wide application of this technique, there remain some significant but unresolved questions. Which patients are most likely to benefit from undergoing the procedure? Is there a demonstrable benefit in terms of clinical signs or survival after undergoing such a procedure, i.e. are the patients we put through these procedures living longer than they otherwise would have done had they gone untreated?

Two papers have been published recently that go some way to answering some of these questions and significantly contribute to the argument in favour of carrying out balloon valvuloplasty for pulmonic stenosis with both improvements in clinical signs and survival.

INTERPRETATION. Both papers refer to a group of 40 dogs with severe pulmonic stenosis (defined in this case as having an instantaneous transvalvular pressure gradient derived from Doppler echocardiography as greater than or equal to 80 mmHg) treated with balloon valvuloplasty. The first paper reports in detail on the outcome in this group with respect to the long-term improvements in pressure gradients and clinical signs. The second paper, by comparing this group with a 'control' untreated group and using sophisticated statistical analysis, determines the hazards associated with various factors in a population of dogs with pulmonic stenosis and analyses treated and untreated populations for differences in outcome.

In the treated group, 79% of dogs had clinical signs prior to balloon valvuloplasty. The procedure was completed successfully in 93% of the animals. There were three fatalities during the procedure; all of the animals that died had a concurrent abnormality of some form. There was a mean reduction in gradient evident in the short term of about 45% that was sustained in the long term. Only three of the dogs evaluated showed significant evidence of restenosis. Eighty per cent of the dogs that had clinical signs prior to valvuloplasty experienced a resolution of their clinical signs following the procedure. The six dogs that were in heart failure when they underwent the procedure all ultimately died. Five of these deaths were considered related to the underlying heart disease. This may suggest that the prognosis for this subpopulation is not as good.

In the paper where the group undergoing valvuloplasty is compared with a control population that did not undergo valvuloplasty (usually because of financial constraints) some interesting conclusions emerge. A number of factors were shown to be significantly associated with an increased risk of death from heart failure. Two of the main factors discovered were (i) the magnitude of the pressure gradient (every 1 mmHg increase in pressure gradient was associated with a 3% increase in risk), and (ii) the presence of clinical signs at presentation was associated with a 16-fold increase in risk (confidence intervals 4–60.2). The presence of tricuspid valve regurgitation and right ventricular hypertrophy were significant univariate risk factors but when combined in a multivariate model did not remain significant.

Figure 13.2 shows the clearly divergent survival curves of the group undergoing valvuloplasty and the group that did not when corrected for differences in the prevalence of clinical signs between the two groups at presentation.

It was shown in this study that undergoing balloon valvuloplasty was associated with a 53% reduction in risk of adverse outcome (interestingly a similar figure to the reduction in magnitude of gradient seen above).

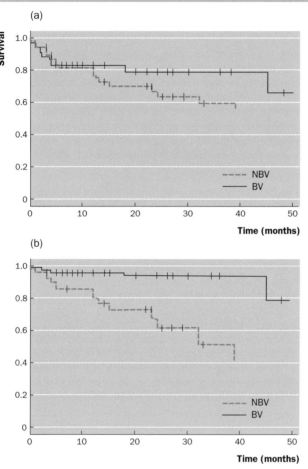

Fig. 13.2 Survivor curves comparing time to death associated with heart failure, including sudden death for dogs treated with balloon valvuloplasty (BV), and dogs in the non-treatment group (NBV). (a) Without adjustment for other variables. (b) Following adjustment of the model for clinical signs, gradient pressure, and age at presentation. The crosses represent censoring times (i.e. the times at which dogs were lost to follow-up). The survivor curves are not displayed beyond 50 months because of the small number of dogs followed up for this length of time. No deaths were in the BV group beyond 40 months, and only 2 deaths were in the BV group beyond 50 months. Source: Johnson et al. (2004).

Comment

This combination of papers is a valuable contribution to our collective knowledge regarding the utility and validity of balloon valvuloplasty for the management of congenital pulmonic stenosis in the dog. On the basis of these data we can say that those animals at greatest risk of developing heart failure and dying as a consequence of their disease are those with the greater pressure gradient and those with clinical signs at the time of presentation. We can also advise that there is a clear and significant reduction in risk of this adverse outcome when valvuloplasty is performed.

One might consider that this improvement in outcome with a reduction in gradient is intuitively obvious but one only needs to look at the study reporting the outcome of dogs with aortic stenosis by Orton *et al.* |19| to see that a reduction in gradient does not always translate into an improvement in survival. By contrast in patients with pulmonic stenosis these studies fortunately show that improvement in gradient mirrors an improvement in outcome and this information can now be used as the basis of a clear evidence-based recommendation that patients with severe stenosis should undergo this procedure where possible.

Long-term follow-up of dogs with patent ductus arteriosus

Van Israel N, Dukes-McEwan J, French AT. *J Small Anim Pract* 2003; **44**: 480–90

BACKGROUND. Patent ductus arteriosus is consistently reported as one of the two most common congenital heart conditions encountered in dogs. Surgical and other interventional techniques have been used to achieve closure of the patent ductus arteriosus in affected patients for many years. The first reports of successful surgical closure are now nearly 40 years old |21|. Studies documenting the outcome of dogs with patent ductus arteriosus have previously been published and differences in outcome according to whether or not closure was undertaken have been shown |22|. Since the advent of echocardiography, cases of patent ductus arteriosus can undergo a more detailed evaluation both prior to and following surgery.

INTERPRETATION. This paper evaluates a number of parameters in dogs before and after closure of their patent ductus arteriosus. There are a number of different parameters compared and a wide array of results, both descriptive and statistical, is generated. The paper confirms, unsurprisingly, that outcome is better in animals in which the ductus is closed (or at least closure is attempted and volume of ductal flow is reduced). What is perhaps more surprising is that three of the eight dogs that did not undergo closure survived over 100 months (8 years) even though they ultimately died of cardiac-related problems.

Significant changes in electrocardiographic variables were seen with the reduction in R-wave amplitude following attempted or successful closure. Interestingly, there was no demonstrable reduction in vertebral heart score in the 18 animals for which pre- and post-closure radiographs were available. Some echocardiographic indices showed significant reductions including the systolic and diastolic diameters of the left ventricle. The fractional shortening of the myocardium decreased significantly. Although a reduction in fractional shortening might be considered to indicate impairment of ventricular systolic function, in this case it probably represents a resolution of the significant volume load associated with a patent ductus arteriosus.

No difference in the prevalence of persistent ductal flow was seen according to the technique of closure used but this analysis was somewhat hampered by three different techniques being compared and relatively small numbers of animals in the study overall.

There was a trend toward a worse outcome in those animals with evidence of mitral insufficiency at original examination compared with those without but this failed to reach statistical significance ($P = 0.052$).

Comment

This paper is highly complicated. There are a large number of variables analysed; clinical, electrocardiographic, echocardiographic, radiographic and outcome parameters are all assessed. This leads to a large number of results being generated, many of which show non-significant variability. Does this paper add valuably to our body of knowledge regarding this condition? There are a few points that are of considerable value. First, despite a high frequency of residual flow or recanalization the outcome is improved by closure or at least attentuation of the ductus. Although this information is not necessarily new it adds further weight to our recommendation that ductal closure is usually to be advised. This paper also shows that dogs that do not undergo ductal closure may in some circumstances survive for prolonged periods. This is a fascinating finding and suggests to me that there are some dogs that will benefit more than others from ductal closure; equally there may be some dogs in which ductal closure can be delayed or may not even be necessary. After all what is the difference between moderate residual flow and a small untreated ductus arteriosus? Haemodynamically they are identical.

Finally, this paper suggests that failure of reduction in radiographic size of the cardiac silhouette should not be interpreted as failure of the procedure, and that a fall in fractional shortening is not always a bad thing.

Therapy for heart disease and failure

A wide array of treatments for heart failure in small animal patients is available. Until the publication of studies documenting efficacy of the angiotensin-converting enzyme inhibitors |23,24| there was a distinct lack of an evidential basis for the use of many of these compounds. We should therefore welcome any more critical evaluation of therapy for the management of heart disease and failure.

Over the last 18 months there have been few placebo-controlled evidence-based studies published in the veterinary literature. A number of abstracts have been presented at scientific meetings that suggest further publications may be forthcoming but rather than review this relatively sparse information we should first await peer-review and publication in paper form. As one of the few (if not the only) well conducted placebo-controlled treatment studies published in the last 18 months the following paper deserves consideration in this chapter.

Effect of thyroid hormone supplementation on survival of euthyroid dogs with congestive heart failure due to systolic myocardial dysfunction: a double-blind, placebo-controlled trial

Tidholm A, Falk T, Gundler S, Svensson H, Ablad B, Sylven C. *Res Vet Sci* 2003; **75**: 195–201

BACKGROUND. It has long been noted that a proportion of dogs with cardiac disease, and particularly dilated cardiomyopathy, may also suffer from hypothyroidism. Whether these are comorbid conditions that simply have a high prevalence in some breeds or whether there is a causal link between the two has resulted in some considerable debate |25–27|. The multitude of cardiovascular effects of thyroid hormone on the cardiovascular system |28| begs the question whether therapy with thyroid hormone would have a directly beneficial effect on patients with cardiac disease and failure irrespective of whether or not they have subnormal thyroid hormone production.

INTERPRETATION. In this study a group of 19 dogs with echocardiographic evidence of impaired systolic function and ventricular dilatation was identified. These dogs were randomized to receive either levothyroxine or placebo in addition to standard background therapy with furosemide, digoxin and propranolol. The groups were compared with respect to a number of parameters at the inception of the study and then after 2 months of treatment. The only parameter that differed significantly between the groups after 2 months of treatment was, not surprisingly, the total T_4 level! Most importantly, there was no significant difference in the survival times for the two groups. Figure 13.3 shows the survival curves for the two groups demonstrating the lack of divergence.

Comment

This is a study that is limited by the small number of animals included. The authors describe it as a 'pilot' study, although whether it will be repeated by a larger similar study remains to be seen. It is easy to criticize others' work and therefore I will concentrate on the positive. Limited attempts to provide an evidential basis for treatment of veterinary patients with heart disease and failure are better than no attempts at all. It is difficult for a study, whatever the size, to prove that a therapy has no effect. It always remains possible that there is a small effect that has not been detected because of the size of the sample of the population included in the study. What a small study can do, however, is show that there is no substantial effect of therapy on outcome. There are studies in the veterinary literature where as few as 10 dogs randomized to two groups resulted in the detection of a significant difference in outcome |29|. Thus what we can say as a result of this study is that if a difference in outcome exists as a consequence of utilization of levothyroxine in the management of patients with systolic heart failure it is not large.

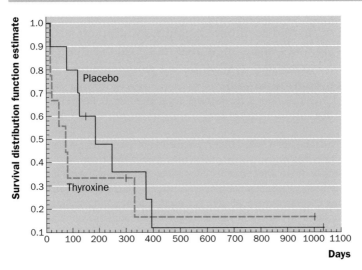

Fig. 13.3 Survival curves based on the Kaplan–Meier method for dogs with dilated cardiomyopathy treated with furosemide, digoxin, propranolol, and placebo ($n = 10$) (—) or thyroxine ($n = 9$) (----). The four dogs that were euthanized for reasons unrelated to heart disease (i.e. pyometra, diabetes mellitus, myiasis and behavioural problems) were censored in the statistical analysis and are represented by vertical bars. Source: Tidholm *et al.* (2003).

Furosemide and the progression of left ventricular dysfunction in experimental heart failure

McCurley JM, Hanlon SU, Wei SK, Wedam EF, Michalski M, Haigney MC.
J Am Coll Cardiol 2004; **44**: 1301–7

BACKGROUND. This paper cannot be regarded as 'clinical', nor is it about small animals; however, it is worthy of brief mention. Human evidence-based cardiology is littered with studies that have challenged widely held dogmas regarding the benefits of therapies for heart failure or arrhythmias and have subsequently shown those dogmas to be wrong. Two shining examples of this are the CAST (Cardiac Arrhythmia Suppression Trial) study and the PROMISE (Prospective RandOmized Milrinone Survival Evaluation) study |30,31|. One remaining and largely unchallenged dogma in the management of heart disease is the long-term benefit, and relatively wide safety margin associated with the use of loop diuretics in the management of heart failure. The above study uses a model of pacing induced heart failure in pigs to look for evidence of a potentially detrimental effect of loop diuretics on the progression of myocardial systolic failure.

INTERPRETATION. In this study 32 pigs with pacing induced cardiac disease were randomized to two groups of 16. Both groups were managed similarly with the exception that one group received a daily injection of furosemide and the other group did not (the others received a daily placebo injection). The pigs were then monitored for the development of systolic myocardial failure by serial echocardiography. The predetermined definition of systolic failure was when the fractional shortening had reached 16%. Figure 13.4 illustrates the relative rates at which the two groups developed systolic myocardial failure. The group receiving furosemide appeared to develop systolic failure earlier.

Another and less surprising finding of the study is that the aldosterone level in the furosemide-treated group was considerably higher after treatment, probably reflecting the increased stimulation of the renin–angiotensin–aldosterone system associated with volume and sodium depletion.

Comment

Whether the elevated aldosterone simply reflects a result with a common cause (i.e. the administration of furosemide), or whether there is a causal relationship between the elevated aldosterone and progression of myocardial failure is unclear. What is clear is that we should look more critically at our current strategies for diuresis and where possible explore combination therapy to minimize the dose of potent diuretics necessary and ameliorate the harmful effects these agents may be having. There is insufficient conclusive evidence to advocate the widespread cessation of the use of furosemide. This would, in my opinion, harm a considerably greater numbers of animals than it would help. What is suggested, however, is the potential benefit of more careful and considered use of such potent agents.

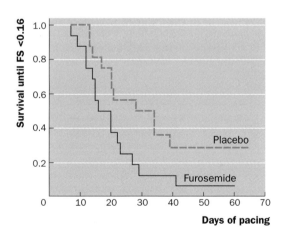

Fig. 13.4 Cumulative probability of the development of severe systolic dysfunction as defined as a fractional shortening (FS) of <0.16 in placebo-treated (dashed line) and furosemide-treated animals (solid line) ($n = 16$ for both groups). $P = 0.038$ from log-rank statistics. Source: McCurley et al. (2004).

Conclusion

It is not possible in a review chapter to do justice to the wide variety of articles published over a 12 to 18-month period. The choice of the above articles is as much a reflection of my own areas of interest and bias as it is the individual significance of the articles chosen for review.

What we can see is a number of strands developing in small animal cardiology, some of which I predict will become much more widely accepted and widespread in years to come. For those reading this article who feel their work has been either missed out or misrepresented I apologize. For those of you who have gleaned some useful and interesting information from the above I am pleased.

References

1. Biomarkers Definitions Working Group. Biomarkers and surrogate endpoints: preferred definitions and conceptual framework. *Clin Pharmacol Ther* 2001; **69**: 89–95.
2. de Bold AJ, Borenstein HB, Veress AT, Sonnenberg H. A rapid and potent natriuretic response to intravenous injection of atrial myocardial extract in rats. *Life Sci* 1981; **28**: 89–94.
3. Levin ER, Gardner DG, Samson WK. Natriuretic peptides. *N Engl J Med* 1998; **339**: 321–8.
4. Haggstrom J, Hansson K, Kvart C, Pedersen HD, Vuolteenaho O, Olsson K. Relationship between different natriuretic peptides and severity of naturally acquired mitral regurgitation in dogs with chronic myxomatous valve disease. *J Vet Cardiol* 2000; **2**: 7–16.
5. Schober KE, Cornand C, Kirbach B, Aupperle H, Oechtering G. Serum cardiac troponin I and cardiac troponin T concentrations in dogs with gastric dilatation-volvulus. *J Am Vet Med Assoc* 2002; **221**: 381–8.
6. Herndon WE, Kittleson MD, Sanderson K, Drobatz KJ, Clifford CA, Gelzer A, Summerfield NJ, Linde A, Sleeper MM. Cardiac troponin I in feline hypertrophic cardiomyopathy. *J Vet Intern Med* 2002; **16**: 558–64.
7. DeFrancesco TC, Atkins CE, Keene BW, Coats JR, Hauck ML. Prospective clinical evaluation of serum cardiac troponin T in dogs admitted to a veterinary teaching hospital. *J Vet Intern Med* 2002; **16**: 553–7.
8. Caragher TE, Fernandez BB, Jacobs FL, Barr LA. Evaluation of quantitative cardiac biomarker point-of-care testing in the emergency department. *J Emerg Med* 2002; **22**: 1–7.
9. Sleeper MM, Clifford CA, Laster LL. Cardiac troponin I in the normal dog and cat. *J Vet Intern Med* 2001; **15**: 501–3.
10. Alpert JS, Thygesen K, Antman E, Bassand JP. Myocardial infarction redefined—a consensus document of The Joint European Society of Cardiology/American College of

Cardiology Committee for the redefinition of myocardial infarction. *J Am Coll Cardiol* 2000; **36**: 959–69.

11. Calvert CA. Dilated congestive cardiomyopathy in Doberman Pinschers. *Comp Cont Ed* 1986; **8**: 417–30.

12. Brownlie SE, Cobb MA. Observations on the development of congestive heart failure in Irish wolfhounds with dilated cardiomyopathy. *J Small Anim Pract* 1999; **40**: 371–7.

13. Tidholm A, Jonsson L. Dilated cardiomyopathy in the Newfoundland: a study of 37 cases (1983–1994). *J Am Anim Hosp Assoc* 1996; **32**: 465–70.

14. Meurs KM. Boxer dog cardiomyopathy: an update. *Vet Clin North Am Small Anim Pract* 2004; **34**: viii, 1235–44.

15. Richardson P, McKenna W, Bristow M, Maisch B, Mautner B, O'Connell J, Olsen E, Thiene G, Goodwin J, Gyarfas I, Martin I, Nordet P. Report of the 1995 World Health Organization/International Society and Federation of Cardiology Task Force on the Definition and Classification of cardiomyopathies. *Circulation* 1996; **93**: 841–2.

16. Meurs KM, Spier AW, Wright NA, Atkins CE, DeFrancesco TC, Gordon SG, Hamlin RL, Keene BW, Miller MW, Moise NS. Comparison of the effects of four antiarrhythmic treatments for familial ventricular arrhythmias in Boxers. *J Am Vet Med Assoc* 2002; **221**: 522–7.

17. Harpster NK. Boxer cardiomyopathy. A review of the long-term benefits of antiarrhythmic therapy. *Vet Clin North Am Small Anim Pract* 1991; **21**: 989–1004.

18. Fox PR, Maron BJ, Basso C, Liu SK, Thiene G. Spontaneously occurring arrhythmogenic right ventricular cardiomyopathy in the domestic cat: a new animal model similar to the human disease. *Circulation* 2000; **102**: 1863–70.

19. Orton EC, Herndon GD, Boon JA, Gaynor JS, Hackett TB, Monnet E. Influence of open surgical correction on intermediate-term outcome in dogs with subvalvular aortic stenosis: 44 cases (1991–1998). *J Am Vet Med Assoc* 2000; **216**: 364–7.

20. Buchanan JW, Anderson JH, White RI. The 1st balloon valvuloplasty: an historical note. *J Vet Intern Med* 2002; **16**: 116–17.

21. Buchanan JW. Symposium: Thoracic surgery in the dog and cat—III: patent ductus arteriosus and persistent right aortic arch surgery in dogs. *J Small Anim Pract* 1968; **9**: 409–28.

22. Eyster GE, Eyster JT, Cords GB, Johnston J. Patent ductus arteriosus in the dog: characteristics of occurrence and results of surgery in one hundred consecutive cases. *JAVMA* 1976; **168**: 435–8.

23. Pouchelon JL, Martignoni L, King JN, for the BENCH (BENazepril in Canine Heart disease) study group. The effects of benazepril on survival times and clinical signs of dogs with congestive heart failure: results of a multicenter, prospective, randomized, double-blinded, placebo-controlled, long-term clinical trial. *J Vet Card* 1999; **1**: 7–18.

24. The COVE Study Group. Controlled clinical evaluation of enalapril in dogs with heart failure: results of the Cooperative Veterinary Enalapril Study Group. *J Vet Intern Med* 1995; **9**: 243–52.

25. Calvert CA, Jacobs GJ, Medleau L, Pickus CW, Brown J, McDermott M. Thyroid-stimulating hormone stimulation tests in cardiomyopathic doberman pinschers: a retrospective study. *J Vet Intern Med* 1998; **12**: 343–8.

26. Panciera DL. An echocardiographic and electrocardiographic study of cardiovascular function in hypothyroid dogs. *J Am Vet Med Assoc* 1994; **205**: 996–1000.

27. Gerritsen RJ, van den Brom WE, Stokhof AA. Relationship between atrial fibrillation and primary hypothyroidism in the dog. *Vet Q* 1996; **18**: 49–51.

28. Klein I, Ojamaa K. Thyroid hormone and the cardiovascular system. *N Engl J Med* 2001; **344**: 501–9.

29. Luis Fuentes V, Corcoran B, French A, Schober KE, Kleeman R, Justus C. A double-blind, randomized, placebo-controlled study of pimobendan in dogs with dilated cardiomyopathy. *J Vet Intern Med* 2002; **16**: 255–61.

30. Echt DS, Liebson PR, Mitchell LB, Peters RW, Obias-Manno D, Barker AH, Arensberg D, Baker A, Friedman L, Greene HL, *et al.* Mortality and morbidity in patients receiving encainide, flecainide, or placebo. The Cardiac Arrhythmia Suppression Trial [see comments]. *N Engl J Med* 1991; **324**: 781–8.

31. Packer M, Carver JR, Rodeheffer RJ, Ivanhoe RJ, DiBianco R, Zeldis SM, Hendrix GH, Bommer WJ, Elkayam U, Kukin ML. Effect of oral milrinone on mortality in severe chronic heart failure. The PROMISE Study Research Group. *N Engl J Med* 1991; **325**: 1468–75.

14

Pharmacology

MARK PAPICH

Introduction

In the past several months, most of the discussion of recent developments and changes in veterinary small animal practice has centred on the availability of new drugs. There have been three areas in which the most significant changes have taken place: anti-inflammatory/analgesic therapy, immunosuppressive therapy and antibiotic therapy. This chapter will focus on the changes and relevant literature pertaining to these developments.

Non-steroidal anti-inflammatory drugs

Most of the discussed anti-inflammatory/analgesic drugs in small animal veterinary medicine have been the non-steroidal anti-inflammatory drugs (NSAIDs). There have been many new additions to the list of approved drugs to treat osteoarthritis in the USA. The NSAIDs have been the most rapidly expanding group of drugs. In addition to carprofen (Rimadyl) and etodolac (EtoGesic), we now have several new additions such as deracoxib (Deramaxx), firocoxib (Previcox), tepoxalin (Zubrin) and meloxicam (Metacam). In other countries, additional drugs are available, such as tolfenamic acid (Tolfedine), nimesulide and ketoprofen (Anafen).

The pharmacological action of the NSAIDs have been reviewed in other articles [1–4]. There have been several new developments in the NSAIDs in the last few years, including new drugs for use in dogs. The most recent development in understanding the mechanism of action of NSAIDs is the inhibition of the isoenzymes of cyclo-oxygenase (COX; prostaglandin [PG] endoperoxide synthase). PG synthase-1 (COX-1) is a constitutive enzyme expressed in tissues [1–4]. PGs, prostacyclin and thromboxane synthesized by this enzyme are responsible for normal physiological functions. PG synthase-2 (COX-2), on the other hand, is inducible and synthesized by macrophages and inflammatory cells after stimulation by cytokines and other mediators of inflammation. In some tissues, COX-2 may be constitutive. The target of recently developed NSAIDs has been COX-2, with the goal of producing analgesia and suppressing inflammation without inhibiting physiologically important prostanoids [5].

In some instances, the mechanism of action may not be entirely known. For example, carprofen appears to be a COX-1 sparing drug |5|, but there is no agreement among investigators on whether or not it also inhibits COX-2 *in vivo*. Although there is evidence for inhibitory effects on the enzyme cyclooxygenase in some models, carprofen did not show an *in vivo* anti-PG effect in dogs |6|, which may explain the low rate of gastrointestinal (GI) adverse effects at approved doses. In one recent study, the investigators were unable to show that carprofen inhibited either COX-1 or COX-2 |7|. When one examines the other drugs registered for veterinary medicine, there is also confusion in the literature. For example, deracoxib is considered a highly selective COX-2 inhibitor based on an assay performed in purified enzymes |8|. In this study, the COX-1/COX-2 ratio was 1275; much higher than other drugs tested. But when tested in canine whole blood and compared with other NSAIDs, deracoxib had a ratio of only 12 (carprofen had a ratio of 6–7) |9|.

Some of the confusion regarding understanding the action of the veterinary NSAID is that *in vitro* studies to examine their relative effects on COX-1 versus COX-2 have varied in their techniques and the cell system used. For example, in a study using canine enzyme systems, carprofen had a COX-1/COX-2 ratio of 129 |5|. In another study, using cell lines of another species (sheep and rodent) the ratio was 1.0 |1|, and in a study using canine macrophages, the ratio was 1.75 |10|. Yet another study on carprofen showed a ratio of 5.3 and that it was 1000 times less potent in whole blood than in cell culture |11|. This emphasizes the effect of protein binding on *in vitro* assays.

There have been conflicting results when other drugs have been examined. The ratios for etodolac, another NSAID approved for dogs, has a COX-1/COX-2 ratio of 8.1 in humans, but 0.52–0.53 in dogs. Another study with etodolac showed that the selectivity for COX-2 was 10 times greater in people than dogs |8,12|. Dr Vane, a pre-eminent expert on COX inhibition, concludes that the inhibitory activity of a drug for COX-1 compared to its inhibitory activity for COX-2 can vary according to whether tests are done on pure enzymes, cell homogenates, intact cells or with the types of cells used |1|. According to Dr Lees, one of the leading investigators of NSAIDs in veterinary medicine, there are several unexplored questions to be answered for veterinary drugs |13|.

Although for most NSAIDs we assume that PG inhibition is the most important mechanism of action, there may be other mechanisms (some not fully understood) that may also explain the actions of these drugs. For example, some NSAIDs, including salicylates have been suggested to inhibit nuclear factor κB (NF-κB). NF-κB is an important promoter for inflammatory mediators. Veterinary drugs, such as carprofen and others, may also act through inhibition of the activation of NF-κB |7|.

Is there an advantage for cyclo-oxygenase-2 inhibitors?

Recently, drugs for human use that are highly COX-2 specific have become available: celecoxib (Celebrex), valdecoxib (Bextra) and rofecoxib (Vioxx, now discontinued) |14|. These are often referred to as the COXIBs and they are among the top-selling prescription drugs of any category in human medicine. Deracoxib is the first veterinary drug in this group. Other COX-2-specific drugs will probably follow. The newest in this class is firocoxib (Previcox), sponsored by Merial Ltd. It is more specific for COX-2 than deracoxib, but at this time it has not yet been marketed.

Evaluations of these new drugs show that they are not necessarily more effective than older drugs, but they may be safer for the GI tract |15|. However, the studies demonstrating safety in people have been criticized |16|. Some sceptics have proposed that selective COX-2 inhibitors may not be appropriate for all patients because COX-2 enzyme products may be involved in actions other than inflammation. For example, COX-2 products may be biologically important for angiogenesis, renal function, regulation of bone resorption, reproductive function and healing of gastro-duodenal ulcers |17|. COX-2 selective drugs may also cause a higher risk of cardio-vascular problems in people because they preserve COX-1, which may promote platelet aggregation and vasoconstriction |18|. This is the reason that the popular drug rofecoxib (Vioxx) has been voluntarily taken off the market. There have been serious concerns expressed about the events that led up to this withdrawal. Some experts believe that the high COX-2 selectivity of this drug led to this increased risk |19|.

Dual inhibitors

There have been older drugs promoted to be 'dual inhibitors' of arachidonic acid metabolites, but none were commercially successful. Dual inhibitor drugs effectively inhibit both COX and lipoxygenase (LOX). Therefore, they inhibit synthesis of both inflammatory PGs and leukotrienes. Interest in a dual inhibitor has focused on the potential benefits in inhibiting LOX, which may include higher GI safety, and greater analgesic efficacy |20. LOX metabolites are involved in hyperalgesia, and inflammatory responses |21|. Older drugs thought to have dual inhibitor capability were benoxaprofen and ketoprofen. Benoxaprofen was taken off the market, and the evidence for ketoprofen acting as a dual inhibitor is weak. Corticosteroids have been shown to be dual inhibitors in some studies because they inhibit phosphodiesterase A_2 the enzyme that forms arachidonic acid from cell membranes. However, the corti-costeroid inhibition of both leukotrienes and PG may not be clinically relevant.

Recently, a new drug was approved in Europe and the USA that acts as a dual inhibitor. Tepoxalin (Zubrin) acts as both LOX and COX inhibitor. The metabolite is active, but only acts as a COX inhibitor. The COX inhibitor functions are more specific for COX-1 than COX-2, although this was not a canine-specific assay (data from Schering-Plough). Nevertheless, tepoxalin has a good GI safety profile that matches other more selective COX-2 inhibitors. Tepoxalin has been shown to be effective in dogs with osteoarthritis and showed GI safety at several times the label dose. The only question remaining about tepoxalin is the duration of the LOX inhibit-ory effect. As shown in Table 14.1, the half-life for the LOX inhibitor parent drug is much shorter than the metabolite, which has little LOX inhibition. The other question remaining to be answered for tepoxalin is the contribution of anti-LOX action on the overall therapeutic effect. Studies in osteoarthritis in dogs (the regis-tered indication for tepoxalin) have not revealed whether or not it is the COX or the

Table 14.1 Features of commonly used drugs in dogs

Drug	Half-life in dogs	Dose in dogs
Aspirin	8 hours	10–20 mg/kg q8–12h, oral
Carprofen	8 hours (range 4.5–10)	4.4 mg/kg q24h, or 2.2 mg/kg q12h, oral
Deracoxib	3 hr at 2–3 mg/kg 19 hr @ 20 mg/kg	3–4 mg/kg q24h, oral
Etodolac	7.7 hrs fasted; 12 hr non-fasted	10–15 mg/kg q24h, oral
Flunixin	3.7 hr	1 mg/kg, oral or i.m., once
Meloxicam	12–36 hours	0.2 mg/kg initial, then 0.1 mg/kg q24h, oral
Naproxen	74 hr	5 mg/kg initial, then 2 mg/kg q48h, oral
Phenylbutazone	6 hours	15–22 mg/kg q12h, oral
Piroxicam	40 hours	0.3 mg/kg, q24h, or q48h, oral
Tepoxalin	1.6 hrs parent drug; 13 hr for active metabolite	20 mg/kg initial; then 10 mg/kg q24h, oral

LOX inhibition (or possibly some other mechanism) that is responsible for a favourable clinical effect. Whether or not the dual inhibition action of tepoxalin will be effective for other inflammatory diseases (for example, respiratory disease, dermatitis) has not been reported.

Gastrointestinal toxicity of non-steroidal anti-inflammatory drugs

Among the adverse reactions caused by NSAIDs, GI problems are the most frequent reason to discontinue NSAID therapy or consider alternative treatment. In animals, GI effects range from mild gastritis and vomiting, to severe GI ulceration, bleeding and even deaths. These effects have been documented for the past three decades in the veterinary literature. GI toxicity is caused by two mechanisms: direct irritation of the drug on the GI mucosa and the result of PG inhibition |17|. Direct irritation occurs because the acidic NSAIDs become more lipophilic in the acid milieu of the stomach and diffuse into the gastric mucosa where they cause injury. PGs have a cytoprotective effect on the GI mucosa and inhibition of these compounds results in decreased cytoprotection, diminished blood flow, decreased synthesis of protective mucus and inhibition of mucosal cell turnover and repair. In healthy dogs, COX-1 is the primary COX enzyme that produces PGs (primarily PGE_2) |10|. An examination of published reports of GI toxicity from the administration of NSAIDs in animals indicates that the most serious problems are caused from doses that are higher than recommended, but toxicity also has been observed from relatively mild doses in susceptible individuals. Some factors may increase the risk of GI toxicosis, including concurrent corticosteroids, and other GI diseases.

The most recently approved NSAIDs in the USA for dogs are carprofen, etodolac, meloxicam, deracoxib and tepoxalin. A few other drugs are approved in Canada and Europe (tolfenamic acid and ketoprofen for example). For the newer veterinary registered NSAIDs, the GI safety profile, in comparison with older drugs, has contributed to their popularity in veterinary medicine. However, there is no evidence in the published literature using controlled clinical trials to show that one is safer or more effective than another. In a study in which carprofen, meloxicam and ketoprofen were compared in dogs after endoscopic evaluation after 7 and 28 days of administration, there was no statistical difference among the drugs with respect to development of gastroduodenal lesions [22].

Meloxicam safety profile is supported by the lack of effect on GI PGs. It had a sparing effect on GI PGs (COX-1 mediated) compared with aspirin [23], but it was a potent inhibitor of lipopolysaccharide-induced PG synthesis (COX-2 mediated).

In a study that compared the GI effects of recommended doses of carprofen, etodolac and aspirin on the canine stomach and duodenum for 28 days, etodolac and carprofen produced significantly fewer lesions than aspirin [24]. Lesion scores in these treated groups were no different than administration of placebo. The safety data for all the approved veterinary drugs available from the Food and Drug Administration (FDA)'s Freedom of Information (FOI) Summary also documents their safety.

The putative explanation for this degree of safety of carprofen, etodolac, deracoxib and meloxicam is that these drugs have preferential inhibitory action for COX-2 than COX-1 (high COX-1/COX-2 ratio). Perhaps a more accurate description of these drugs is that they have a COX-1 sparing effect [15]. However, as discussed earlier, COX-1/COX-2 ratios may not necessarily correlate with GI safety, and the calculated ratios may vary from study to study, and from species to species. Some drugs may lose their COX-2 specificity at doses used clinically. The dose dependence was shown for etodolac. At the label dose it was safe, but at higher doses, (2.7 × dose) it produced GI lesions, and, at the high dose (5.3 × dose), caused death. Etodolac loses some of its COX-2 selectivity at high doses [17] and this may be one explanation for these observations at doses that are higher than the label recommendation. At high doses, meloxicam also has demonstrated some GI toxicity. The sponsors of this drug in Europe recommended reducing the original approved dose from 0.2 to 0.1 mg/kg because of some initial GI problems [22].

Renal toxicity

In the kidney, PGs play an important part in modulating the tone of blood vessels and regulating salt and water balance. Renal injury caused by NSAIDs has been described in people, and horses, but has not been well documented in small animals. Reported cases of toxicity occurred when high doses were used or when there were other complicating factors. Renal injury occurs as a result of inhibition of renal PG synthesis [25]. In animals that have decreased renal perfusion caused by dehydration, anaesthesia, shock, or pre-existing renal disease, this leads to renal ischaemia [26].

Additional information is needed with regard to the safety of currently available COX-2 inhibitors on the kidney. Some of the PGs that play an important part in salt and water regulation and haemodynamics in the kidney are synthesized by COX-2 enzymes [27]. Constitutive COX-2 is found in various sections of the kidney and administration of drugs that are selective for COX-2 may adversely affect the kidney in some situations. Administration of a specific COX-2 inhibitor to salt-depleted people decreased renal blood flow, glomerular filtration rate and electrolyte excretion [27]. Of the currently available NSAIDs, carprofen's effect on renal function has been the most extensively studied. Because carprofen is registered for use in perioperative situations in an injectable formulation (Rimadyl injectable 50 mg/ml) investigations were performed to determine if there was any evidence of renal toxicity, particularly during conditions of anaesthesia. In one study, carprofen, ketorolac and ketoprofen were examined in healthy dogs undergoing surgery, but without i.v. fluid administration. There were minor increases in renal tubular epithelial cells on urine sediment, but overall carprofen had no adverse effects on renal function [28]. Some ketorolac- and ketoprofen-treated dogs had transient azotaemia. In other studies, administration of carprofen to anaesthetized healthy dogs had no adverse effects on renal function [29,30]. Renal effects from deracoxib were reported by the manufacturer. At high doses, there is a dose-dependent effect on renal tubules. It is well tolerated in most dogs up to 10 mg/kg for 6 months, but there is a potential for a dose-dependent renal tubular degeneration/regeneration at doses of 6 mg/kg or higher. (Clinically approved dose for long-term treatment is 1–2 mg/kg per day.) Tepoxalin was evaluated in anaesthetized, healthy, normotensive, normovolaemic dogs at a dose of 10 mg/kg (currently registered dose) using renal scintigraphy. There were no adverse effects on renal function detected [31].

Hepatic safety

As pointed out in a recent review, any NSAID has the potential for causing hepatic injury [32]. The author states that NSAIDs as a class have been associated with considerable hepatotoxicity. Hepatic toxicity caused by NSAID can be either idiosyncratic (unpredictable, non-dose related) or intrinsic (predictable and dose related) [33,34]. Toxicity to acetaminophen and aspirin are intrinsic; reactions to other drugs tend to be idiosyncratic and unpredictable. Administration of NSAID to animals with hepatic disease has been questioned because of the role of the liver in metabolizing these drugs, but there is no evidence that prior hepatic disease predisposes a patient to NSAID-induced liver injury. Drug enzyme systems are remarkably preserved in hepatic disease and pre-existing hepatic disease is not a contraindication for administration of an NSAID. Patients with liver disease may be more prone to GI ulceration, and there is concern that administration of NSAIDs could increase the risk of this complication.

Carprofen was approved by FDA in October 1996 for relief of pain and inflammation in dogs. Before this approval, it was registered for treatment of dogs in Europe (Zenecarp), and was evaluated in clinical trials. In studies in dogs with arthritis, it was effective and had a low incidence of adverse effects [35]. In longer-term studies in which carprofen was administered from 2 weeks to 5 years, the incidence of adverse reactions was only 1.3%. Vomiting, diarrhoea, anorexia and lethargy were the most common adverse reactions documented. Attention has focused on the hepatic toxicity caused by carprofen because of a report in the published literature [36]. In this report, 21 dogs were described in which carprofen was associated with acute, idiosyncratic hepatotoxicosis. Affected dogs had diminished appetites, vomited and were icteric with elevations in hepatic enzymes and bilirubin. Dogs received the usual recommended dose and developed signs an average of 19 days after therapy was initiated. No predisposing conditions were identified. Most dogs recovered without further consequences. Many of the dogs in that report were Labrador retrievers, but there is no follow-up evidence to show that this breed of dogs has an increased risk of carprofen hepatotoxicity. Other NSAIDs used in veterinary medicine also have potential for causing liver injury. Idiosyncratic reactions are rare (1/1000–1/10 000 patients). But, any unexplained increase in hepatic enzymes or bilirubin 7–90 days after initiating NSAID administration should be investigated.

Clinical drug selection for NSAIDs

For acute pain, such as peri-operative use, veterinarians have administered some of the injectable NSAIDs with good results. Drugs used in these instances include ketoprofen, flunixin meglumine, carprofen, meloxicam, tolfenamic acid (Tolfedine, available outside the USA) and ketorolac tromethamine (Toradol). These drugs have been used short-term, 1 or 2 days, to decrease fever and decrease pain from surgery or trauma. Pre-operative injections of carprofen to dogs were shown to be beneficial to decrease post-operative pain in dogs after ovariohysterectomy |37|. Meloxicam has been evaluated in two published studies for peri-operative use and was shown to be superior to butorphanol in some of the pain assessments that were measured. Carprofen and meloxicam are the only registered injectable NSAIDs for dogs in the USA.

Oral NSAIDs also may be used for acute treatment of myositis, arthritis and post-operative pain, or they may be administered chronically for osteoarthritis. Drugs that have been administered in the USA to small animals in these cases include aspirin, phenylbutazone, ketoprofen, carprofen, etodolac, piroxicam, naproxen and meclofenamic acid. The most recently approved drugs are carprofen, etodolac, meloxicam, tepoxalin and deracoxib. Doses are listed in the accompanying table. For long-term use there are no controlled studies that compare which is the most effective. When drugs are compared with one another, it is difficult, using subjective measurements, to demonstrate differences between these drugs for reducing pain in animals.

In summary, there are several choices for treating dogs with osteoarthritis with NSAID. Like people, there may be greater differences among individuals in their response than there are differences among the drugs. When selecting drugs, veterinarians sometimes select aspirin as an initial drug because it is inexpensive and familiar to most pet owners. However, GI problems can be common with aspirin especially at high doses. Other veterinarians prefer to select a drug that is approved by the FDA such as the newer etodolac, carprofen, meloxicam, tepoxalin or deracoxib for treatment in dogs. Many veterinarians use a rotating schedule of two or more drugs to identify which drug is better tolerated and effective in each patient. Outside the USA ketoprofen and tolfenamic acid have been used. The newer drugs may have a greater safety profile with respect to gastroduodenal lesions compared with aspirin, at least during the initial stages of treatment. Carprofen has been shown to lack significant renal effects when administered to anaesthetized healthy dogs and is safe in the peri-operative period. For treatment of pain in cats using NSAID, there are fewer choices that have been shown to be safe. Ketoprofen and meloxicam is approved in some countries for the treatment of cats and have been used safely. Doses for the clinical use of the NSAIDs are listed in Table 14.1 as well as in published references |**38**|.

Cyclosporin

The other important anti-inflammatory drug that has gained more veterinary recognition this past year has been cyclosporin (Atopica). It has been used by veterinarians as the human drug (Neoral), but now an approved veterinary formulation has stimulated more interest in its use.

Cyclosporin is a fat-soluble, cyclic polypeptide fungal product with potent immunosuppressive activity. In North America, the United States Pharmacopeia lists the drug name as *cyclosporine*, whereas the UK nomenclature spells it as *cyclosporin*. It has been an important drug used in humans, primarily to produce immunosuppression in organ transplant patients. This drug binds to a specific cellular receptor on calcineurin and inhibits the T-cell receptor-activated signal transduction pathway. Particularly important are its effects to suppress interleukin-2 and other cytokines, and inhibit proliferation of activated T lymphocytes. The action of cyclosporin is more specific for T cells as compared with B cells. One important advantage in comparison with other immunosuppressive drugs is that it does not cause significant myelosuppression or suppress non-specific immunity.

Clinical use

Cyclosporin has been used for a number of diseases in veterinary medicine. Many of these diseases have been dermatological, as reviewed in a recent paper by Robson and Burton |**39**|. In dogs, when used in the treatment of perianal fistulas |**40,41**| an 85% healing rate was found in one study |**40**| (2.5–6 mg/kg per day); in sebaceous adenitis, good response was reported in one case |**42**|; and in idiopathic sterile nodular panniculitis, excellent results were seen in two reported cases which were followed for 6 months following discontinuance of the cyclosporin |**43**|.

Immune-mediated diseases

Cyclosporin has been used for treatment of a variety of immune-mediated diseases, that include immune-mediated haemolytic anaemia, inflammatory bowel disease, immune-mediated polyarthritis, and aplastic anaemia, as well as others. For these diseases, the true efficacy has not been measured on the basis of controlled clinical studies. Results are primarily anecdotal. It is generally accepted that the dose should be in the range of at least 10 mg/kg per day, and perhaps twice a day to produce clinical effects. Trough blood cyclosporin concentrations should be at least 600 ng/ml.

For immune-mediated skin diseases, in small pilot studies results for treating pemphigus foliaceous in dogs have been disappointing |**44,45**|. It did not help any patients with mycosis fungoides. In a study in which five dogs with pemphigus foliaceus were treated, there was little benefit |46|. The dogs with pemphigus foliaceus were initially treated with the 'atopy dose' of 5 mg/kg per day. If there was no response the dose was increased to 10 mg/kg per day. At the end of the trial, it was concluded that at 5–10 mg/kg per day cyclosporin was unable to produce complete remission in any of the five dogs. In a case study of immune-mediated polyarthritis in dogs |47|, dogs were treated with prednisolone and various other immune-modifying drugs. Three dogs treated with cyclosporin at 5 mg/kg per day did not respond.

Atopic dermatitis

In people it has been used successfully for treatment of atopic dermatitis |48|. Because of this efficacy, the use of cyclosporin for treating canine atopic dermatitis has been investigated in dogs |49|. In a pilot study, cyclosporin was effective in 13 of 14 dogs with atopic dermatitis |50|. In another trial of 30 dogs treated with either cyclosporin (5 mg/kg per day) or prednisolone (0.5 mg/kg per day), the efficacy of cyclosporin was not statistically different than prednisolone |51–53|. Reductions in mean lesion scores were 60% and 59% in prednisolone and cyclosporin groups, respectively. Reduction in mean pruritus scores were 81% and 78% in prednisolone and cyclosporin groups, respectively. In another published study from the same author, 91 dogs with atopic dermatitis were treated with cyclosporin. Two doses were examined, 2.5 mg/kg per day and 5 mg/kg per day. The formulation used was Neoral (formulations to be discussed below). There was a dose-dependent effect. Dogs treated with 5 mg/kg had a statistically significant reduction in pruritus scores (45%) and skin lesions (67%). The dose of 2.5 mg/kg was not statistically different from placebo. In another study, however, it was demonstrated that some dogs may benefit from lower doses |54|. In this study, administration of cyclosporin (5 mg/kg) was compared with methylpred-nisolone (0.75 mg/kg) for treatment of canine atopic dermatitis. The response was not different between the drugs, but there was an overall better assessment of efficacy with cyclosporin. There were more GI problems in dogs treated with cyclosporin. In the cyclosporin-treated dogs, the dose was started at 5 mg/kg per day for 4 weeks, but eventually half of the dogs were adjusted to an every-other-day dose, and one-quarter of the dogs were given cyclosporin at 5 mg/kg only twice a week.

Use in cats

For organ transplantation in cats |55| a dose of 3 mg/kg every 12 h was used to achieve blood concentrations of 300–500 ng/ml. At North Carolina State University (NCSU) we routinely administer 25 mg/cat for suppression of immunity for transplantation, and modify as needed with monitoring. For treatment of inflammatory disease in cats, including eosinophilia granuloma complex, lower doses are possible. A good response to a dose of 25 mg/cat was seen in six cases of eosinophilic plaque and three cases of oral eosinophilic granuloma |56|. Because the smallest Neoral capsule is 25 mg, the most common dose is 25 mg/cat, once daily. (Smaller capsules are now available for veterinary use—see below.) The most common adverse effects are anorexia, vomiting and refusal to eat their food if cyclosporin is mixed with food. Toxoplasmosis has been reported in cats treated with cyclosporin, presumably due to the immunosuppression.

Formulations and pharmacokinetics

The pharmacokinetics of cyclosporin are complicated because of the differences between dosage forms, presence of many metabolites, influence of drug interactions and variability in oral absorption. The formulation, Sandimmune, has been used for many years. Although effective, it exhibits variable rate and extent of oral absorption. The newer formulation is a microemulsion called Neoral and has a much more consistent rate and extent of absorption that is less affected by influences such as feeding than Sandimmune. With administration of Neoral, oral absorption is not improved if patients were already showing good absorption with Sandimmune, but poor absorbers of Sandimmune will have higher and more consistent absorption after switching to Neoral.

The introduction in late 2003 of Atopica represents the first oral veterinary formulation of cyclosporin. The formulation is exactly the same as Neoral (micro-emulsion), except that there is a greater variety of capsule sizes available (10, 25, 50 and 100 mg). Absorption, kinetics and dissolution is expected to be the same as for Neoral. There are at least two generic formulations available for clinical use in the USA. The bioequivalence between these formulations and Atopica has not been determined for animals.

Cyclosporin is metabolized in the gut and liver to several metabolites. Twenty-five to 30 such metabolites have been identified. The prehepatic intestinal enzymes account for significant metabolism of cyclosporin [57] and systemic absorption in dogs is only 20–30% [58]. Systemic absorption in cats is similar at 25–29% [59]. The intestinal metabolism by cytochrome P-450 enzymes and the efflux caused by intestinal P-glycoprotein (P-gp) account for most of the loss in systemic availability after oral administration. One explanation for higher oral absorption from Neoral than Sandimmune formulation is that P-gp is inhibited by Neoral and less cyclosporin is transported back to the intestine [60]. Drug enzyme inhibitors, such as ketoconazole, diltiazem or the flavonoids in grapefruit juice, can inhibit the pre-systemic metabolism and produce a profound increase in systemic availability of cyclosporin. For example, 5–10 mg/kg of ketoconazole once daily can decrease the dose of cyclosporin because clearance is reduced by 85% [58].

Administration and monitoring

A common oral dose in people is 5–10 mg/kg per day to achieve targeted whole blood concentrations of 150–400 ng/ml. In people, dosages are adjusted to meet the needs of the individual patient on the basis of clinical response and monitoring trough plasma concentrations. For animals, doses of 10–20 mg/kg per day were frequently cited in older publications, but more recent recommendations, in which newer formulations have been used cited lower doses. For organ transplantation in cats [55] a dose of 3 mg/kg every 12 h of the Neoral formulation (dose was doubled for Sandimmune formulation) was used to achieve trough blood concentrations of 300–500 ng/ml. At NCSU we routinely administer 25 mg/cat for suppression of immunity for transplantation, and modify as needed with monitoring. For organ transplant in dogs, 10 mg/kg every 12 h to achieve concentrations of 500–600 ng/ml has been used |**61**|. A report on treating perianal fistulas in dogs |**62**| found that an average dose of 6 mg/kg every 12 h was needed to achieve a targeted blood concentration of 400–600 ng/ml. However, this recommendation was later modified to 2.5–6 mg/kg per day (3 mg/kg every 12 h) to achieve an effective blood concentration of 100–300 ng/ml. For dogs when treating perianal fistulas we have achieved adequate blood concentrations, without producing toxicity at a dose of 3 mg/kg every 12 h.

As cited in the clinical trials above, for treating dermatitis in dogs, the effective dose has been 5 mg/kg per day. Some clinicians have been able to lower the dose, or administer the dose every other day, and still maintain clinical remission. However, lower doses are usually not effective. The pharmacokinetics of cyclosporin in treated animals has been examined |**63**|. In their study, they found that routine monitoring of cyclosporin in dogs with atopic dermatitis was not necessary. When animals were administered a dose of 5 mg/kg per day, there did not appear to be a strong correlation between blood concentration achieved and clinical response.

Cyclosporin is available in human formulation capsules of 25 and 100 mg, 20 mg/ml oral solution and 50 mg/ml injection. The veterinary brand (Atopica) is available as 10, 25, 50 and 100 mg. There are also generic preparations available, but their absorption and pharmacokinetics have not been reported for animals. Some comparisons have not demonstrated that the generic formulations are significantly less expensive than brand name products.

Because of wide individual variation in cyclosporin pharmacokinetics, monitoring has been used to determine the optimum dose for each patient. According to one paper, clinical benefits have not been observed when trough concentrations have fallen below 50 ng/ml, therefore blood testing of patients failing therapy was suggested to reveal inadequate dosing |**39**|. However, as mentioned earlier, another study |**63**| failed to show a correlation between clinical response and blood concentration.

One must be cognisant of the assay used when monitoring cyclosporin. Plasma values will be lower than whole-blood assays because as much as 50–60% and 10–20% of the dose is concentrated in erythrocytes and leucocytes, respectively. Non-specific assays will report higher values than a more specific [monoclonal or high performance liquid chromatography (HPLC)] assay. Despite the hypothesized higher specificity when using the monoclonal assay, important discrepancies between these assays and the more specific HPLC assay have been reported |**64**|. For example, in people the difference between HPLC and the commonly used fluorescence polarization immunoassay (FPIA by TDx, Abbott Laboratories, Abbott Park, Illinois, USA) monoclonal immunoassay was 57%. In cats, we found that the TDx assay overestimated the true cyclosporin concentration by a factor of approximately twofold. (That is, TDx assay reporting 500 ng/ml corresponded to an actual value of 250 ng/ml.). In dogs, the TDx assay overestimates the true cyclosporin concentrations by a factor of 1.5–1.7 |**63**|. When using a specific radioimmunoassay or HPLC, true concentrations are measured. But, when using a TDx fluorescence polarization assay (monoclonal whole blood), multiply the feline concentrations by 0.5 to get the true concentration and multiply the canine concentration by 0.6 to get the true concentration.

Most current recommendations are based on trough blood sample monitoring. Trough samples are collected immediately before the next scheduled dose; therefore, the sample is either 12 or 24 h after the last dose. These recommendations are being modified in human medicine to a recommendation of a 2-h sample (C_2). Apparently, there is evidence that a C_2 blood sample value correlates better with clinical results than trough samples [65,66]. In cats, levels are approximately twice as high at 2 h compared with the levels at 12 h [59].

Adverse effects and precautions

Cyclosporin can cause vomiting, diarrhoea, anorexia, secondary infections, hair loss (hirsutism in people) and gingival hyperplasia [67]. Tremors or shaking have been observed in dogs administered high doses. One reference noted few adverse effects as long as blood concentrations were kept within accepted limits [62].

The most common clinical problems with cyclosporin in dogs that have been cited in the clinical trials discussed previously [51–54,68] are gastrointestinal. Vomiting, anorexia and diarrhoea can be seen. When anorexia and vomiting are reported, veterinarians have tried various interventions such as lowering the dose, or administration of the dose with some food. However, whether this decreases the efficacy of the drug should be considered. Feeding will reduce the amount of cyclosporin absorbed in dogs by 15–20%, but it is unlikely that this decrease will be severe enough to affect efficacy.

Nephrotoxicity, once a problem with older forms, is rare with current formulations. Secondary malignancies are a possible complication to long-term therapy.

Interactions

Several drugs may interact with cyclosporin. For example, co-administration of ketoconazole in people to treat secondary fungal infections will decrease metabolism of cyclosporin [58]. Ketoconazole has been used deliberately to reduce the need for cyclosporin in some investigations [69] and clinically doses have been reduced by one-third of the original dose when administered with ketoconazole. In one study with cyclosporin in the treatment of perianal fistulae, the dose of 1 mg/kg cyclosporin combined with 10 mg/kg ketoconazole was used. The author felt that a dose of 0.5 mg/kg combined with 10 mg/kg ketoconazole could also be used [70]. Erythromycin, grapefruit juice and diltiazem also may inhibit cyclosporin metabolism and increase blood concentrations. Cyclosporin does not reduce cyclosporin clearance.

Antibiotics

There have been new antibiotics added to the human market during the past year. These represent, in some cases, new classes of drugs. They are aimed primarily at treating Gram-positive cocci that cause infections that are resistant or difficult to treat with older drugs. Such new antibiotics include cephalosporins and other β-lactams.

Cephalosporins

Veterinarians are familiar with the cephalosporins commonly referred to as the first-generation cephalosporins represented by the oral drugs cephalexin (Keflex) and cefadroxil (Cefa-Tabs, Cefa-Drops), and the injectable drug cefazolin. These drugs have a spectrum of activity that includes staphylococci, streptococci and many of the enteric Gram-negative bacilli. However, resistance among Gram-negative bacteria develops easily, primarily from synthesis of β-lactamase enzymes that can hydrolyse these drugs. Extended-spectrum cephalosporins include cephalosporins from the second, third and fourth generation. Traditionally, in veterinary medicine the use of extended-spectrum cephalosporins has been reserved for treatment of bacterial infections that are resistant to other drugs. The bacteria often identified in these resistance problems have been *Escherichia coli*, *Klebsiella pneumoniae*, *Enterobacter* species, *Proteus* species (especially indole-positive) and *Pseudomonas aeruginosa*. However, there is now an approved extended-spectrum cephalosporin registered for routine use available for once-daily treatment in dogs. New developments are discussed below.

Of the second-generation cephalosporins, the ones used most often in veterinary medicine are cefoxitin and cefotetan. Their use has been valuable for treating organisms resistant to the first-generation cephalosporins or in cases in which there are anaerobic bacteria present. Anaerobic bacteria such as those of the *Bacteroides fragilis* group can become resistant by synthesizing a cephalosporinase enzyme. Cefoxitin and cefotetan, which are in the cephamycin group, are resistant to this enzyme and may be active against these bacteria. Therefore, these drugs may be valuable for some cases such as septic peritonitis that may have a mixed population of anaerobic bacteria and Gram-negative bacilli.

The third-generation cephalosporins are the most active of the cephalosporins against Gram-negative bacteria, especially enteric bacteria that are resistant to other cephalosporins. Most drugs in this group (exceptions discussed below) are intended for i.v. or i.m. administration. For convenience, some have been administered to animals s.c. But one should be warned that the i.m. or s.c. administration of these drugs could be irritating and painful. One of the most frequently administered drugs in this group is cefotaxime (Claforan) because of its potency and activity against most enteric Gram-negative bacteria and some streptococci. Compared with other cephalosporins, ceftazidime is the most active against *Pseudomonas*, against which all of the other cephalosporins, except cefoperazone, have little or no activity. Doses have been derived for ceftazidime in dogs based on pharmacokinetic data [71]. Doses vary depending on the indication, but 30 mg/kg every 8 h i.m., s.c. or i.v. will maintain effective concentrations for many infections.

As the drugs mentioned are all injectable, there has been a need for an oral extended-spectrum cephalosporin. Of the human drugs available, cefixime (Suprax) has been used in dogs because it is one of the few third-generation cephalosporins that can be administered orally. Doses have been derived from pharmacokinetic studies [72,73]. The doses have ranged from 5 to 10 mg/kg twice daily orally. Another oral third-generation cephalosporin is cefpodoxime proxetil. This drug has been used off-label in its human form (Vantin) by veterinarians for several years, but now there is a veterinary formulation (Simplicef). This drug has a longer half-life than most other cephalosporins. To treat the indications for which it is registered in dogs (skin infections), it can be given once a day orally at a dose of 5–10 mg/kg. Its absorption from oral administration is good (63%) compared with other oral third-generation cephalosporins and it is excreted mostly in the urine with a half-life of 5.6–6 h. For more serious or refractory infections against bacteria that may have high minimal inhibitory concentration (MIC) values (off-label indications), or for treating immuno-suppressed animals with Gram-negative infections, this author suggests that veterinarians consider twice a day frequency instead of the labelled frequency of once a day in order to maintain the drug concentration above the MIC for a longer period. As cefpodoxime is excreted in the urine, it may have efficacy against urinary tract infections, but clinical results have not been reported. Cefpodoxime proxetil is not registered for use in cats. Other cephalosporins have been used safely in cats, with doses extrapolated from dogs, but there are no data reported for cefpodoxime.

Cefpodoxime is more active than many other third-generation cephalosporins against staphylococcus. However, it is not active against *Pseudomonas aeruginosa*, enterococcus, or methicillin-resistant staphylococcus. One should be aware that the break-point for susceptibility is lower than for other third-generations cephalo-sporins. Therefore, it is possible for a bacterial isolate to be sensitive to cefotaxime or ceftazidime (breakpoint 8 μg/ml) but resistant to cefpodoxime (breakpoint 2 μg/ml) |74|. Specific disks are suggested for testing bacterial isolates, rather than relying on the results from other cephalosporins.

The most recent development in this class is the fourth-generation cephalo-sporins. The first fourth-generation cephalosporin is cefepime (Maxipime). It is unique from other cephalosporins because of its broad spectrum of activity that includes Gram-positive cocci, enteric Gram-negative bacilli and *Pseudomonas*. It has the advantage of activity against some extended-spectrum β-lactamase producing strains of *Klebsiella* and *Escherichia coli* that have become resistant to many other β-lactam drugs and fluoroquinolones. Except for one investigation in dogs, adult horses and foals, the use of cefepime has been limited in veterinary medicine |75|.

Carbapenems

The carbapenems are β-lactam antibiotics that include imipenem-cilastatin sodium (Primaxin), meropenem (Merrem) and most recently, ertapenem (Invanz). Imi-penem is administered with cilastatin to decrease renal tubular metabolism. Cila-statin does not affect the antibacterial activity. Imipenem has become a valuable antibiotic because it has a broad spectrum that includes many bacteria resistant to other drugs |76|. Imipenem is not active against methicillin-resistant staphylococci or resistant strains of *Enterococcus faecium*. The high activity of imipenem is attributed to its stability against most of the β-lactamases (including extended-spectrum β-lactamase) and ability to penetrate porin channels that usually exclude other drugs |77|. The carbapenems are more rapidly bactericidal than the cephalosporins and less likely to induce release of endotoxin in an animal from Gram-negative sepsis. Resist-ance to carbapenems has been extremely rare in veterinary medicine.

Some disadvantages of imipenem are the inconvenience of administration, short shelf-life after reconstitution and high cost. It must be diluted in fluids prior to administration. A common dose for small animals is 10 mg/kg every 8 h or 5 mg/kg every 6 h. This dose must be given by constant rate infusion over 30–60 min, but it has been administered subcutaneously. One of the adverse effects caused from imipenem therapy is seizures. Another problem is the risk of renal injury, which should be minimized by the addition of cilastatin |78|. Meropenem, one of the newest of the carbapenem class of drugs has antibacterial activity approximately equal to, or greater than imipenem. Other characteristics are similar to imipenem. Its advantage over imipenem is that it is more soluble and can be administered in less fluid volume and more rapidly. For example, small volumes can be administered subcutaneously with almost complete absorption. There is also a lower incidence of adverse effects to the central nervous system, such as seizures |76|. Based on pharmacokinetic experiments in our laboratory |79|, the recommended dose is 12 mg/kg every 8 h s.c., or 24 mg/kg i.v., every 8 h. Organisms with lower MIC values can be treated twice a day instead of every 8 h and for sensitive organisms in the urinary tract, 8 mg/kg, s.c., every 12 h can be used. In our experience, these doses have been well tolerated except for slight hair loss over some of the s.c. dosing sites.

Ertapenem is the newest drug in this class. It has a longer half-life in people and can be administered once a day. Experiments are underway in animals to determine the optimum dosing. Ertapenem has good activity against most Gram-negative organisms, except *Pseudomonas aeruginosa*.

Fluoroquinolones

The fluoroquinolones approved in the USA for animals include enrofloxacin, marbofloxacin, difloxacin and orbifloxacin. In the USA, all of these drugs are approved for dogs; orbifloxacin, marbofloxacin and enrofloxacin are approved for cats. Enro floxacin 100 mg/ml injection and danofloxacin (A180) injection are approved for cattle. A topical formulation of enrofloxacin and silver sulphadiazine (Baytril Otic) is registered for treating otitis in dogs. There are several other fluoroquinolones approved for use in human medicine (ciprofloxacin, lomefloxacin, enoxacin, ofloxacin), but their used has been limited in veterinary medicine, except for ciprofloxacin.

The mechanisms of action and important pharmacological properties have been reviewed elsewhere |80|. These drugs have as their advantages: (i) spectrum of activity that includes most Gram-negative bacteria and many Gram-positive bacteria, including staphylococci; (ii) oral and injectable administration; and (iii) good safety profile. Important deficiencies in the spectrum of activity include Gram-positive cocci, especially enterococci (*Enterococcus faecalis* and *Enterococcus faecium*) and anaerobic bacteria. The newest generations of fluoroquinolones (referred to by some authors as the third-generation fluoroquinolones) include trovafloxacin, grepafloxacin, gatifloxacin, gemifloxacin and moxifloxacin. Two of these, trovafloxacin and grepafloxacin, have already been discontinued for use in people because of adverse effects (abnormal cardiac rhythms and hepatic injury). The new generation of fluoroquinolones, with substitutions at the C-8 position, (C-8 methoxy for example) have as their advantage a broader spectrum that includes anaerobic bacteria and Gram-positive cocci. The difference in spectrum of activity is largely caused by increased activity against the DNA-gyrase of Gram-positive bacteria, rather than activity against topoisomerase i.v., which is the target in Gram-positive bacteria for the older quinolones |81,82|. Premafloxacin, a veterinary third-generation quinolone is one of this class for which reports are available on its potential in veterinary medicine |83|, but this drug will probably not be developed for veterinary use. Pradofloxacin has been evaluated in dogs and cats, but the experience thus far is limited to a few research abstracts |84,85|. It was more active than other fluoroquinolones against bacterial isolates from dogs and cats |84|. At a dose of 3 mg/kg orally it was effective for treatment of urinary tract infections in dogs |85|. Moxifloxacin (Avelox) is a human drug of this group and has been used on a limited basis for the treatment of infections in dogs and cats caused by bacteria that have been refractory to other drugs.

Of the currently available fluoroquinolones, all have a similar spectrum of activity, but they may vary in potency. Against some Gram-negative bacilli, especially *Pseudomonas aeruginosa*, the human drug ciprofloxacin is more active than veterinary quinolones. Enrofloxacin in small animals is metabolized to ciprofloxacin, which may account for 10–20% of the total quinolone maximum plasma concentrations (C_{MAX}) and as much as 35% of the total area under the curve |86|. Orbifloxacin and marbofloxacin have little or no active metabolites, but they are well absorbed and achieve higher plasma concentrations after equivalent doses compared with enrofloxacin and difloxacin. Generally, all of the veterinary fluoroquinolones attain good concentrations in tissues, with tissue/plasma concentration ratios approaching, or greater than 1.0 |87|.

Fluoroquinolones have had a good safety record after administration to animals. Central nervous system effects, such as seizures, may occur at high doses but are rare. In young animals, especially dogs and foals, arthropathy of the developing cartilage is possible, leading to joint injury and lameness. Recently, blindness in cats caused by fluoroquinolones has attracted attention. The labelled dose for enrofloxacin (Baytril) use in cats in the USA was recently changed by the drug manufacturer (Bayer Corporation). Because of dose-related ocular toxicosis, the dose in cats should not exceed 5 mg/kg per day. The mechanism for the toxicity is not understood, but degenerative lesions in the retina have been identified. In studies performed by the manufacturer, there were no adverse effects observed in cats treated with 5 mg/kg per day of enrofloxacin. However, the administration of enrofloxacin at 20 mg/kg or greater, caused salivation, vomiting and depression. At doses of 20 mg/kg or greater, there were mild to severe fundic lesions on ophthalmological examination including changes in the fundus and retinal degeneration. There were also abnormal electroretinograms, including blindness. Ocular problems have not been reported in other species.

Besides enrofloxacin, the other fluoroquinolones registered for use in cats are orbifloxacin (Orbax) and marbofloxacin (Zeniquin). The current approved dose of orbifloxacin for cats is 2.5–7.5 mg/kg per day. In a published study |88| orbifloxacin oral liquid was administered to cats at 0, 15, 45 and 75 mg/kg for at least 30 days (eight cats/group). This represents six, 18 and 30 times the lowest label dosage. No ocular lesions were observed in any cats treated with 15 mg/kg. At the higher doses (18 and 30 times the dose) there was tapetal hyperreflectivity in the area centralis and minimal photoreceptor degeneration. When marbofloxacin was administered to cats at 5.55, 16.7 and 28 mg/kg, representing two, six and 10 times the lowest label dose, for 6 weeks there were no ocular lesions in cats (manufacturer's data). At 55.5 mg/kg (10 times the lowest label dose) for 14 days there were also no lesions from marbofloxacin.

References

1. Vane JR, Botting RM. New insights into the mode of action of anti-inflammatory drugs. *Inflamm Res* 1995; **44**: 1–10.

2. Papich MG. Pharmacologic considerations for opiate analgesic and non-steroidal anti-inflammatory drugs. *Vet Clin North Am Small Anim Pract* 2000; **30**(4): 815–37.

3. Meade EA, Smith WL, DeWitt DL. Pharmacology of prostaglandin endoperoxide synthase isozymes-1 and -2. *Ann N Y Acad Sci* 1994; **714**: 136–42.

4. Laneuville O, Breuer DK, Dewitt DL, Hla T, Funk CD, Smith WL. Differential inhibition of human prostaglandin endoperoxide synthases-1 and -2 by non-steroidal anti-inflammatory drugs. *J Pharmacol Exp Ther* 1994; **271**(2): 927–34.

5. Ricketts AP, Lundy KM, Seibel SB. Evaluation of selective inhibition of canine cyclo-oxygenase 1 and 2 by carprofen and other nonsteroidal anti-inflammatory drugs. *Am J Vet Res* 1998; **59**: 1441–6.

6. McKellar QA, Delatour P, Lees P: Stereospecific pharmacodynamics and pharmacokinetics of carprofen in the dog. *J Vet Pharmacol Ther* 1994; **17**: 447–54.

7. Bryant CE, Farnfield BA, Janicke HJ. Evaluation of the ability of carprofen and flunixin meglumine to inhibit activation of nuclear factor kappa B. *Am J Vet Res* 2003; **64**: 211–15.

8. Gierse JK, Staten NR, Casperson GF, Koboldt CM, Trigg JS, Reitz BA, Pierce JL, Seibert K. Cloning, expression, and selective inhibition of canine cyclooxygenase-1 and cyclooxygenase-2. *Vet Ther* 2002; **3**(3): 270–80.

9. McCann ME, Andersen DR, Zhang D, Brideau C, Black WC, Hanson PD, Hickey GJ. *In vitro* effects and *in vivo* efficacy of a novel cyclo-oxygenase-2 inhibitor in dogs with experimentally induced synovitis. *Am J Vet Res* 2004; **65**: 503–12.

10. Kay-Mugford P, Benn SJ, LaMarre J, Conlon P. *In vitro* effects of non-steroidal anti-inflammatory drugs on cyclooxygenase activity in dogs. *Am J Vet Res* 2000; **61**: 802–10.

11. Wilson JE, Chandrasekharan NV, Westover KD, Eager KB, Simmons DL. Determination of expression of cyclooxygenase-1 and -2 isozymes in canine tissues and their differential sensitivity to non-steroidal anti-inflammatory drugs. *Am J Vet Res* 2004; **65**: 810–18.

12. Glaser KB. Cyclooxygenase selectivity and NSAIDs: cyclooxygenase-2 selectivity of etodolac (Lodine). *Inflammopharmacology* 1995; **3**: 335–45.

13. Lees P. Pharmacology of drugs used to treat osteoarthritis in veterinary practice. *Inflammopharmacology* 2003; **11**: 385–99.

14. FitzGerald GA, Patrono C. The Coxibs, selective inhibitors of cyclooxygenase-2. *N Engl J Med* 2001; **345**: 433–42.

15. Peterson WL, Cryer B. COX-1-sparing NSAIDs: is the enthusiasm justified? *J Am Med Assoc* 1999; **282**: 1961–3.

16. Malhotra S, Shafiq N, Pandhi P. COX-2 inhibitors: a CLASS act, or just VIGORously promoted. *MedGenMed* 2004; **6**(1): 6.

17. Wolfe MM, Lichtenstein DR, Singh G. Gastrointestinal toxicity of non-steroidal anti-inflammatory drugs. *N Engl J Med* 1999; **340**: 1888–99.

18. Mukherjee D, Nissen SE, Topol EJ. Risk of cardiovascular events associated with selective COX-2 inhibitors. *JAMA* 2001; **286**: 954–9.

19. Topol EJ. Failing the public health—rofecoxib, Merck and the FDA. *N Engl J Med* 2004; **351**: 1707–9.

20. Trang T, McNaull B, Quirion R, Jhamandas K. Involvement of spinal lipoxygenase metabolites in hyperalgesia and opioid tolerance. *Eur J Pharmacol* 2004; **491**: 21–30.

21. Bertolini A, Ottani A, Sandrini M. Dual acting anti-inflammatory drugs: a reappraisal. *Pharmacol Res* 2001; **44**: 437–50.

22. Forsyth SF, Guilford WG, Haslett SJ, Godfrey J. Endoscopy of the gastroduodenal mucosa after carprofen, meloxicam and ketoprofen administration in dogs. *J Small Anim Pract* 1998; **39**: 421–4.

23. Jones CJ, Streppa HK, Harmon BG, Budsberg SC. In vivo effects of meloxicam and aspirin on blood, gastric mucosal, and synovial fluid prostanoid synthesis in dogs. *Am J Vet Res* 2002; **63**: 1527–31.

24. Reimer ME, Johnston SA, Leib MS, Duncan RB Jr, Reimer DC, Marini M, Gimbert K. The gastroduodenal effects of buffered aspirin, carprofen, and etodolac in healthy dogs. *J Vet Intern Med* 1999; **13**(5): 472–7.

25. Brown SA. Renal effects of non-steroidal anti-inflammatory drugs. In: Kirk RW (ed). *Current Veterinary Therapy X*. Philadelphia: WB Saunders Co., 1989; pp. 1158–61.

26. Mathews KA. Non-steroidal anti-inflammatory analgesics in pain management in dogs and cats. *Can Vet J* 1996; **37**: 539–45.

27. Rossat J, Maillard M, Nussberger JU, Brunner HR, Burnier M. Renal effects of selective cyclooxygenase-2 inhibition in normotensive salt-depleted subjects. *Clin Pharmacol Ther* 1999; **66**: 76–84.

28. Lobetti RG, Joubert KE. Effect of administration of non-steroidal anti-inflammatory drugs before surgery on renal function in clinically normal dogs. *Am J Vet Res* 2000; **61**(12): 1501–7.

29. Ko JCH, Miyabiyashi T, Mandsager RE, Heaton-Jones TG, Mauragis DF. Renal effects of carprofen administered to healthy dogs anesthetized with propofol and isoflurane. *Am J Vet Med Assoc* 2000; **217**: 346–9.

30. Boström IM, Nyman GC, Lord PF, Haggstrom J, Jones BE, Bohlin HP. Effects of carprofen on renal function and results of serum biochemical and hematologic analyses in anesthetized dogs that had low blood pressure during anesthesia. *Am J Vet Res* 2002; **63**(5): 712–21.

31. Gogny M, Fusellier M, Delpong V, Marescaux L, Desfontis J-C. *Renal Scintigraphy. Application to the Study of the Renal Tolerability of Tepoxalin (Zubrin) in the Anesthetized Dog.* Presented at the Worldwide Zubrin Symposium, Athens, Greece; October 2003.

32. Lee WM. Drug induced hepatotoxicity. *N Engl J Med* 2003; **349**: 474–85.

33. Tolman KG. Hepatotoxicity of non-narcotic analgesics. *Am J Med* 1998; **105**(Suppl 1B): 13–17S.

34. Bjorkman D. Nonsteroidal anti-inflammatory drug-associated toxicity of the liver, lower gastrointestinal tract, and esophagus. *Am J Med* 1998; **105**(Suppl 5A): 17–21S.

35. Vasseur PB, Johnson AL, Budsberg SC, Lincoln JD, Toombs JP, Whitehair JG, Lentz EL. Randomized, controlled trial of the efficacy of carprofen, a nonsteroidal antiinflammatory drug, in the treatment of osteoarthritis in dogs. *J Am Vet Med Assoc* 1995; **206**(6): 807–11.

36. MacPhail CM, Lappin MR, Meyer DJ, Smith SG, Webster CR, Armstrong PJ. Hepatocellular toxicosis associated with administration of carprofen in 21 dogs. *J Am Vet Med Assoc* 1998; **212**(12): 1895–901.

37. Lascelles BDX, Cripps PJ, Jones A, Waterman-Pearson AE. Efficacy and kinetics of carprofen, administered preoperatively or postoperatively, for the prevention of pain in dogs undergoing ovariohysterectomy. *Vet Surg* 1998; **27**(6): 568–82.

38. Papich MG. *Handbook of Veterinary Drugs.* Philadelphia: WB Saunders Co, 2002; 551 pages.

39. Robson DC, Burton GG. Cyclosporine: applications in small animal dermatology. *Vet Dermatol* 2003; **14**: 1–9.

40. Mathews KA, Sukhiani HR. Randomized controlled trial of cyclosporine for treatment of perianal fistulas in dogs. *J Am Vet Med Assoc* 1997; **211**: 1249–53.

41. Griffiths LG, Sullivan M, Borland WW. Cyclosporine as the sole treatment for anal furnculosis: preliminary results. *J Small Anim Pract* 1999; **40**: 569–72.

42. Carothers MA, Kwochka KW, Rojko JL. Cyclosporine responsive granulomatous sebaceous adenitis in a dog. *J Am Vet Med Assoc* 1991; **198**: 1645–8.

43. Guaguere E. Efficacy of cyclosporine in the treatment of idiopathic sterile nodular panniculitis in two dogs. *Vet Derm* 2000; **11**(Suppl 1): 22.

44. Rosenkrantz W. Immunomodulating drugs in dermatology. In: Kirk RW (ed). *Current Veterinary Therapy X.* Philadelphia: WB Saunders Co., 1989; pp. 570–7.

45. Rosenkrantz WS, Griffin CE, Barr RJ. Clinical evaluation of cyclosporine in animal models with cutaneous immune-mediated disease and epitheliotropic lymphoma. *J Am Anim Hosp Assoc* 1989; **25**: 377–84.

46. Olivry T, Rivierre C, Murphy KM. Efficacy of cyclosporine for treatment of induction of canine pemphigus foliaceus. *Vet Record* 2003; **152**: 53–4.

47. Clements DN, Gear RN, Tattersall J, Carmichael S, Bennett D. Type I immune-mediated polyarthritis in dogs: 39 cases (1997–2002). *J Am Vet Med Assoc* 2004; **224**: 1323–7.

48. Camp RDR, Reitamo S, Friedmann PS, Ho V, Heule F. Cyclosporin A in severe, therapy-resistant atopic dermatitis: Report of an international workshop. *Br J Dermatol* 1993; **129**(2): 217–20.

50. Fontaine J, Olivry T. Cyclosporine for the management of atopic dermatitis in dogs: a pilot clinical trial. *Vet Rec* 2001; **148**: 662–3.

51. Olivry T, Rivierre C, Jackson HA, Murphy KM, Sousa CA. Cyclosporin-A decreases skin lesions and pruritus in dogs with atopic dermatitis: a prednisolone-controlled blinded trial. *Vet Dermatol* 2000; **11**(Suppl 1): 47.

52. Olivry T, Rivierre C, Jackson HA, Murphy KM, Davidson G, Sousa CA. Cyclosporine decreases skin lesions and pruritus in dogs with atopic dermatitis: a blinded randomized prednisolone-controlled trial. *Vet Dermatol* 2002; **13**: 77–87.

53. Olivry T, Steffan J, Fisch RD, Prelaud P, Guaguere E, Fontaine J, Carlotti DN; European Veterinary Dermatology Cyclosporine Group. Randomized controlled trial of the efficacy of cyclosporine in the treatment of atopic dermatitis in dogs. *J Am Vet Med Assoc* 2002; **221**(3): 370–7.

54. Steffan J, Alexander D, Brovedani F, Fisch RD. Comparison of cyclosporine A with methylprednisolone for treatment of canine atopic dermatitis: a parallel, blinded, randomized controlled trial. *Vet Dermatol* 2003; **14**: 11–22.

55. Mathews KG, Gregory CR. Renal transplants in cats: 66 cases (1987–1996). *J Am Vet Med Assoc* 1997; **211**: 1432–6.

56. Guaguère E, Prélaud P. Efficacy of cyclosporine in the treatment of 12 cases of eosinophilic granuloma complex. *Vet Derm* 2000; 11(Suppl 1): 31.

57. Wu C-Y, Benet LZ, Hebert MF, Gupta SK, Rowland M, Gomez DY, Wacher VJ. Differentiation of absorption and first-pass gut and hepatic metabolism in humans: studies with cyclosporine. *Clin Pharmacol Ther* 1995; **58**(5): 492–7.

58. Myre SA, Schoeder TJ, Grund VR, Wandstrat TL, Nicely PG, Pesce AJ, First MR. Critical ketoconazole dosage range for ciclosporin clearance inhibition in the dog. *Pharmacology* 1991; **43**(5): 233–41.

59. Mehl ML, Kyles AE, Craigmill AL, Epstein S, Gregory CR. Disposition of cyclosporine after intravenous and multi-dose oral administration in cats. *J Vet Pharmacol Ther* 2003; **26**(5): 349–54.

60. Lown KS, Mayo RR, Leichtman AB, Hsiao HL, Turgeon DK, Schmiedlin-Ren P, Brown MB, Guo W, Rossi SJ, Benet LZ, Watkins PB. Role of intestinal P-glycoprotein (mdr-1) in interpatient variation in the oral bioavailability of cyclosporine. *Clin Pharmacol Ther* 1997; **62**(3): 248–60.

61. Mathews KA, Holmberg DL, Miller CW. Kidney transplantation in dogs with naturally occurring end-stage renal disease. *J Am Anim Hosp Assoc* 2000; **36**: 294–301.

62. Mathews KA, Sukhiani HR. Randomized controlled trial of cyclosporine for treatment of perianal fistulas in dogs. *J Am Vet Med Assoc* 1997; **211**: 1249–53.

63. Steffan J, Strehlau G, Maurer M, Rohlfs A. Cyclosporin A pharmacokinetics and efficacy in the treatment of atopic dermatitis in dogs. *J Vet Pharmacol Ther* 2004; **27**: 231–8.

64. Steimer W. Performance and specificity of monoclonal immunoassays for cyclosporine monitoring: how specific is specific? *Clin Chem* 1999; **45**: 371–81.

65. Levy G, Thervet E, Lake J, Uchida K; Consensus on Neoral C(2): Expert Review in Transplantation (CONCERT) Group. Patient management by Neoral C2 monitoring: an international consensus statement. *Transplantation* 2002; **73**(9 Suppl): S12–18.

66. Nashan B, Cole E, Levy G, Thervet E. Clinical validation studies of Neoral C2 monitoring: a review. *Transplantation* 2002; **73**(Suppl): S3–11.

67. Vaden SL. Cyclopsorine. In: Bonagura JD (ed). *Current Veterinary Therapy XII*. Philadelphia: WB Saunders, 1995; pp. 73–7.

68. Guaguère E, Steffan J, Olivry T. Cyclosporin A: a new drug in the field of canine dermatology. *Vet Derm* 2004; **15**: 61–74.

69. Patricelli AJ, Hardie RJ, McAnulty JF. Cyclosporine and ketoconazole for the treatment of perianal fistulas. *J Am Vet Med Assoc* 2002; **220**: 1009–16.

70. Mouatt J. Cyclosporine and ketoconazole interaction for treatment of perianal fistulas in the dog. *Aust Vet J* 2002; **80**(4): 207–11.

71. Moore KW, Trepanier LA, Lautzenhiser SJ, Fialkowski JP, Rosin E. Pharmacokinetics of ceftazidime in dogs following subcutaneous administration and continuous infusion and the association with in vitro susceptibility of Pseudomonas aeruginosa. *Am J Vet Res* 2000; **61**(10): 1204–8.

72. Bialer M, Wu WH, Look AM, Silber BM, Yacobi A. Pharmacokinetics of cefixime after oral and intravenous doses in dogs: bioavailability assessment for a drug showing nonlinear serum protein binding. *Res Commun Chem Pathol Pharmacol* 1987; **56**: 21–32.

73. Lavy E, Ziv G, Aroch I, Glickman A. Clinical pharmacologic aspects of cefixime in dogs. *Am J Vet Res* 1995; **56**: 633–8.

74. NCCLS. *Performance Standards for Antimicrobial Disk and Dilution Susceptibility Tests for Bacteria Isolated from Animals; Approved Standard*, 2nd edn. NCCLS document M31-A2. Wayne, Pennsylvania: NCCLS, 2002.

75. Gardner SY, Papich MG. Comparison of cefepime pharmacokinetics in neonatal foals and adult dogs. *J Vet Pharmacol Ther* 2001; **24**(3): 187–92.

76. Edwards JR, Betts MJ. Carbapenems: the pinnacle of the beta-lactam antibiotics or room for improvement? *J Antimicrob Chemother* 2000; **45**: 1–4.

77. Livermore DM. Of Pseudomonas, porins, pumps, and carbapenems. *J Antimicrob Chemother* 2001; **47**: 247–50.

78. Barker CW, Zhang W, Sanchez S, Budsberg SC, Boudinot FD, McCrackin Stevenson MA. Pharmacokinetics of imipenem in dogs. *Am J Vet Res* 2003; **64**(6): 694–9.

79. Bidgood T, Papich MG. Plasma pharmacokinetics and tissue fluid concentrations of meropenem after intravenous and subcutaneous administration in dogs. *Am J Vet Res* 2002; **63**(12): 1622–8.

80. Papich MG, Riviere JE. Fluoroquinolone antimicrobial drugs. In: Adams HR (ed). *Veterinary Pharmacology and Therapeutics*, 8th edn. Ames, IA: Iowa State University Press, 2001; pp. 898–917.

81. Pestova E, Millichap JJ, Noskin GA, Peterson LR. Intracellular targets for moxifloxacin: a comparison with other fluoroquinolones. *J Antimicrob Chemother* 2000; **45**: 583–90.

82. Hooper DC. Mechanisms of action and resistance of older and newer fluoroquinolones. *Clin Infect Dis* 2000; **31**(Suppl 2): S24–8.

83. Watts JL, Salmon SA, Sanchez MS, Yancey RJ. *In vitro* activity of premafloxacin, a new extended-spectrum fluoroquinolone, against pathogens of veterinary importance. *Antimicrob Agents Chemother* 1997; **41**: 1190–2.

84. de Jong A, Stephan B, Friederichs S. *Antibacterial Activity of Pradofloxacin Against Canine and Feline Pathogens Isolated from Clinical Cases* [abstract]. Antimicrobial Agents In Veterinary Medicines (AAVM), Ottawa, Canada, June 2004.

85. Stephan B, Roy O, Skowronski V, Edingloh M, Greife H. *Clinical Efficacy of Pradofloxacin in the Treatment of Canine Urinary Tract Infections* [abstract]. AAVM, Ottawa, Canada, June 2004.

86. Cester CC, Schneider M, Toutain P-L. Comparative kinetics of two orally administered fluoroquinolones in dog: enrofloxacin versus marbofloxacin. *Revue Méd Vét* 1996; **147**: 703–16.

87. Bidgood T, Papich MG. Pharmacokinetics of enrofloxacin and marbofloxacin and tissue concentrations in dogs. (Accepted *J Vet Pharmacol Therap*, in press 2005).

88. Kay-Mugford PA, Ramsey DT, Dubielzig RR, Tuomar DL, Turck PA. *Ocular Effects of Orally Administered Orbifloxacin in Cats* [Abstract]. American College of Veterinary Ophthalmologists 32nd Annual Meeting 2001: 9–13 October.

15

Small animal reproduction

JOHN VERSTEGEN, KARINE ONCLIN

Introduction

Small animal reproduction (SAR) is a new and rapidly evolving field in veterinary medicine. There were only a few years between the initial master works of the few so-called fathers of SAR (PW Concannon, W Jochle, K Arbeiter or V Shille and G Staben-feld), followed by few yearly published data available in the seventies and eighties, to the tremendously exciting number of publications produced today. During 2003–2004, many new studies were either presented at the main 5th International Symposium on Canine and Feline Reproduction held in Brazil, the 2nd ACCD International Sympo-sium on Non-Surgical Contraceptive Methods for Pet Population Control, the 5th EVSSAR European Congress or published as part of the scientific literature.

Clinic and biotechnology, molecular biology, cryobiology and *in vitro* technolo-gies are among the fields already developed in many mammal species, which are see-ing a continuous and promising development in dogs and cats, often used as models for exotic carnivores or endangered species. SAR is also beginning to benefit from comparative studies, including human medicine for which dogs and cats are used as models for different reproductive diseases including mammary tumours, pregnancy-associated diabetes mellitus or prostate diseases. Fortunately, in line with the growing interest in pets and their social role in our society as well as endangered species' preservation, institutional and private funding for SAR particularly in fields related to the control of reproduction are slowly developing. Owners' and breeders' concerns are being echoed in research and educational institutions. Now with high-quality services, it is also offered not only in specialized private practices but also in univer-sities which are slowly integrating SAR in essential teaching objectives as in other medicine-related fields. All this is reflected in an increased number of high-quality scientific and clinical publications. One major observation is the internationalization of research with an increased number of high-quality publications coming from all over the world, including South America, Eastern countries and Japan. Being a new science, the main and essential questions in basic reproductive physiology are slowly being answered. During the last years, at least three main fields have seen a dramatic increase in high-quality publications: fundamental endocrine and physiological research in dogs and cats; control of reproduction with the development of new alternatives to surgical contraception; and *in vitro* biotechnologies of reproduction in the female and the male, including cryobiology and cloning.

The control of reproduction in dogs and cats assumes that fundamental research will help to understand the mechanisms underlying the peculiar reproductive physiology of these species. In dogs, many basic questions remain and still need to be studied further, including: (i) regulation of corpus luteum function and anoestrus; (ii) determination of the optimal time for artificial insemination with fresh but mainly frozen semen, which is still of moderate quality after thawing; and (iii) control of reproduction using alternatives to surgery. In dogs and cats, the basic, practical aspects of *in vitro* biotechnologies need to be answered to allow for the development of these medically assisted technologies, e.g. how and when to inseminate, etc. Some of these questions have been approached in SAR publications over the last year and are opening up interesting perspectives for the future, both in clinical and fundamental research.

Control of reproduction in dogs and cats

The control of reproduction in the dog and cat to respond to major society-raised questions regarding pet over-population can be approached through the prevention of the reproductive cycle or the induction of abortion.

Adding non-surgical contraception to the arsenal of sterilization methods will increase control over breeding in dogs and cats and improve population management. The prevention of reproduction in both species is nowadays either obtained through irreversible, ethically questionable, surgical neutering or through the use of contraceptive agents such as progestins. Both these approaches have advantages but also have side effects that make it necessary to look for alternatives because of both social and medical concerns. Interestingly, and reflecting the social concerns of alternatives to actual contraceptive methods, three different approaches were proposed during 2003–2004. Junaidi *et al.* propose the use of gonadotrophin-releasing hormone (GnRH) agonist contraceptive implants to prevent reproduction in male animals. Ferro *et al.* suggest the use of GnRH vaccines in male dogs, whereas Verstegen *et al.* propose the use of steroid-based contraceptive implants for long-term contraception in female dogs and cats.

The induction of abortion is an alternative to cycle prevention in terms of control of reproduction. Even if less ethical or questionable, this approach is often the only available alternative for pets, wild animals or zoo animals where no efficacious preventive contraceptive methods are available.

The development in Europe of RU38478 (aglepristone), a specific progesterone antagonist, is certainly a major advancement in pharmaceutical research over the last few years. However, there are still many questions remaining concerning its mode of action, particularly in the control of anoestrus duration. Indeed, aglepristone administration during early or mid-pregnancy is known to shorten significantly the interoestrus interval. Galac *et al.* proposed an original approach for studying this interesting observation using di-oestrus non-pregnant animals.

Use of a new drug delivery formulation of the gonadotrophin-releasing hormone analogue Deslorelin for reversible long-term contraception in male dogs

Junaidi A, Williamson PE, Cummins JM, Martin GB, Blackberry MA, Trigg TE.
Reprod Fertil Dev 2004; **15**(6): 317–22

BACKGROUND. In this study the effect of treatment with a slow-release implant containing the GnRH agonist Deslorelin(™) (Peptech Animal Health Australia, North Ryde, NSW, Australia) on pituitary and testicular function in mature male dogs was studied. Four dogs were treated with Deslorelin (6-mg implant) and four were used as controls (blank implant). In control dogs, there were no significant changes over the 12 months of the study in plasma concentrations of luteinizing hormone (LH) or testosterone, or in testicular volume, semen output or semen quality. In Deslorelin-treated dogs, plasma concentrations of LH and testosterone were undetectable after 21 and 27 days, testicular volume fell to 35% of pre-treatment values after 14 weeks and no ejaculates could be obtained after 6 weeks. Concentrations returned to the detectable range for testosterone after 44 weeks and for LH after 51 weeks and both were within the normal range after 52 weeks (Fig. 15.1).

Semen characteristics had recovered completely by 60 weeks after implantation. At this time, the testes and prostate glands were similar histologically to those of control dogs.

INTERPRETATION. In the present study, the authors tested the effects of treatment with a slow-release implant containing Deslorelin on pituitary and testicular function in mature male dogs. They conclude that a single slow-release implant containing 6 mg Deslorelin has potential as a long-term, reversible antifertility agent for male dogs.

Comment

The initial stimulatory effect of GnRH agonist administration is observed in male as well as in female dogs where an initial stimulation of FSH and LH is also observed after the administration of a GnRH agonist implant. Here however, contrary to what is observed in female dogs where an unwanted oestrus cycle is induced after the initial stimulation, this stimulatory effect (Fig. 15.2) is of no clinical consequence and the prolonged inhibition observed in the following days or weeks, allows for reversible contraception of the male dog. The induced control of reproduction in the male dog lasts an average of 10 to 12 months. However, data are limited, information is missing concerning possible escape mechanisms in some animals and long-term safety studies are needed. Indeed, broad distribution of GnRH receptors in extrapituitary tissues and organs has been demonstrated |**1–2**| and through these observations the study of extrapituitary GnRH systems has become one of the important topics regarding the physiological significance of GnRH. In addition to potential direct effects of GnRH on gonads, it has been reported that GnRH may act as a neuromodulator or an immunomodulator |**3–5**|. There are interesting *in vitro* studies about the

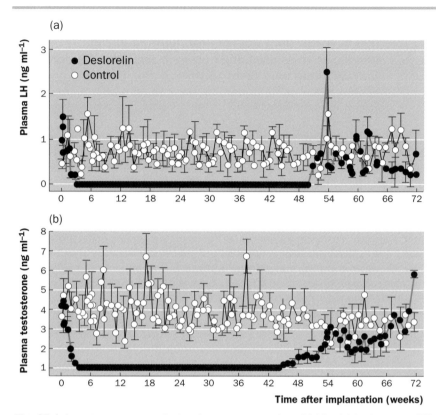

Fig. 15.1 Long-term responses in the plasma concentration of (a) luteinizing hormone (LH) and (b) testosterone to a subcutaneous slow-release implant containing 6 mg Deslorelin™ (Peptech Animal Health Australia, North Ryde, NSW, Australia) in male dogs (●). ○, control. Data are the mean ± SEM (n = 4). Source: Junaidi *et al.* (2004).

diverse functions of GnRH, and GnRH was demonstrated to promote or inhibit cell proliferation depending on the cell type (thymocytes, splenocytes, lymphocytes), to interfere with cell adhesion, cell migration, and to interfere with cytoskeletal remodelling. What would be the effect of long-term extrapituitary GnRH receptor down-regulation? This needs to be further analysed. However, and even if preliminary, this is an interesting approach to the problem of contraception in dogs; new developments, including control in the female, are long awaited and will probably soon be offering an alternative treatment to surgical sterilization.

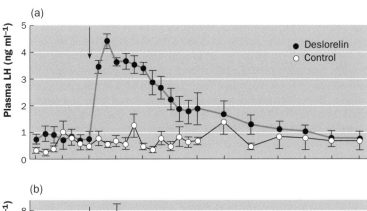

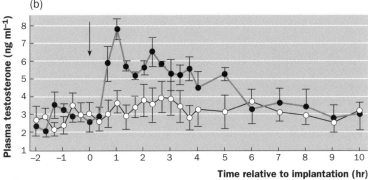

Time relative to implantation (hr)

Fig. 15.2 Acute responses in the plasma concentration of (a) luteinizing hormone (LH) and (b) testosterone following the implantation of a subcutaneous slow-release implant (arrow) containing 6 mg Deslorelin™ (Peptech Animal Health Australia, North Ryde, NSW, Australia) in male dogs (●). ○, control. Data are the mean ± SEM (n = 4). Source: Junaidi et al. (2004).

Efficacy of an anti-fertility vaccine based on mammalian gonadotrophin releasing hormone (GnRH-I)—a histological comparison in male animals

Ferro VA, Khan MAH, McAdam D, et al. Vet Immunol Immunopathol 2004; **101**: 73–86

BACKGROUND. An N-terminal modified GnRH-I (tetanus toxoid-CHWSYGLRPG-NH$_2$) conjugate was evaluated histologically in a number of male animal species (mice, dogs and sheep). The immunogen has previously been shown to be highly effective in rats, by suppressing both steroidogenesis and spermatogenesis. However, cross-species efficacy of peptide vaccines is known to be highly variable. Therefore, a comparative evaluation of reproductive tissues from animals immunized against this immunogen adsorbed on to an alum-based adjuvant was made. Sheep and dogs were chosen, as use of antifertility vaccines in these species is important in farming and veterinary practice. Changes in testicular size were measured during the immunization period and the greatest alteration (attributed to gonadal atrophy) was observed in the rat. Following euthanasia, testicular tissue was evaluated for spermatogenesis. The most susceptible species to GnRH-I ablation was the rat, which showed significant ($P < 0.0001$) arrest in spermatogenesis compared with untreated controls. Testicular sections taken from treated animals were completely devoid of spermatozoa or spermatids, in comparison with 94% of the untreated controls showing evidence of spermatogenesis. The immunized mice and rams also showed significant arrest ($P < 0.0001$). There was a 30–45% decrease in spermatogenesis and total azoospermia was not apparent. However, the least responsive were the dogs, which showed little significant variation compared with untreated animals and only a 5% decrease in activity (Fig. 15.3). A comparison of the specific IgG response with GnRH-I indicated that in sheep and dogs the response was

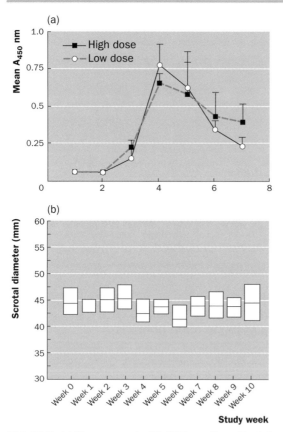

Fig. 15.3 (a) Measurement of GnRH-I specific antibody levels in dogs immunized at week 0, 2, 4 and 6. (b) Measurement of the mean scrotal diameters in dogs immunized with TT-CHWSYGLRPG-NH$_2$ at week 0, 2, 4 and 6. The pre-treatment measurement was used as the untreated control. Source: Ferro et al. (2004).

not maintained, unlike in rodents, suggesting that suppression of fertility may be due to differences in immune responses in different animal species.

INTERPRETATION. The main hindrance to progression and advancement of antifertility vaccines based on GnRH is related to lack of efficacy. Production of high-affinity antibodies against GnRH (immuno-neutralization) has been demonstrated in many species but with varying success in fertility disruption. Antibody titre is not necessarily a good indicator of vaccine efficacy and did not correlate well with histological and clinical observations. Immunization in the dog caused little response against spermatogenesis. Furthermore, the endocrine efficacy should be clearly tested taking into account the diurnal and seasonal variations.

Comment

The development of a veterinary contraceptive with total disruption of spermatogenesis using vaccines as the approach remains a challenge. Early attempts to raise GnRH antisera produced gonadal atrophy in some animals, presumably by interrupting LH and follicle-stimulating hormone secretion as proposed by Arimura *et al.* |6|. These observations suggested the potential clinical application of GnRH for immunoneutralization in domestic animals. However, more than 30 years later, the results are still disappointing. The choice of adjuvant seems to be critical as success clearly appears to vary with the carrier, but is questionable in terms of practicability and safety. Indeed, the most potent adjuvant actually available is generally the one mainly associated with side effects, preventing their use in companion animals. Lastly, the results are inconsistent and not reliable enough to allow this to be proposed as a valuable contraceptive solution. The classical vaccine approach, as previously described in dogs and cats, appears to have a poor future and applicability in controlling reproduction in carnivores.

Long term (>2 years), reversible, and side effect-free contraception with a co-extruded silastic-based progestin implant in dogs and cats: an efficient alternative to immunocontraception

Verstegen J, Boisrame B, Onclin K. Proceedings of the 2nd ACCD Conference, Betteridge, Colorado; August 2004, 145–54

BACKGROUND. Many technologies have been explored and proposed for the development of a long-acting, non-surgical contraceptive for dogs and cats. This approach should not be expensive to allow the widest use possible. It should be easy to administer and reversible to allow the owner to change his or her mind or to better organize and control reproduction of his or her pet. Particularly important is that it should be devoid of significant side effects. The authors' goal was to develop a device responding to these requirements and, by using available technologies, to reduce development costs. After 4 years of development, they produced a 2-year contraceptive implant, effective both in dogs and cats, and devoid of significant side effects during a 4-year follow-up study. Its contraceptive effects were reversible.

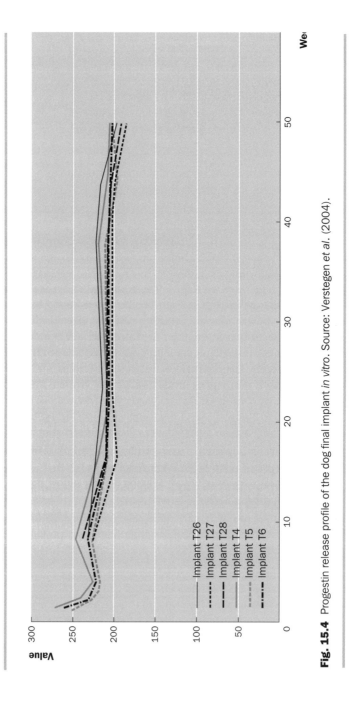

Fig. 15.4 Progestin release profile of the dog final implant *in vitro*. Source: Verstegen *et al.* (2004).

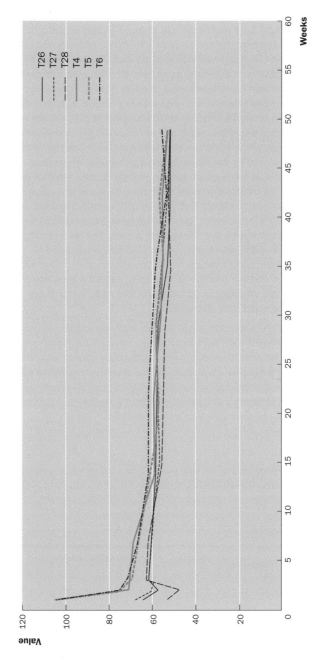

Fig. 15.5 Progestin release profile of the cat final implant *in vitro*. Source: Verstegen *et al.* (2004).

The development of these implants was executed in phases: (i) phase 1—*in vivo* determination of the minimum effective progestin dose (MED) to control oestrus cycles in dogs and cats; (ii) phase 2—definition of a prototype formulation (*in vitro* and *in vivo* releases; Figs. 15.4 and 15.5); (iii) phase 3—clinical trials; (iv) phase 4—*in vitro* optimization of the implant; and (v) phase 5—*in vivo* efficacy and tolerance studies. Efficacy in controlling reproduction was evaluated by observing the occurrence of oestrus periods, vaginal smears every week, and blood samples to test oestradiol and progesterone every week in the absence of oestrus and to check the quality of the oestrus every other day when oestrus signs were present; bitches were allowed to mate every other day when the oestrus cycle was detected. The queens were freely living with tom cats during the entire study period and mating occurrence was checked; intervals from s.c. implantation to first oestrus were noted. When the animals had mated, fertility was assessed by the ultrasonography diagnosis of pregnancy conducted every week to detect the occurrence of and the normal development of pregnancy.

The side effects of the treatments were controlled by monthly evaluation of body weight, palpation of mammary glands and detection of possible lesions, including signs of pseudopregnancy or tumours. Ultrasonographic examinations were conducted every month to check the uterus and ovaries, and blood samples were taken every month to monitor blood glucose, cortisol and insulin and every 3 months to check biochemistry and haematology. Mammary glands and uterine biopsies were taken at initiation and termination of the study. After a 4-year observation period, the implants were considered as fully effective and devoid of any significant side effects in both dogs and cats (Table 15.1).

INTERPRETATION. This study approaches the control of reproduction by continuous slow release of low doses of progestins. It demonstrates, using low doses, the possibility of controlling reproduction for a minimum of two years and without side effects. The classically described side effects of progestins are proposed to be related to chronic overdosing in past studies, whereas the use of a very low dose that is still efficacious in controlling oestrus cycles does not seem to induce any of these side effects of progestins (e.g. cystic endometrial hyperplasia, glucose intolerance, mammary lesions, etc.).

Comment

The interest in this study not only lies in the prevention of reproduction but in showing that clear dose-related studies are needed for many 'older' drugs; up till now

Table 15.1 Mean inhibition of oestrus cycle in dogs and cats

	Treated animal	Control animal
Mean duration of action of dog implant (interval implantation return in oestrus)		
Beagle dogs	26 ± 4 months	6.8 ± 2 months
Mongrel dogs	29 ± 5.8 months	9.1 ± 3 months
Mean duration of action of cat implant (interval implantation return in oestrus)		
European queens	27 ± 3.1 months	NA

Source: Verstegen *et al.* (2004).

their use has been based on data developed in other large animal species, but without real pharmacokinetic data in the target species. Further, it demonstrates the interest of new delivery technologies that are now available, which will improve treatment of animals in the future. However, long-term efficacy and toxicity data are not yet available concerning the developed and proposed implants. Just as for the GnRH agonist implant, the long-term effects of this new technology need to be further described. More studies are certainly warranted before such concepts are available in practice. A revisited use of the progestin may open new perspectives in terms of contraception and alternatives to surgery. This may represent a cheap and easy way to control reproduction in the dog and the cat and, if confirmed, the potential protective effects of low-dose contraceptive treatment with progestins may be of major interest in protecting animals against the development of mammary tumours and uterine diseases. Similarly, the interest of such formulation in the treatment and prevention of male prostatic diseases deserves more attention.

Effects of aglepristone, a progesterone receptor antagonist, administered during the early luteal phase in non-pregnant bitches

Galac S, Kooistra HS, Dieleman SJ, Cestnick V, Okkens AC. *Theriogenology* 2004; **62**: 494–500

BACKGROUND. Aglepristone, a progesterone receptor antagonist, was administered to six non-pregnant bitches during the early luteal phase in order to determine its effects on the duration of the luteal phase, the interoestrus interval, and plasma concentrations of progesterone and prolactin. Aglepristone was administered subcutaneously once daily on two consecutive days in a dose of 10 mg/kg body weight, beginning 12 ± 1 days after ovulation. Blood samples were collected before, during and after administration of aglepristone for the determination of plasma progesterone and prolactin concentrations. The differences in mean plasma concentration of progesterone and of prolactin before, during and after treatment were not significant. Also, the duration of the luteal phase in the six treated bitches (72 ± 6 days) did not differ significantly from that in untreated control dogs (74 ± 4 days). However, the intervals during which plasma progesterone concentration exceeded 64 and 32 nmol/l were significantly shorter in the six treated bitches than in untreated control dogs (Fig. 15.6). The interoestrus interval was significantly shorter in beagle bitches treated with aglepristone (158 ± 16 days) than in the same group prior to treatment (200 ± 5 days).

INTERPRETATION. This study has shown that administration of aglepristone during the luteal phase in the non-pregnant bitch affects progesterone secretion but not sufficiently to shorten the luteal phase. Plasma prolactin concentration was not affected. The interoestrus interval was shortened in animals treated with aglepristone during the non-pregnant dioestrus (interoestrus length of 158 ± 16 days) when compared with untreated animals (interoestrus length of 200 ± 5 days) suggesting that in the early luteal phase aglepristone influences the hypothalamic–pituitary–ovarian axis and facilitates oestrus recurrence.

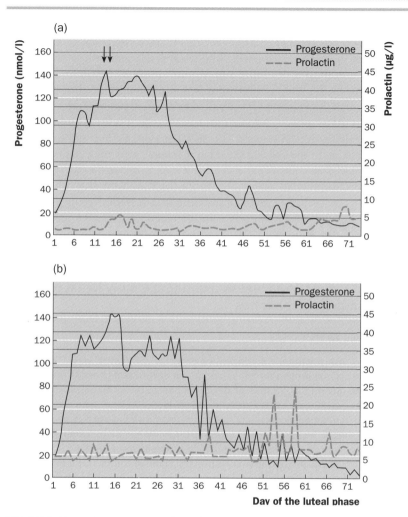

Fig. 15.6 Mean plasma concentrations of progesterone and prolactin in six beagle bitches treated with aglepristone (a) and three control beagle bitches (b), starting from the day of ovulation (day 1) to the end of the luteal phase. Aglepristone was administered on two consecutive days beginning 12 days after ovulation (arrows), subcutaneously in a dose of 10 mg/kg body weight once daily. Source: Galac *et al.* (2004).

Comment

The shortening effects of aglepristone on the post-treatment interoestrus in animals where the duration of the luteal phase was not modified, was analysed by the authors as being the consequence of an effect of aglepristone on the hypothalamic–pituitary–ovarian axis. To ascertain this observation the authors related it to the continuous increase of GnRH release and pituitary responsiveness to GnRH during anoestrus correlated to the observed increase in follicle-stimulating hormone seen in the bitch during anoestrus by Kooistra and Okkens |7| and Onclin et al. |8|. However, taking into account the short half-life of aglepristone it is difficult to directly correlate these two short-acting injections with hypothalamic–pituitary–endocrine events occurring more than 45–50 days later. As suggested by Hoffman et al. |9| and Onclin and Verstegen |10|, it is postulated by the present authors that the aglepristone mode of action is at the ovarian level taking off the local paracrine/autocrine progesterone inhibiting tone on follicular wave development thus allowing the resumption of an otherwise progesterone-inhibited follicular wave. Indeed, progesterone receptors are known to be present not only at the central nervous system level but also at nearly every reproductive organ level, particularly that of the ovary, and the paracrine role of progesterone on follicular growth and corpus luteum function has been long demonstrated (Rothschild, 1996 |11|). However, this still needs to be validated and demonstrates that a large amount of fundamental research is still needed in this field.

Fundamental and clinical research in canine reproduction

Many fundamental and clinical aspects of male and female dog reproduction still need to be studied and explained. In clinical situations, the veterinarians are still requesting answers to fundamental questions: When do we need to inseminate bitches, and when is the best time for artificial insemination with fresh or frozen semen? Even if many studies have tried to answer these questions the results and interpretations are still controversial. In this section, Tsumagari et al., in a very well developed research study, have new evidence that canine artificial insemination with frozen semen can successfully be achieved using vaginal insemination on days 5 and 7 post-LH surge. Less fundamental but still of clinical interest, Seyrek-Intas et al. confirmed that cornuectomy in bitches can be safely performed in pathological conditions and that further fertility is preserved.

In the male dog reproduction, the effects of drugs and improvement on semen quality represent an essential part of most significant papers published recently. The effects of blood adjunction, aromatase inhibitors or drugs, such as griseofulvin, on semen quality and preservation, have been described in papers of clinical significance. The confirmation that Percoll gradient centrifugation is useful in improving poor quality semen was also demonstrated. Lastly, a more fundamental scientific study analysed the acrosome and hyper-reactivity protective effects of prostatic lectin, and demonstrated for the first time an essential role, other than dilution and volume, of prostatic fluid in male dog ejaculation.

Optimal timing for canine artificial insemination with frozen semen and parentage testing by microsatellite markers in superfecundency

Tsumagari S, Ichikawa Y, Torium H, et al. *J Vet Med Sci* 2003; **65**(9): 1003–5

BACKGROUND. Parentage testing was performed in 16 litters from canine artificial inseminations with frozen semen from different sires on days 5 and 7 after the LH surge. It became apparent that only 25% of dams had superfecundation but 43.8% of dams were whelped after inseminations only on day 5 after the LH surge, and 31.3% of dams after insemination only on day 7. Of the total 87 puppies, 46% were born after insemination on days 5, and 54 after insemination on day 7.

INTERPRETATION These results strongly suggested that canine artificial insemination with frozen semen could be sufficiently successful on days 5 and 7 after the LH surge.

Comment

The results that were presented in the summary of the study need to be clarified and enhanced. Indeed, not enough attention was given to some essential aspects, deserving to be further discussed for their clinical implications. The authors achieved an 80% conception rate using frozen semen in two artificial inseminations using vaginal deposition! This confirmed that using vaginal deposition of frozen semen with a balloon-tipped catheter and a large volume high conception rate similar or superior to that obtained using intra-uterine insemination can be achieved. These results are in agreement with those obtained by Verstegen *et al.* |**12**| using only one insemination but they demonstrated that an equivalent conception rate can be obtained using vaginal and uterine insemination when a balloon-tipped catheter and a large volume is used. This mimics what naturally occurs in the dog with a cranial vagina semen deposition, but with a copulatory tie, which ensures that the semen is forced through the cervix opening during natural mating by the large prostatic fluid volume ejaculated during the third part of the ejaculation process. In fact the dog can be considered as an intrauterine semen depositor, which is mimicked in this study and already demonstrated by the author and his team in 1996 |**12**|. The 80% pregnancy rate obtained in this study using frozen semen is superior to that generally described using frozen semen and is even superior to that naturally observed in the dog. The microsatellite analysis study indicates that the fertilization period may vary from animal to animal, with some animals being fertile at day 5, whereas some were fertile at day 7 after the LH surge. The fertilization period may be longer than is usually accepted as some animals were pregnant from both inseminations realized at day 5 and day 7, giving a fertilization period of minimum 48 h; on the other hand, this may be a sign of non-synchronized ovulation. Interestingly, more pups were obtained from the insemination performed at day 7 than at day 5 and litter size apparently was larger when inseminations were successful at days 5 and 7, or 7 only. This may indicate that day 5 could be the beginning of the fertilization period and too early in some animals thus making days 6 and 7 probably better for fertilization to occur or that, again, ovulation is not synchronous and extends over more than 2 days. Interestingly, days 7 and 8 are also the days when cervical closure was described by the present author |12| as occurring in beagle bitches and was shown to be a limiting factor for vaginal fertilization. Pregnancies have been obtained with transcervical inseminations realized after day 8. This again raised the question of the duration of the fertilization period or the character sychronous versus asynchronous of ovulation in the dog. However, more bitches were pregnant from insemination realized at day 5 (43.8%) than at day 7 (31.3%). All these results open up interesting perspectives. If further confirmed, the excellent results obtained with vaginal deposition of frozen semen may dramatically change the way artificial insemination with frozen semen is performed in the dog making this technology more readily available for practitioners.

Unilateral hysterectomy (cornuectomy) in the bitch and its effect on subsequent fertility
Seyrek-Intas K, Wehrend A, Nak A, et al. Theriogenology 2004; **61**: 1713–17

BACKGROUND. During caesarean section of bitches the early stages of tissue necrosis of the uterus is often encountered. These alterations mostly require an ovariohysterectomy, which means the end of breeding life. The aim of this study was to create a model of unilateral hysterectomy during dystocia and to evaluate subsequent fertility. Unilateral cornuectomy was performed in 18 clinically healthy bitches of different ages, breeds and at different stages of the sexual cycles. Four bitches were not available for follow-up examinations. Twelve bitches were mated at the first obvious oestrus period post-operatively and 10 pregnancies were diagnosed. Nine bitches delivered one to five puppies (mean 3.8) after a gestation period of 63–67 days. The puppies were in very good condition and showed high viability.

INTERPRETATION. Unilateral cornuectomy of the uterus had no adverse effects and post-operative mating revealed pregnancy without complications and normal parturition. In the case of pathological changes in one uterine horn during a caesarean section unilateral hysterectomy seems to be an alternative to ovariohysterectomy.

Comment

This is a straightforward observation of clinical importance. Unilateral cornuectomy, even if not demonstrated in this study, may also be important in unilateral pyometra, which is often seen, where medical treatment is not possible or available.

Disappearance of the PHA-E lectin binding site on the surface of ejaculated sperm and sperm capacitation in the dog

Kawakami A, Sato T, Hirano T, Hori T, Tsutsui T. *J Vet Med Sci* 2004a; **66**(5): 495–500

BACKGROUND. Ejaculated semen and cross-sections of the cauda epididymides collected from three normal dogs were smeared or stamped on glass slides, and the sperm on the slides was stained with seven different fluorescein isothiocyanate-lectins (Con A, DBA, GS-1, PHA-E, PSA, UEA-1, WGA) to examine the relation between sperm-binding glycoprotein derived from the canine prostate and sperm capacitation. The only lectin that stained the ejaculated sperm but not the cauda epididymal sperm was PHA-E. The sperm ejaculated by five other dogs was incubated for 4 h in fluid flushed from the uterine horns or oviducts of oestrus bitches, and then the percentages of actively motile sperm and hyperactivated sperm (HA-sperm) were determined. The percentages of PHA-E-labelled sperm and sperm labelled with fluoresceinated calcium indicator to assess the influx of calcium into the sperm were also evaluated. The mean percentages of actively motile sperm, HA-sperm, and calcium-labelled sperm after 4 h of incubation in the uterine flush fluid and oviductal flush fluid were significantly higher than in the control medium (P <0.05, 0.01), but the mean percentages of PHA-E-labelled sperm were lower (both P <0.01). The percentages of PHA-E-unlabelled sperm correlated with the percentages of both HA-sperm and Ca-labelled sperm (r^2 = 0.787 and 0.812, respectively; Table 15.2). The results indicate that loss of the glycoprotein secreted by the canine prostate on

Table 15.2 Changes in the mean (±SE) percentages of motile sperm, hyperactivated (HA) sperm, acrosome-reacted (AR) sperm, PHA-E lectin-labelled sperm, and fluoresceinated calcium indicator in sperm ejaculated by five dogs and incubated for 4 h in control MEM (Eagle's minimum essential medium), uterine flush MEM and oviductal flush MEM

Incubation period (h)	Motile sperm (%)	HA-sperm (%)	AR-sperm (%)	PHA-E-labelled sperm (%)	Ca-labelled sperm (%)
0 (Control MEM)	88.0 ± 3.0	0	0	100.0 ± 0.0	0
4 (Control MEM)	57.0 ± 4.4	18.2 ± 2.0	7.2 ± 1.2	71.8 ± 3.0	24.6 ± 5.5
4 (Uterine flush)	69.0 ± 2.2*‡	24.2±1.0*	9.0 ± 1.4	50.4±1.9**‡	51.8±2.4†‡
4 (Oviductal flush)	72.0 ± 1.8*‡	62.2 ± 2 7†‡§	10.4 ± 1.4	22.6 ± 1.8**‡§	73.0 ± 2 7†‡§

* P <0.05
† P <0.01.
‡ In comparison with control MEM after 4 h of incubation.
§ In comparison with uterine flush MEM.
Source: Kawakami *et al.* (2004a).

the sperm surface induces the influx of calcium into the sperm, and then hyperactivation of the sperm.

INTERPRETATION. The glycoproteins produced by the prostate protect canine semen against early capacitation. They are lost as a result of the action of uterine and oviductal proteolytic enzymes and then sperm capacitation may be promoted. The loss of these glycoproteins secreted by the canine prostate, and acting as decapacitation factors on the sperm surface, induces the influx of calcium into the sperm, and then hyperactivation.

Comment

The proposal, however indirectly demonstrated in this study, that canine prostate, as in other species, secretes glycoproteins which bind to sperm cell receptors and protect the sperm against capacitation, is one of the first demonstrations, other than dilution, of the role of prostatic fluid in dog sperm function. As the canine semen is supposed to survive several days in the female genital tract, the development of protective methods against early semen activation, capacitation and hyperreactivity seems essential. The role of uterine and oviductal proteins in preventing early capacitation has already been demonstrated in different species and oviductal epithelium interaction with sperm cells is one of the mainly characterized protection processes |13|. The demonstration in dogs of the role of prostatic glycoproteins opens up further development in semen cryoprotection and also has clear clinical implications with regard to the reduced fertility observed in many old dogs also known to be prone to prostatic diseases and thus potential abnormalities in the production of these important glycoproteins.

Effect of blood admixture on the *in vitro* survival of chilled and frozen-thawed canine spermatozoa

Rijselaere T, Van Soom A, Maes D, Verberckmoes S, de Kruif A. *Theriogenology* 2004; **61**: 1589–602

BACKGROUND. Haematospermia in the dog usually occurs secondary to benign prostatic hypertrophy or trauma of the penis or prepuce during semen collection. Regarding the difficulty of removing blood cells from a haematospermic sample, the present study was performed to determine whether blood contaminated ejaculates can still be chilled (4°C) or frozen (–196°C) without an additional decrease in sperm quality. In the first experiment, blood additions of up to 10% exerted no negative effects on the functional characteristics of canine spermatozoa cooled (4°C) and stored for 4 days in an egg-yolk–Tris extender (Table 15.3).

In contrast, in experiment 2, blood admixtures of 4% or more to semen before freezing clearly had negative effects on cryopreserved (–196°C) spermatozoa, mainly on the motility parameters, on the membrane integrity and on the acrosomal status of the spermatozoa (Fig. 15.7).

In experiment 3, it was seen that these negative effects of blood admixture on cryopreserved spermatozoa were mainly associated with the red blood cells (RBCs),

Table 15.3 Mean (+SD) motility, progressive motility, percentage spermatozoa with an intact plasma membrane integrity (intact plasma membrane; SYBR14-PI staining), percentage spermatozoa with normal morphology (normal spermatozoa; eosin/nigrosin staining) and percentage spermatozoa with an intact acrosome (intact acrosome; PSA-staining) after 4 days of storage at 4°C for dog semen samples with 0, 1, 2, 4 and 10% (v/v) blood admixture

Sperm quality parameter	Blood admixture (%, v/v)				
	0	1	2	4	10
Motility (%)	78.8 ± 4.8	82.5 ± 2.9	77.5 ± 5.0	80.0 ± 0.0	80.0 ± 0.0
Progressive motility (%)	76.3 ± 4.8	81.3 ± 2.5	76.3 ± 4.8	78.8 ± 2.5	77.5 ± 2.9
Intact plasma membrane (%)	81.0 ± 7.4	80.8 ± 7.6	83.0 ± 6.0	81.3 ± 1.7	81.8 ± 5.4
Normal spermatozoa (%)	75.0 ± 7.4	78.0 ± 3.4	77.3 ± 6.2	73.5 ± 9.3	75.3 ± 7.2
Intact acrosome (%)	89.0 ± 2.1	92.5 ± 1.9	90.3 ± 1.5	92.0 ± 2.9	93.0 ± 2.6

No significant differences were found for all the evaluated semen characteristics ($P > 0.05$).
Source: Rijselaere et al. (2004).

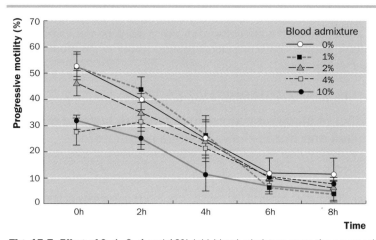

Fig. 15.7 Effect of 0, 1, 2, 4 and 10% (v/v) blood admixture upon the progressive motility of frozen–thawed canine spermatozoa during storage for 8 h at 37°C. Source: Rijselaere et al. (2004).

whereas the addition of plasma, serum or inactivated serum exerted little or no negative effect. Moreover, in experiment 4, it was seen that 58.3 ± 11.6% of the RBCs haemolysed after a freeze–thaw process. In experiment 5, a clear and negative effect of haemoglobin on cryopreserved canine spermatozoa was observed.

INTERPRETATION. The authors conclude that the presence of up to 10% of blood is not detrimental for the storage of chilled canine spermatozoa and that the detrimental effect of blood on cryopreserved spermatozoa are at least partially attributable to the high amount of haemoglobin originating from the RBC haemolysis observed after freezing and thawing.

Comment

This study is interesting as it is generally believed that the quality of semen may be affected by contamination with not only urine or purulent exudate but also blood. The presence of blood in dog semen is relatively common and may be related to the collection procedure, penis, urethral or prostatic abnormalities and pathologies. This, well defined study, clearly demonstrated that the presence of blood up to 10% in the ejaculate immediately diluted in an egg-yolk extender is of no importance on the semen quality and probably fertility after several days of preservation at 4°C. This is not surprising as at the time of mating or insemination many bitches still present bloody vaginal discharges. However, in earlier studies, England and Allen |**14**| have demonstrated the deleterious effects of admixture of blood in fresh undiluted semen. This study expanded the possibility of preserving bloody semen if rapidly extended in an egg-yolk extender which by its membrane protecting effects probably protects the RBC membrane and prevents the deleterious effects of haemoglobin originating from the RBC haemolysis. The presence of RBC when semen is frozen is of concern as egg yolk is not able to prevent RBC haemolysis and the toxic effects of haemo-globin on sperm cells. This study confirms the need for separation protocols when bloody semen needs to be frozen. Interestingly, separation protocols are described in the following paper.

Separation of canine epididymal spermatozoa by Percoll gradient centrifugation

Hishinuma M, Sekine J. *Theriogenology* 2004; **61**: 365–72

B ACKGROUND. The objective was to characterize the separation of canine epididymal spermatozoa on a Percoll gradient. Epididymal spermatozoa were overlaid on a 45 and 90% discontinuous Percoll gradient and centrifuged at 700 μg for 20 min. The Percoll column was separated into six fractions (top to bottom, A–F) after centrifugation. Fractions A–C contained few spermatozoa. Spermatozoa with bent or folded tails and a large amount of granular debris were observed in fraction B. Fraction D contained many non-motile spermatozoa, erythrocytes and round epithelial cells. Spermatozoa in fraction E had significantly lower motility than those in the initial layer. Spermatozoa in fraction F had motility similar to those before separation; it contained 40.6% of the motile spermatozoa layered and 67.5% of all motile spermatozoa recovered. There was no significant difference between fraction F and the initial layer in sperm membrane integrity. In the sperm–oocyte penetration assay, spermatozoa from fraction F had a significantly higher penetration rate into the immature homologous oocytes than those from fraction E. Although the recovery rate of the motile spermatozoa was low, the canine epididymal spermatozoa with motility, membrane integrity and penetrating capability could be separated by two-layer discontinuous Percoll gradient centrifugation (Table 15.4).

Table 15.4 Characteristics of canine epididymal spermatazoa after separation by Percoll gradient centrifugation

Fraction	Volume (ml)	Total number of spermatazoa[1] ($\times 10^6$)	Motility[2] (%)	Membrane integrity (%)	
				Eosin staining	Water test
Initial	6.0 ± 0	50.0 ± 0 (100)	63.9 ± 2.3[a] (100)	84.1 ± 3.1[a]	73.2 ± 10.0[a]
A	1.8 ± 0.1[a]	0.1 ± 0.1[a] (0.2)	NE	NE	NE
B	1.0 ± 0.1[b]	1.2 ± 1.3[a] (2.4)	32.0 ± 23.9[c] (1.2)	48.1 ± 7.1[d]	39.9 ± 9.7[b]
C	0.9 ± 0.1[c]	2.7 ± 1.7[ab] (5.4)	20.0 ± 2.4[c] (1.7)	51.0 ± 15.0[d]	35.9 ± 6.4[b]
D	1.0 ± 0.1[bc]	10.1 ± 6.5[c] (20.2)	19.7 ± 1.5[c] (6.3)	58.1 ± 11.9[cd]	28.9 ± 11.7[b]
E	1.1 ± 0.1[b]	7.0 ± 2.0[bc] (14.0)	47.6 ± 5.0[b] (10.4)	70.1 ± 8.8[bc]	35.6 ± 14.3[b]
F	0.3 ± 0.1[d]	21.7 ± 4.2[d] (43.4)	59.8 ± 3.1[ab] (40.6)	79.0 ± 4.8[ab]	66.0 ± 19.3[a]
Total	6.0 ± 0	42.8 ± 4.9 (85.6)	(60.2)	–	–

Two ml sperm suspension containing 5×10^7 spermatozoa were layered on to 4 ml Percoll gradient. Data are expressed as means ±SD of five dogs (three replicates for each dog). NE, not examined. a–d, values with different superscripts in the same column were different. $P < 0.05$.

Source: Hishinuma and Sekine (2004).

INTERPRETATION. Canine spermatozoa, in this case from epididymis, can be separated by two-layer discontinuous Percoll gradient centrifugation. The recovery rate is about 65% of all motile spermatozoa but poorly motile, erythrocytes, epithelial cell debris have been clearly discarded.

Comment

This is an easy protocol that can be readily applied to poor quality semen contaminated with cell debris, erythrocytes or to improve motility characteristics before semen freezing. Similarly this protocol can be used to remove seminal plasma or extenders after thawing. The recovery rate should probably be improved by further optimization studies.

Influence of griseofulvin treatment on semen quality in the dog

von Heimendahl A, England GCW, Sheldon IM. *Anim Reprod Sci* 2004; **80**: 175–81

BACKGROUND. Griseofulvin is used to treat dermatomycosis in many species and causes oligospermia in suprapharmacological doses. The aim of the present study was to evaluate the effect of griseofulvin administered at therapeutic doses on semen quality in dogs. Four dogs were treated with griseofulvin (25 mg/kg per day) for 30 days. Semen collections and analyses were performed before, during and for 100 days after treatment for the griseofulvin group and 10 untreated control dogs. Semen analyses included mean percentage of forward progressively motile sperm, total sperm output, normal live sperm and normal dead sperm. There was no significant difference between control and treated dogs for each of the semen quality parameters (Fig. 15.8).

INTERPRETATION. Therapeutic doses of griseofulvin had no deleterious effect upon semen quality in dogs, although this does not preclude potential embryotoxic and teratogenic effects.

Comment

Many drugs are assumed or said to have deleterious effects on spermatogenesis and maturation. However, few pharmaceutical companies have up to now included the dog and the assessment of drug effects on spermatogenesis in their safety trials before drug registration. As more and more concerns are presented regarding endocrine disrupters and their potential effects on fertility, these kinds of studies are certainly of significant interest. This is not a great or clinically highly significant study but it clearly demonstrates the interest of dog semen evaluation in toxicological studies not only for the animal *per se* but also for other species. Dog spermatogenesis is very similar to that observed in other species; because the dog is an easy animal to collect from and to assess, the use of this animal as a model for other species, including endangered species of carnivores and humans, is of major interest.

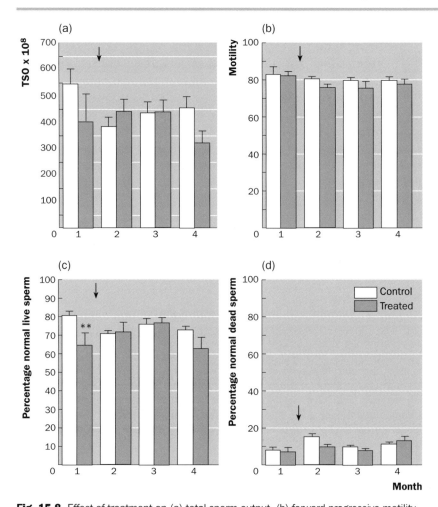

Fig. 15.8 Effect of treatment on (a) total sperm output, (b) forward progressive motility, (c) percentage of normal live sperm and (d) percentage of normal dead sperm ($P < 0.01$). Source: von Heimendahl et al. (2004).

Therapeutic effects of aromatase inhibitors in two azoospermic dogs with high plasma estradiol 17 beta levels

Kawakami E, Taguchi N, Hirano T, Hori T, Tsutsui T. J Vet Med Sci 2003; **65**(12): 1343–5

Improvement in spermatogenic function after subcutaneous implantation of a capsule containing an aromatase inhibitor in four oligozoospermic dogs and one azoospermic dog with high plasma estradiol 17 beta concentrations

Kawakami E, Taguchi N, Hirano T, Hori T, Tsutsui T. *Theriogenology* 2004b; **62**: 165–78

BACKGROUND. In Kawakami *et al.* (2003) two azoospermic dogs with high plasma oestradiol-17β (E2) levels were subcutaneously injected with an aromatase inhibitor, 4-androstene-4-ol-3,17-dione, 2 mg every other day for 4 weeks. Before the aromatase inhibitor treatment the plasma E2 levels of the two dogs (21 and 22 pg/ml, respectively) were higher than those of two normal dogs (8.1 and 12.3 pg/ml), and they fell to 11–17 pg/ml between 1 and 4 weeks after the start of aromatase inhibitor treatment. The plasma testosterone levels after the start of aromatase inhibitor treatment had increased to 2.1–3.1 ng/ml. A small number of sperm were detected in the semen of the two dogs between 3 and 6 weeks after the start of aromatase inhibitor treatment.

In Kawakami *et al.* (2004b), a capsule containing an aromatase inhibitor (4-androsten-4-ol-3,17-dione) was subcutaneously implanted in four oligozoospermic beagle dogs and one azoospermic beagle dog with high plasma E2 concentrations (15–19 pg/ml) and low plasma testosterone concentrations (0.6–0.8 ng/ml) for 8 weeks and the effect of the aromatase inhibitor on spermatogenic dysfunction was assessed. Plasma E2 and testosterone concentrations and semen quality were examined at 1 week intervals from 3 weeks before to 12 weeks after the start of treatment. Testicular biopsies were done twice (capsule implantation and removal). Plasma E2 concentrations of all dogs decreased (9–14 pg/ml) and plasma testosterone concentrations increased (2.0–2.6 ng/ml) from 3 weeks after capsule implantation to capsule removal (Fig. 15.9).

The mean number of spermatozoa ejaculated by all four oligozoospermic dogs between 4 and 9 weeks after implantation was higher (127×10^6 to 205×10^6) than before implantation (20×10^6 to 38×10^6) ($P <0.05$ and 0.01). Very low numbers (2×10^4 to 4×10^4) of immotile spermatozoa were observed between 7 and 8 weeks after implantation in the semen collected from the dog with azoospermia (Fig. 15.10).

Before implantation, a few spermatozoa were seen in only one-fifth of the seminiferous tubules in this dog; 8 weeks after implantation, the mean diameter and mean number of round spermatids in the seminiferous tubules in all five dogs were higher than before implantation ($P <0.05$).

INTERPRETATION. In the two studies (4 weeks of injections every other day of an aromatase inhibitor, or 8 weeks with a subcutaneously implanted capsule releasing an aromatase inhibitor), treatment in infertile dogs with an initially high plasma concentration of E2 improved their spermatogenic function, concurrent with a decrease in plasma oestradiol and increase in plasma testosterone concentrations.

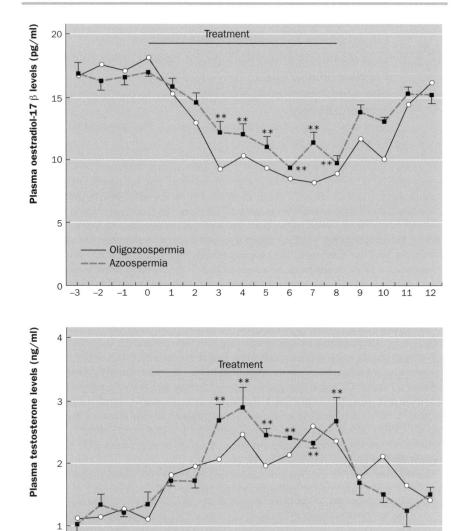

Fig. 15.9 Mean (±SE) plasma concentrations of oestradiol-17β (top) and testosterone (bottom) in four dogs with oligozoospermia (solid line) and one dog with azoospermia (dashed line) given an implant containing an aromatase inhibitor (treatment). Source: Kawakami et al. (2004).

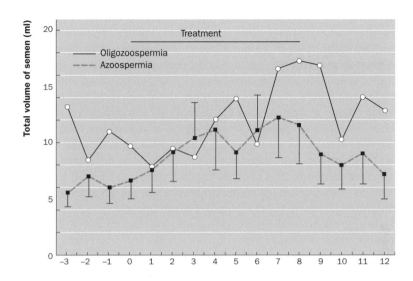

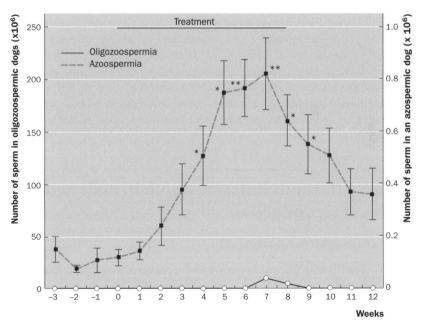

Fig. 15.10 Mean (±SE) total semen volume and total number of spermatozoa in four dogs with oligozoospermia (solid line) and one dog with azoospermia (dashed line) given an implant containing an aromatase inhibitor (treatment). Source: Kawakami *et al.* (2004).

Comment

In the first study, two azoospermic dogs with high plasma E2 were treated sub-cutaneously every other day for 4 weeks with an aromatase inhibitor. The treatment was of short duration; however, a rapid increase in testosterone plasma concentration was observed correlated with a decreased E2 plasma concentration. An increase in sperm volume and cells were observed even after this short period of treatment, as well as a decrease in abnormal cells inversely correlated with an increased motility. In the second study, in order to treat the animals for a longer period of time, a subcutaneous slow-release capsule active for 8 weeks was administered to four oligo-zoospermic dogs and one azoospermic dog. The treatment significantly improved fertility in all treated dogs with maximum results observed in the oligozoospermic animals. As E2 significantly affects spermatogenesis during the second part of the cycle (54 days in total), particularly when associated with a decreased level of plasma testosterone, plasma E2 should be determined in all infertile male dogs particularly in aged animals where subclinical Sertoli cell tumours may be responsible for a shift in the steroidogenesis with an increased E2/testosterone ratio. Similarly in young dogs, genetic factors may be responsible for abnormal steroidogenesis and reduced fertility. Ideally all young dogs where there is a genetic origin for their infertility should be withdrawn from the selection programme. Evaluation of E2 may be proposed as a diagnostic clinical tool and aromatase inhibitor treatments warrant further evaluation. The interest of new formulations of existing drugs is confirmed in this study as demonstrated earlier in the Junaidi *et al.* and Verstegen *et al.* studies concerning contraceptive implants. The availability of different implant formulations now allows for the release of drugs at low concentrations devoid of side effects for long periods. This is certainly a new field of development with many possible applications from antibiotic to antiparasitic or hormone to anti-inflammatory drug administration.

Fundamental and clinical research in male and female cat reproduction

Testis morphometry, seminiferous epithelium cycle length, and daily sperm production in domestic cats
Franca LR, Godinho CL. *Biol Reprod* 2003; **68**: 1554–61

BACKGROUND. There is very little information regarding the testis structure and function in domestic cats; most data are related to the seminiferous epithelium cycle and sperm production. The testis weight in cats investigated in the present study was 1.2 g. Compared with most mammalian species investigated, the value of 0.08% found for testes mass related to the body mass (gonadosomatic index) in cats is very low. The tunica albuginea volume density (%) in these animals was relatively high and comprised about 19% of the testis. Seminiferous tubule and Leydig cell volume density (%) in cats were approximately 90% and 6%, respectively. The mean tubular diameter was 220 μm, and 23 m of seminiferous tubule were found per testis and per gram of testis (Table 15.5).

The frequencies of the eight stages of the cycle, characterized according to the tubular morphology system, were as follows: stage 1, 24.9%; stage 2, 12.9%; stage 3, 7.7%; stage 4, 17.6%; stage 5, 7.2%; stage 6, 11.9%; stage 7, 6.8%; and stage 8, 11 %. The premeiotic and postmeiotic stage frequency was 46% and 37%, respectively. The duration of each cycle of seminiferous epithelium was 10.4 days and the total duration of spermatogenesis based on 4.5 cycles was 46.8 days (Fig. 15.11).

The number of round spermatids for each pachytene primary spermatocyte (meiotic index) was 2.8, meaning that significant cell loss (30%) occurred during the two meiotic divisions. The total number of germ cells and the number of round spermatids per each Sertoli cell nucleolus at stage 1 of the cycle were 9.8 and 5.1, respectively. The Leydig cell volume was approximately 2000 μm^3 and the nucleus volume 260 μm^3. Both Leydig and Sertoli cell numbers per gram of testis in cats were approximately 30 million. The daily sperm production per gram of testis in cats (efficiency of spermatogenesis) was approximately 16 million.

INTERPRETATION. This is the first investigation to perform a detailed and comprehensive study of the testis structure and function in domestic cats. This study shows for the first time

Table 15.5 Biometric and morphometric data in sexually mature cats

Parameter (n = 9)	Mean ± SEM
Body weight (kg)	3.1 ± 0.2*
Testis weight (g)†	1.17 ± 0.07*
Right testis	1.16 ± 0.09
Left testis	1.18 ± 0.10
Gonadosomatic index (%	0.078 ± 0.007*
Testis parenchyma volume density (%):	
Seminiferous tubule	88.2 ± 1.2
Tunica propria	4.2± 0.2
Seminiferous epithelium	78 ± 1.5
Lumen	6 ± 0.7
Intertubular compartment	11.8 ± 1.2
Leydig cell	6.0 ± 0.6
Connective tissue	2.9 ± 0.9
Blood vessels	2.6 ± 0.8
Lymphatic vessels	0.3 ± 0.1
Tubular diameter (μm)	223 ± 5
Seminiferous epithelium height (μm)	81 ± 3
Tubular length per gram of testis (meters)	23.1 ± 3.5
Total tubular length per testis (meters)	22.8 ± 3.8

* $n = 13$.
† Right testis plus left testis divided by two. n, number of animals utilized.
Source: Franca and Godinho (2003).

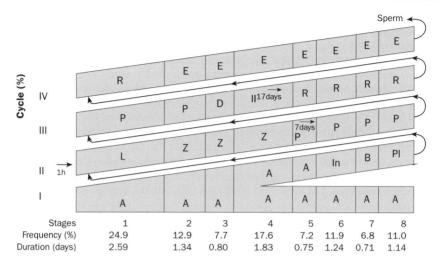

Fig. 15.11 Diagram showing the germ cell composition, the frequencies (%), and the duration in days for each stage of the seminiferous epithelium cycle. Also depicted is the most advanced germ cell type labelled at the eight stages of the cycle at the different time periods (1 h, 7 days and 17 days) following tritiated thymidine injections. The roman numerals indicate the spermatogenic cycle. The space given to each stage is proportional to its frequency and duration. The letters within each column indicate germ cell types present at each stage of the cycle. A, Type A spermatogonia; In, intermediate spermatogonia; B, type B spermatogonia; Pl, preleptotene spermatocytes; L, leptotene; Z, zygotene; P, pachytene; D, diplotene; II, secondary spermatocytes; R, round spermatids; E, elongate spermatids. Source: Franca and Godinho (2003).

Sertoli and Leydig cell number per gram of testis and the daily sperm output in any kind of feline species. In this regard, besides providing a background for comparative studies with other felids, the data obtained in the present work might be useful in future studies in which the domestic cat could be utilized as an appropriate receptor model for the preservation of genetic stock from rare or endangered wild felines using the germ cell transplantation technique.

Comment

The data obtained in this study are most interesting. They define the basic morphometric and functional aspects of the testis in the domestic cat. The gonadosomatic index and morphometric data are low and similar to those observed in humans. The total duration of spermatogenesis is 46.8 days, which is similar to that observed in other mammalian species, including dogs. The daily sperm output per gram of testis is supposed to be about 16 million. Taking into account the fact that the mean testis weight was 1.2 g, the daily sperm output in the cat could be estimated at ±20 million per day. The mean concentration per ejaculate obtained using an artificial vagina ranges from 3 to 143 millions, which corresponds to less than the daily output up to the equivalent of 7 days of production. These data are essential as they set up the basis for domestic cat steroidogenesis analysis and fertility evaluation.

Vaginal and cervical anatomic modifications during the oestrus cycle in relation to transcervical catheterisation in the domestic cat

Zambelli D, Buccioli M, Castagnetti C, Belluzzi S. *Reprod Domest Anim* 2004; **39**: 76–80

BACKGROUND. In a previous study it was observed that it is possible to reach the cervix in all queens with a 1 mm diameter probe only. Therefore the authors developed both a new technique and a catheter (1 mm diameter) to allow transcervical insemination (Zambelli and Castagnetti 2001 |15|). The aims of this study were to investigate vaginal and cervical anatomic modifications during the various stages of the oestrus cycle and to test the previously described technique of transcervical catheterization during various stages of the oestrus cycle. In experiment 1, silicon impression moulds were obtained from the reproductive tracts of 21 queens' cadavers, and vaginal and cervical measures were taken. The results showed that there are some significant anatomic modifications during the various stages of the oestrus cycle in vaginal and cervical anatomy, principally related to the dorsal medial fold increase induced by the follicular phase. In experiment 2, transcervical catheterization was attempted in 95 queens at various stages of the oestrus cycle both during a reproductive and non-reproductive season. After catheterization, methylene blue solution was injected through the cervical catheter. Successful catheterization was assessed during surgery, when colour was observed in the uterine horns. It was possible to perform transcervical catheterization: (i) during a non-reproductive season in 16 of 20 anoestrus queens and in 12 of 15 induced oestrus queens, and (ii) during a reproductive season in 9 of 21 interoestrus queens, in 8 of 13 di-oestrus/pregnancy queens, in 4 of 18 oestrus queens and in 7 of 8 queens in first oestrus during lactation.

INTERPRETATION. Vaginal anatomy in the cat is similar to that observed in the dog with a large posterior vagina associated with a narrow cranial vagina limited in diameter by the presence of a dorsomedial fold, which anatomy changes during the oestrus cycle. Transcervical catheterization is limited by the diameter of the cranial vagina and the dorso-oblic shape of the cervix during oestrus. Catheterization required a catheter of limited diameter, the maximum being about 2 mm. As in the dog, catheterization is easier in anoestrus than during oestrus; in this study successful catheterization occurred in 80% of the anoestrus queens against about 45% of the oestrus animals.

Comment

In the cat, semen deposition is realised in the cranial vagina and not in the uterus as opposed to the dog. However, as the semen volume is naturally reduced (mean 10–120 µl), intrauterine insemination seems to be of clinical interest. This is particularly true when poor quality or even further reduced volume/concentration is concerned. However, this observation will only be correct if, contrary to human or other species with vaginal deposition of semen, the cervix is not involved in semen maturation. This study outlines vaginal anatomy in the domestic queen and gives some indications regarding the development of the artificial insemination technique in this species often used as a model for endangered species of felines. Certainly one of the main goals in this species and in this field is to be able to develop, as in the dog, transcervical insemination, which prevents the need for surgical insemination with its associated anaesthesia risks and ethical concerns.

Development of *in vitro* maturated, *in vitro* fertilised domestic cat embryos following cryopreservation, culture and transfer

Gomez MC, Pope E, Harris R, Mikota S, Dresser BL. *Theriogenology* 2003; **60**: 239–51

BACKGROUND. The ability of embryos to survive cryopreservation successfully is dependent on both morphological and developmental characteristics. Domestic cat oocytes matured *in vitro* exhibit alterations in nuclear and cytoplasmic maturation that may affect developmental competence, particularly after cryopreservation. In experiment 1, we evaluated the developmental competence of *in vitro* produced (IVM/IVF) cat embryos after cryopreservation on days 2, 4 or 5 of IVC. In experiment 2, *in vivo* viability was examined by transfer of cryopreserved embryos into recipient queens. Oocytes recovered from minced ovaries were cultured in TCM-199 with human/equine chorionic gonadotrophin and epidermal growth factor at 38°C in 5% oxygen, 5% carbon dioxide, 90% nitrogen for 24 h. In experiment 1, after IVM/IVF, on day 2 ($n = 56$), day 4 ($n = 48$) and day 5 ($n = 42$) of IVC, embryos were equilibrated for 10 min at 22°C in HEPES (15 mmol/l) Tyrode's (HeTy) with 1.4 ml/l propylene glycol (PG), 0.125 ml/l sucrose, 10% dextran and 10% fetal bovine serum, loaded into 0.25 ml straws, cooled at 2.0°C/min to –6.0°C and held for 10 min. After seeding, cooling resumed at 0.3°C/min to –30°C and, after a 10-min hold, straws were plunged into liquid nitrogen. Straws were thawed in air for 2 min and cryoprotectant was removed by a five-step rinse consisting of 3 min each in HeTY with 0.95 mol/l PG/0.25 mol/l sucrose; 0.95 mol/l PG/0.125 mol/l sucrose; 0.45 mol/l PG/0.125 mol/l sucrose; 0 PG/0.125 mol/l sucrose; 0 PG/0.0625 mol/l sucrose. Contemporary IVM/IVF embryos were used as non-frozen controls (day 2, $n = 14$; day 4, $n = 26$; day 5, $n = 35$). After 8 days of IVC, the number of embryos developing to blastocysts was recorded and blastocyst cell numbers were counted after staining with Hoechst 33342. In experiment 1, developmental stage did not affect the survival rate after thawing (day 2, 79%; day 4, 90%; day 5, 98%) and was not different from that of controls (day 2, 89%; day 4, 88%; day 5, 96%). Blastocyst development was similar among days both after cryopreservation (day 2, 59%; day 4, 54%; day 5, 63%) and in controls (day 2, 55%; day 4, 54%; day 5, 58%). Mean (±SD) cell number of blastocysts was slightly lower (ns) in cryopreserved embryos (day 2, 152 ± 19; day 4, 124 ± 20; day 5, 121 ± 24) than in controls (day 2, 141 ± 25; day 4, 169 ± 21; day 5, 172 ± 19) (Fig. 15.12).

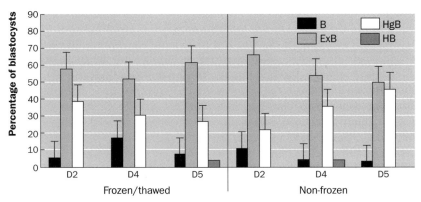

Fig. 15.12 Stages of blastocyst development on day 8 of culture of non-frozen and frozen–thawed embryos on days 2, 4 or 5. B, blastocyst; ExB, expanded; HgB, hatching; HB, hatched. Source: Gomez *et al.* (2003).

In experiment 2, embryos frozen on day 2 (*n* = 68), day 4 (*n* = 49) or day 5 (*n* = 73) were thawed and cultured for 3, 1 or 0 days before transfer by laparotomy to five (mean = 12.6 ± 2.4), 4 (mean = 12.2 ± 3.7) and six (mean = 12.0 ± 1.6) recipients, respectively. Four recipients were pregnant on day 21; two from embryos frozen on day 4 and two from day 5. Two live kittens were born at 66 days, a third kitten died during parturition at 64 days and a fourth pregnancy aborted by day 45.

INTERPRETATION. This study demonstrated that a controlled rate cryopreservation technique can be successfully applied to cat embryos produced by IVM/IVF. *In vitro* development to the blastocyst stage was not affected by the age of embryos at cryopreservation. The birth of live kittens after embryo transfer of cryopreserved embryos is additional validation of progress toward applying assisted reproductive technology to the preservation of endangered felids.

Comment

These results demonstrate that pregnancies may be established and live kittens obtained after transfer of domestic cat embryos produced by IVM/IVF and cryopreserved. Survival rate is still low and needs to be improved, but the birth of live kittens validates progress toward application of assisted reproductive technology to the conservation of endangered or highly valuable species.

Conclusion

SAR is an evolving field of clinical and fundamental research. Surprisingly, while we are now seeing in dogs and cats, as previously in other species, the development of the most sophisticated biotechnology of reproduction techniques (cloning, IVF, etc.), we also see the need to complete fundamental endocrine or physiological studies to set up the strong basis from which SAR will evolve. Up to recently, the tendency was to try to mimic what was being done in other well-known species without spending time to develop the necessary basic knowledge that would allow the understanding of the differences between dogs and cats and the former studied species. Fortunately, this is changing. The cat is a relatively easy species in comparison with the dog, which explains why certain techniques have been more successful in this species than in the dog. The domestic cat as a model for all endangered species of wild felids has already been studied in great detail and many aspects of basic physiology are better understood because of this large number of studies. Many fundamental studies are still needed, however, such as those by Franca and Godhino who study the basis of spermatogenesis in domestic cats.

In the dog, the gap in knowledge is greater and it is only recently that new basic physiology and endocrinology data have been provided to complement the previously available fundamental data, using the newly available technologies or assays. Without a better understanding of basic concepts, such as the fertilization period or control of di-oestrus/anoestrus periods, past mistakes will be made and trials, for example, to clone the dog, will still be unsuccessful. The dog is not a small cow nor is the cat a small dog, and trying to transfer technologies directly from one species to another will not get results. A clear example was given by the immunization trials with GnRH in dogs. These were efficacious in rodents but up to now have been disappointing in the dog. Similarly, the use of many drugs needs to be redefined for dogs and cats. Progestin side effects are probably more related to their misuse in these species than to the fundamental properties of these agents; the use of long-acting slow-release implants may open up new perspectives in their use without associated side effects or with reduced side effects, but will still have clinical efficacy. Drugs said to be toxic need to be characterized in these target species as would any new drugs tested for their potential detrimental effects on fertility, and dogs can be an interesting and easy model to study for other species.

New and interesting developments are now proposed in terms of dog and cat contraception. The availability of implants in the near future to control not only male but also female reproduction are promising and open up new perspectives in contraception. Unique surgical proposals will see alternative techniques developing and may be challenged not only scientifically but politically, especially with increasing ethical concerns. It will not be long before safe and efficacious alternatives will be fully available and surgical neutering will be banned for ethical reasons just as cropping ears and tail docking are now banned in the main countries and breeds except for medical reasons. The Scandinavian countries, Germany and the UK, countries with strong ethical concerns and a powerful public opinion regarding animal welfare, will certainly lead the way. Lastly, the development of all *in vitro* technologies, from semen freezing to insemination, from IVF to cloning, will continue to raise these ethical concerns and should be developed in parallel with a deep scientific thinking on what can be done and what should be refused. Even if treating oligozoospermic dogs with abnormal oestradiol production is nowadays feasible, we should be able, when genetic background is a concern, to say no. Our scientific and social credibility is certainly there even when just dealing with pets.

References

1. Ikemoto T, Park MK. Identification and characterization of the reptile GnRH-2 gene in the leopard gecko and its evolutionary considerations. *Gene* 2003; **316**: 157–65.

2. Ikemoto T, Enomoto M, Park MK. Identification and characterization of a reptilian GnRH receptor from the leopard gecko. *Mol Cell Endocrinol* 2004; **214**: 137–47.

3. Ford CP, Dryden WF, Smith PA. Neurotrophic regulation of Ca channels by the peptide neurotransmitter GnRH. *J Neuroscience* 2003; **23**: 7169–75.

4. Oka Y. Physiology and release activity of GnRH neurons. *Prog Brain Res* 2002; **141**: 259–81.

5. Chen A, Ganor Y, Rahimipour S, Ben-Aroya N, Koch Y, Levite M. The neuropeptides GnRH II and GnRH I are produced by human T cells and trigger laminin receptor gene expression, adhesion, chemotaxis and homing to specific organs. *Nat Med* 2002; **8**: 1421–26.

6. Arimura A, Sato H, Coy DH, Worobec RB, Schally AV, Yanaihara N, Hashimoto T, Yanaihara N, Sukura N. The antigenic determinant of the LH-releasing hormone for three different antisera. *Acta Endocrinol (Copenh)* 1975; **78**: 222–31.

7. Kooistra HS, Okkens AC. Role of changes in the pulsatile secretion pattern of FSH in initiation of ovarian folliculogenesis in bitches. *J Reprod Fertil* 2001; **57**(Suppl): 11–14.

8. Onclin K, Murphy B, Verstegen JP. Comparisons of estradiol, LH and FSH patterns in pregnant and non-pregnant beagle bitches. *Theriogenology* 2002; **57**(8): 1957–72.

9. Hoffmann B, Busges F, Engel E, Kowalewski MP, Papa P. Regulation of corpus luteum function in the bitch. *Reprod Dom Anim* 2004; **39**: 232–40.

10. Onclin K, Verstegen J. Corpus luteum regulation in the bitch. Proceedings of the Vth International Symposium on Dog and Cat Reproduction, Sao Paulo Brazil, 23.

11. Rothchild I. The corpus luteum revisited: are the paradoxical effects of RU486 a clue to how progesterone stimulates its own secretion? *Biol Reprod* 1996; **55**: 1–4.

12. Verstegen JP, Silva LDM, Onclin K. Determination of the role of cervical closure in fertility regulation after mating or artificial insemination in beagle bitches. *J Reprod Fertil* 2001; **57** (Suppl): 31–4.

13. Petrunkina AM, Simon K, Gunzel-Apel A-R, Topfer-Petersen E. Regulation of capacitation of canine spermatozoa during co-culture with heterologous oviductal epithelial cells. *Reprod Dom Anim* 2003; **38**: 455–63.

14. England GCW, Allen WE. Factors affecting the viability of canine spermatozoa effect of seminal plasma and blood. *Theriogenology* 1992; **37**: 373–81.

15. Zambelli D, Castagnetti C. Transcervical insemination with fresh or frozen semen in the domestic cat: new techniques and preliminary results. 5th Annual Conference of the European Society for Domestic Animal Reproduction (ESDAR), Vienna, Austria. *ESDAR* 2001; **34**.

List of abbreviations

ACD	Australian cattle dog	CSF	cerebrospinal fluid
ACTH	adrenocorticotrophic hormone	CT	computed tomography
		CV	cerebrovascular
AD	atopic dermatitis	CVRI	cerebrovascular resistance index
ANOVA	analysis of variance		
ANP	atrial natriuretic peptide	DLA	dog leucocyte antigen
APACHE	Acute Physiology and Chronic Health Evaluation	DPP	deep pain perception
		DTH	delayed hypersensitivity
BA	bile acid	ECS	English cocker spaniel
BAER	brainstem auditory evoked response	EEN	early enteral nutritional
		ELISA	enzyme-linked immunosorbent assay
BAL	bronchoalveolar lavage		
BALF	bronchoalveolar lavage fluid	EPI	exocrine pancreatic insufficiency
BGA	Bermuda grass allergen		
BNP	B-type natriuretic peptide	EPO	erythropoietin
BT	bull terrier	ES	English setter
CADESI	Canine AD Extent and Severity Index	ET	embryo transfer
		FBD	feline bronchial disease
CAST	Cardiac Arrhythmia Suppression Trial	FeLV	feline leukaemia virus
		FOI	Freedom Of Information
CBC	complete blood count	FVRCP	feline viral rhinotracheitis, calicivirus and parvovirus
CCL	cranial cruciate ligament		
CCS	cutaneous clinical score	GABA	γ-aminobutyric acid
CDR3	third 'complementarity determining regions'	GCP	good clinical practice
		GFR	glomerular filtration rate
CG	chorionic gonadotrophin	GI	gastrointestinal
CI	confidence interval	GN	glomerulonephritis
CIBDAI	canine inflammatory bowel disease activity index	GnRH	gonadotrophin-releasing hormone
CKCS	cavalier King Charles spaniel	HA	hyperactivated
CLAD	canine leucocyte adhesion deficiency	HMW	high molecular weight
		HPLC	high-powered liquid chromatography
CNS	central nervous system		
COX	cyclo-oxygenase	Ht	haematocrit
CPLI	canine pancreatic lipase immunoreactivity	IB	intermittent bolus
		IBD	inflammatory bowel disease
CPV	canine parvovirus		
CRF	chronic renal failure	ICP	intracranial pressure
CRI	constant rate infusion	ICU	intensive care unit
CRIF	clamp rod internal fixator	IFA	indirect fluorescent antibody
CsA	cyclosporin A	IL	interleukin

IMHA	immune-mediated haemolytic anaemia	PCV	packed cell volume
IMTP	immune-mediated thrombocytopenia	PDA	patent ductus arteriosus
		PG	propylene glycol
IV	intravenous	PG	prostaglandin
IVDD	intervertebral disc disease	P-GP	P-glycoprotein
JRT	Jack Russell terrier	P–K	Prausnitz–Küstner
KBr	potassium bromide	PROMISE	Prospective Randomized Milrinone Survival Evaluation
KLH	keyhole limpet haemocyanin		
LH	luteinizing hormone		
LH-R	luteinizing hormone receptor	PUFA	polyunsaturated fatty acid
		PVF	peak vertical force
LOX	lipoxygenase	RBC	red blood cell
LPR	lymphoplasmacytic rhinitis	rcEPO	recombinant canine EPO
LR	Labrador retriever	rhEPO	recombinant human EPO
LRTI	lower respiratory tract infection	RI	resistance index
		ROC	receiver operating curve
MAP	magnesium ammonium phosphate	RT–PCR	reverse transcriptase–polymerase chain reaction
MAT	microscopic agglutination test	SAR	small animal reproduction
		SDS–AGE	sodium dodecyl sulphate–agarose gel electrophoresis
MD	*Malassezia* dermatitis		
MDR	multidrug resistant		
MED	minimum effective dose	SIBO	small intestinal bacterial overgrowth
MHC	major histocompatibility complex		
		sIgA	secretory IgA
MIC	minimum inhibitory concentration	S/Purea	serum or plasma urea
		TAP	trypsinogen activation peptide
MP	methylprednisolone		
MRI	magnetic resonance imaging	TCR	T-cell receptor
MST	median survival time	Th	T helper
NF-κB	nuclear factor κB	TLI	trypsin-like immunoreactivity
NGGA	normalized glottal gap area		
ngl rhBMP-2	non-glycosylated recombinant human bone morphogenetic protein-2	TPA	tibial plateau angle
		TPLO	tibial plateau levelling osteotomy
NSAID	non-steroidal anti-inflammatory drug	TS	total solids
		UTCR	urinary TAP-to-creatinine ratio
PB	phenobarbital		
PBMC	peripheral blood mononuclear cells	VI	vertical impulse
		VMDB	veterinary medical database
PCD	primary ciliary dyskinesia	VTH	veterinary teaching hospital

Index of papers reviewed

Adin CA, Herrgesell EJ, Nyland TG, Hughes JM, Gregory CR, Kyles AE, Cowgill LD, Ling GV. Antegrade pyelography for suspected ureteral obstruction in cats: 11 cases (1995–2001). *J Am Vet Med Assoc* 2003; 222(11): 1576–81. **257**

Adin DB, Taylor AW, Hill RC, Scott KC, Martin FG. Intermittent bolus injection versus continuous infusion of furosemide in normal adult greyhound dogs. *J Vet Intern Med* 2003; 17(5): 632–6. **87**

Albasan H, Lulich JP, Osborne CA, Lekcharoensuk C, Ulrich LK, Carpenter KA. Effects of storage time and temperature on pH, specific gravity, and crystal formation in urine samples from dogs and cats. *J Am Vet Med Assoc* 2003; 222(2): 176–9. **252**

Aper R, Smeak D. Complications and outcome after thoracodorsal axial pattern flap reconstruction of forelimb skin defects in 10 dogs, 1989–2001. *Vet Surg* 2003; 32(4): 378–84. **192**

Bailey D, Erb H, Williams L, Ruslander D, Hauck M. Carboplatin and doxorubicin combination chemotherapy for the treatment of appendicular osteosarcoma in the dog. *J Vet Intern Med* 2003; 17(2): 199–205. **76**

Balkman CE, Center SA, Randolph JF, Trainor D, Warner KL, Crawford MA, Adachi K, Erb HN. Evaluation of urine sulfated and non-sulfated bile acids as a diagnostic test for liver disease in dogs. *J Am Vet Med Assoc* 2003; 222(10): 1368–75. **223**

Barros PS, Safatle AM, Queiroz L, Silva VV, Barros SB. Blood and aqueous humour antioxidants in cataractous poodles. *Can J Ophthalmol* 2004; 39(1): 19–24. **242**

Basso C, Wichter T, Danieli GA, Corrado D, Czarnowska E, Fontaine G, McKenna WJ, Nava A, Protonotarios N, Antoniades L, Wlodarska K, D'Alessi F, Thiene G. Arrhythmogenic right ventricular cardiomyopathy causing sudden cardiac death in boxer dogs: a new animal model of human disease. *Circulation* 2004; 109(9): 1180–5. **283**

Bentley E, Campbell S, Woo HM, Murphy CJ. The effect of chronic corneal epithelial debridement on epithelial and stromal morphology in dogs. *Invest Ophthalmol Vis Sci* 2002; 43(7): 2136–42. **237**

Bentley E, Murphy CJ. Thermal cautery of the cornea for treatment of spontaneous chronic corneal epithelial defects in dogs and horses. *J Am Vet Med Assoc* 2004; 224(2): 250–3. **239**

Blaeser LL, Gallagher JG, Boudrieau RJ. Treatment of biologically inactive non-unions by a limited en bloc ostectomy and compression plate fixation: a review of 17 cases. *Vet Surg* 2003; 32(1): 91–100. **206**

Borenstein N, Behr L, Chetboul V, Tessier D, Nicole A, Jacquet J, Carlos C, Retortillo J, Fayolle P, Pouchelon JL, Daniel P, Laborde F. Minimally invasive patent ductus arteriosus occlusion in 5 dogs. *Vet Surg* 2004; 33(4): 309–13. **186**

Boutilier P, Carr A, Schulman RL. Leptospirosis in dogs: a serologic survey and case series 1996 to 2001. *Vet Ther* 2003; 4(4): 387–96. **264**

Braddock JA, Church DB, Robertson ID, Watson ADJ. Trilostane treatment in dogs with pituitary-dependent hyperadrenocortism. *Aust Vet J* 2003; 81(10): 600–7. **125**

Lipscomb VJ, Hardie RJ, Dubielzig RR. Spontaneous pneumothorax caused by pulmonary blebs and bullae in 12 dogs. *J Am Vet Med Assoc* 2003; **39**(5): 435–45. **111**

Lodmell DL, Parnell MJ, Weyhrich JT, Ewalt LC. Canine rabies DNA vaccination: a single-dose intradermal injection into ear pinnae elicits elevated and persistent levels of neutralizing antibody. *Vaccine* 2003; 21(25–26): 3998–4002. **58**

Lora-Michiels M, Biller DS, Olsen D, Hoskinson JJ, Kraft SL, Jones JC. The accessory lung lobe in thoracic disease: a case series and anatomical review. *J Am Anim Hosp Assoc* 2003; **39**: 452–8. **191**

Lu D, Lamb CR, Pfeiffer DU, Targett MP. Neurologic signs and results of magnetic resonance imaging in 40 cavalier King Charles spaniels with Chiari type 1-like malformations. *Vet Rec* 2003; **153**(9); 260–3. **157**

Macdonald ES, Norris CR, Berghaus RB, Griffey SM. Clinicopathologic and radiographic features and etiologic agents in cats with histologically confirmed infectious pneumonia: 39 cases (1991–2000). *J Am Vet Med Assoc* 2003; 223(8): 1142–50. **105**

MacDonald KA, Kittleson MD, Munro C, Kass P. Brain natriuretic peptide concentration in dogs with heart disease and congestive heart failure. *J Vet Intern Med* 2003; 17(2): 172–7. **276**

Mansfield CS, Jones BR, Spillman T. Assessing the severity of canine pancreatitis. *Res Vet Sci* 2003; 74(2): 137–44. **93 228**

Mason N, Duval D, Shofer FS, Giger U. Cyclophosphamide exerts no beneficial effect over prednisone alone in the initial treatment of acute immune-mediated hemolytic anemia in dogs: a randomized controlled clinical trial. *J Vet Intern Med* 2003; 17(2): 206–12. **40**

Mathews KG, Roe S, Stebbins M, Barnes R, Mente PL. Biomechanical evaluation of suture pullout from canine arytenoid cartilages: effects of hole diameter, suture configuration, suture size, and distraction rate. *Vet Surg* 2004; 33(3): 191–9. **189**

Mazzaferro EM, Greco DS, Turner AS, Fettman MJ. Treatment of feline diabetes mellitus using an α-glucosidase inhibitor and a low carbohydrate diet. *J Feline Med Surg* 2003; 5(3): 183–9. **127**

McCurley JM, Hanlon SU, Wei SK, Wedam EF, Michalski M, Haigney MC. Furosemide and the progression of left ventricular dysfunction in experimental heart failure. *J Am Coll Cardiol* 2004; 44: 1301–7. **290**

Medaille C, Trumel C, Concordet D, Vergez F, Braun JP. Comparison of plasma/serum urea and creatinine concentrations in the dog: a 5-year retrospective study in a commercial veterinary clinical pathology laboratory. *J Vet Med A Physiol Pathol Clin Med* 2004; 51(3): 119–23. **249**

Michiels L, Day MJ, Snaps F, Hansen P, Clercx C. A retrospective study of non-specific rhinitis in 22 cats and the value of nasal cytology and histopathology. *J Feline Med Surg* 2003; 5(5): 279–85. **99**

Mohr AJ, Leisewitz AL, Jacobson LS, Steiner JM, Ruaux CG, Williams DA. Effect of early enteral nutrition on intestinal permeability, intestinal protein loss, and outcome in dogs with severe parvoviral enteritis. *J Vet Intern Med* 2003; 17(6): 791–8. **85 230**

Moore AH. Use of topical povidone-iodine dressings in the management of mycotic rhinitis in three dogs. *J Small Anim Pract* 2003; 44(7): 326–9. **98**

Moore DL, McLellan GJ, Dubielzig RR. A study of the morphology of canine eyes enucleated or eviscerated due to complications following phacoemulsification. *Vet Ophthalmol* 2003; 6(3): 219–26. **245**

Morello E, Vasconi E, Martano M, Peirone B, Buracco P. Pasteurized tumoral autograft and adjuvant chemotherapy for the treatment of canine distal radial osteosarcoma: 13 cases. *Vet Surg* 2003; 32(6): 539–44. **209**

Moritz A, Schneider M, Bauer N. Management of advanced tracheal collapse in dogs using intraluminal self-expanding biliary wallstents. *J Vet Intern Med* 2004; 18(1): 31–42. **91 104 184**

Morris DO, DeBoer DJ. Evaluation of serum obtained from atopic dogs with dermatitis attributable to *Malassezia pachydermatis* for passive transfer of immediate hypersensitivity to that organism. *Am J Vet Res* 2003; 64(3): 262–6. **11**

Murphy S, Sparkes AH, Smith KC, Blunden AS, Brearley MJ. Relationships between the histological grade of cutaneous mast cell tumours in dogs, their survival and the efficacy of surgical resection. *Vet Rec* 2004; 154(24): 743–6. **179**

Norris CR, Byerly JR, Decile KC, Berghaus RD, Walby WF, Schelegle ES, Hyde DM, Gershwin LJ. Allergen-specific IgG and IgA in serum and bronchoalveolar lavage fluid in a model of experimental feline asthma. *Vet Immunol Immunopathol* 2003; 96(3–4): 119–27. **109**

Olby N, Levine J, Harris T, Munana K, Skeen T, Sharp N. Long-term functional outcome of dogs with severe injuries of the thoracolumbar spinal cord: 87 cases (1996–2001). *J Am Vet Med Assoc* 2003; 222(6): 762–9. **168**

Olivry T, Mueller RS and the International Task Force on Canine Atopic Dermatitis. Evidence-based veterinary dermatology: a systemic review on the pharmacotherapy of canine atopic dermatitis. *Vet Dermatol* 2003; 14(3): 121–46. **1**

Penninck D, Smyers B, Webster CR, Rand W, Moore AS. Diagnostic value of ultrasonography in differentiating enteritis from intestinal neoplasia in dogs. *Vet Radiol Ultrasound* 2003; 44(5): 570–5. **66**

Polton GA, Brearley MJ. Anal Sac Adenocarcinoma in the Dog—A Series of 80 Clinical Cases. Scientific Abstracts, 47th Annual British Small Animal Veterinary Association (BSAVA) Congress Proceedings, 2004; p 563. **177**

Preziosi DE, Goldschmidt MH, Greek JS, Jeffers JG, Shanley KS, Drobatz K, Mauldin EA. Feline pemphigus foliaceus: a retrospective analysis of 57 cases. *Vet Dermatol* 2003; 14(6): 313–21. **16**

Proulx DR, Ruslander DM, Dodge RK, Hauck ML, Williams LE, Horn B, Price GS, Thrall DE. A retrospective analysis of 140 dogs with oral melanoma treated with external beam radiation. *J Vet Radiol Ultrasound* 2003; 44(3): 352–9. **75**

Quinnell RJ, Kennedy LJ, Barnes A, Courtenay O, Dye C, Garcez LM, Shaw MA, Carter SD, Thomson W, Ollier WE. Susceptibility to visceral leishmaniasis in the domestic dog is associated with MHC class II polymorphism. *Immunogenetics* 2003; 55(1): 23–8. **38**

Randolph JF, Scarlett J, Stokol T, MacLeod JN. Clinical efficacy and safety of recombinant canine erythropoietin in dogs with anemia of chronic renal failure and dogs with recombinant human erythropoietin-induced red cell aplasia. *J Vet Intern Med* 2004; 18(1): 81–91. **266**

Rayward RM, Thomson DG, Davies JV, Innes JF, Whitelock RG. Progression of osteoarthritis following TPLO surgery: a prospective radiographic study of 40 dogs. *J Small Anim Pract* 2004; 45(2): 92–7. **199**

Rijselaere T, Van Soom A, Maes D, Verberckmoes S, de Kruif A. Effect of blood admixture on the *in vitro* survival of chilled and frozen-thawed canine spermatozoa. *Theriogenology* 2004; 61: 1589–602. **332**

Rinkinen M, Teppo A-M, Harmoinen J, Westermarck E. Relationship between canine mucosal and serum immunoglobulin A (IgA) concentrations:

serum IgA does not assess duodenal secretory IgA. *Microbiol Immunol* 2003; 47(2): 155–9. **221**

Roulet A, Puel O, Gesta S, Lepage JF, Drag M, Soll M, Alvinerie M, Pineau T. MDR 1-deficient genotype in Collie dogs hypersensitive to the P-glycoprotein substrate ivermectin. *Eur J Pharmacol* 2003; 460(2-3): 85–91. **18**

Sævik BK, Bergvall K, Holm BR, Saijonmaa-Kolumies LE, Hedhammer A, Larsen S, Kristensen F. A randomised, controlled study to evaluate the steroid sparing effect of essential fatty acid supplementation in the treatment of canine atopic dermatitis. *Vet Dermatol* 2004; 15(3): 137–45. **6**

Saito M, Olby N, Spaulding K, Munana K, Sharp NJH. Relationship amongst basilar artery resistance index, degree of ventriculomegaly, and clinical signs in hydrocephalic dogs. *Vet Radiol Ultrasound* 2003; 44(6): 687–94. **163**

Saxena BB, Clavio A, Singh M, Rathnam P, Bukharovich EY, Reimers TJ Jr, Saxena A, Perkins S. Effect of immunization with bovine luteinizing hormone receptor on ovarian function in cats. *Am J Vet Res* 2003; 64(3): 292–8. **137**

Schmökel HG, Weber FE, Seiler G, Von Rechenberg B, Schense JC, Schawalder P, Hubbell J. Treatment of non-unions with non-glycosylated recombinant human bone morphogenetic protein-2 delivered from a fibrin matrix. *Vet Surg* 2004; 33(2): 112–18. **206**

Seyrek-Intas K, Wehrend A, Nak A, Basri Tek H, Yilmazbas G, Gokhan T, Bostedt H. Unilateral hysterectomy (cornuectomy) in the bitch and its effect on subsequent fertility. *Theriogenology* 2004; 61: 1713–17. **330**

Shamir M, Goelman G, Chai O. Post-anesthetic cerebellar dysfunction in cats. *J Vet Intern Med* 2004; 18(3): 368–9. **149**

Simpson AM, Ludwig LL, Newman SJ, Bergman PJ, Hottinger HA, Patnaik AK. Evaluation of surgical margins required for complete excision of cutaneous mast cell tumours in dogs. *J Am Vet Med Assoc* 2004; 224(2): 236–40. **181**

Sisson D. Use of a self-expanding occluding stent for non-surgical closure of patent ductus arteriosus in dogs. *J Am Vet Med Assoc* 2003; 223(7): 999–1005. **187**

Steffan J, Alexander D, Brovedani F, Fisch RD. Comparison of cyclosporine A with methylprednisolone for treatment of canine atopic dermatitis: a parallel, blinded, randomized controlled trial. *Vet Dermatol* 2003; 14(1): 11–22. **5 43**

Steiner JM, Williams DA. Development and validation of a radioimmunoassay for the measurement of canine pancreatic lipase immunoreactivity in serum of dogs. *Am J Vet Res* 2003; 64(10): 1237–41. **224**

Stiles J, Honda CN, Krohne SG, Kazacos EA. Effect of topical administration of 1% morphine sulfate solution (MSS) on signs of pain and corneal wound healing in dogs. *Am J Vet Res* 2003; 64(7): 813–18. **239**

Strain GM. Deafness prevalence and pigmentation and gender associations in dog breeds at risk. *Vet J* 2004; 167(1): 23–32. **159**

Swinnen C, Vroom M. The clinical effect of environmental control of house dust mites in 60 house dust mite-sensitive dogs. *Vet Dermatol* 2004; 15(1): 31–6. **8**

Tidholm A, Falk T, Gundler S, Svensson H, Ablad B, Sylven C. Effect of thyroid hormone supplementation on survival of euthyroid dogs with congestive heart failure due to systolic myocardial dysfunction: a double-blind, placebo-controlled trial, *Res Vet Sci* 2003; 75: 195–201. **289**

Trepanier LA, Hoffman SB, Kroll M, Rodan I, Challoner L. Efficacy and safety of once versus twice daily administration of methimazole in cats with hyperthyroidism. *J Am Vet Med Assoc* 2003; 222(7): 954–8. **135**

General index

A

abortion, induction of 318
acarbose in feline diabetes 127–8
Acarex® test 8
accessory lung lobe disease 191–2
acepromazine, effect on laryngeal motion 102, 103
acetaminophen, hepatotoxicity 300
acetaminophen absorption test 232, 233
acid-base balance in feline CRF 270–2, 274
ACTH stimulation test 121, 122, 138
  17-hydroxyprogesterone levels 123–4
acute dyspnoea 98, 114–15
adverse effects
  of cyclosporin 306
  of fluoroquinolones 310
  of non-steroidal anti-inflammatory drugs 298–301
Aelurostrongylus abstrusus LRTIs, feline 107
age
  effect on immune response 49, 51, 55–8
  relationship to cataract prevalence 241–2, 243
aglepristone (RU38478) 318, 327–8
alopecia X, steroid hormone analysis 20–1, 23
aluminium, and post-vaccination sarcoma 73, 74
amylase levels in canine pancreatitis 93–4
anaerobic bacteria, resistance to cephalosporins 307
anaesthetic agents, effect on laryngeal motion 102–4, 117
anal furunculosis 44
anal sac, apocrine carcinoma 71–3, 79–80, 175–8
analgesia, topical, effect on corneal ulcers 239–40
Anaplasma, immune response 34
antegrade pyelography 257–9, 273
antibiotic-responsive enteropathy 218–21
antibiotics
  carbapenems 308–9
  cephalosporins 307–8
  fluoroquinolones 309–11
  topical, effect on corneal ulceration 240–1
antioxidants, protection of lens 243
APACHE scoring system 217
apocrine carcinoma of anal sac 71–3, 79–80, 175–8

aromatase inhibitors, effect in azoospermia 338–41
arrhythmogenic cardiomyopathy 283–4
arthropod-borne infections 33–5, 60
artificial insemination
  blood admixture, effect on sperm quality 332–4
  frozen semen, use in dogs 329–30
  timing in dogs 330
  transcervical insemination in cats 344–5
arytenoid cartilage motion, effect of anaesthetic agents 102–4
arytenoid lateralization 189–91
ascorbic acid concentration, and cataracts 243
aspartate, CSF concentrations in epilepsy 154
aspergillosis, nasal 97, 98–9, 116
aspirin 298, 301
  hepatotoxicity 300
asthma, feline 98, 109–11, 117
atherosclerosis, association with endocrinopathies 132–3, 139
Atopica 304
  see also cyclosporin
atopy
  atopic dermatitis (AD) *see* canine atopic dermatitis
  food allergy 12–15
atrial natriuretic peptide (ANP) 276, 277–8
autoimmune subepidermal blistering dermatoses 30–3
autopsy findings, concurrence with antemortem diagnosis 84–5
axial pattern flaps 192–3
azathioprine, in immune-mediated haemolytic anaemia 41, 42
azithromycin, in hepatopathy associated with *Bartonella* sp. 226
azoospermia, effect of aromatase inhibitors 338–41

B

babesiosis 33–5
bacterial pneumonia, feline 105, 106
balloon valvuloplasty in pulmonic stenosis 284–7